THE AMBULATORY ANESTHESIA HANDBOOK

Compliments of your

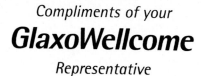

GlaxoWellcome

Representative

D0096006

THE AMBULATORY ANESTHESIA HANDBOOK

Rebecca S. Twersky, M.D.
Associate Professor of Anesthesiology
Director
Division of Ambulatory Anesthesia
SUNY Health Science Center at Brooklyn;
Medical Director
Ambulatory Surgery Unit
The Long Island College Hospital
Brooklyn, New York

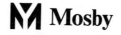 Mosby

St. Louis   Baltimore   Berlin   Boston   Carlsbad   Chicago   London   Madrid
Naples   New York   Philadelphia   Sydney   Tokyo   Toronto

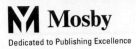

Mosby

Dedicated to Publishing Excellence

Executive Editor: Susan M. Gay
Developmental Editor: Sandra Clark Brown
Project Manager: Gayle May Morris
Editing and Production: Carlisle Publishers Services
Manufacturing Supervisor: Kathy Grone

Copyright © 1995 by Mosby–Year Book, Inc.

Printed in the United States of America
Composition by Carlisle Communications, Ltd.
Printing/Binding by R.R. Donnelley & Sons Company

Mosby–Year Book, Inc.
11830 Westline Industrial Drive
St. Louis, Missouri 63146

Library of Congress Cataloging-in-Publication Data
The ambulatory anesthesia handbook / [edited by] Rebecca S. Twersky.
    p.   cm.
  Includes bibliographical references and index.
  ISBN 0-8151-8847-1
  1. Anesthesia.   2. Ambulatory Surgery.   I. Twersky, Rebecca S.
  [DNLM: 1. Anesthesia.   2. Ambulatory Surgery.   WO 200 A4974 1995]
RD82.A655   1995
617.9′6—dc20
DNLM/DLC
for Library of Congress   94–32505
                                                CIP

95   96   97   98   99   /   9   8   7   6   5   4   3   2   1

Contributors

Frances Chung, M.D., F.R.C.P.C.

Associate Professor in Anesthesiology
Department of Anesthesiology
University of Toronto;
Director
Toronto Western Division
Toronto Hospital
Toronto, Ontario

Hernando De Soto, M.D.

Assistant Professor of Anesthesiology
University of Florida School of Medicine;
Director
Pediatric Anesthesia
University of Florida Medical Center
Jacksonville, Florida

Lucinda L. Everett, M.D.

Assistant Professor of Anesthesiology
Director
Preanesthesia Assessment Clinic
Medical College of Virginia/Virginia Commonwealth University
Richmond, Virginia

Barbara S. Gold, M.D.

Assistant Professor of Anesthesiology
Department of Anesthesiology
University of Minnesota
Minneapolis, Minnesota

Carmen R. Green, M.D.

Assistant Professor of Anesthesiology
Department of Anesthesiology
University of Michigan Medical Center
Ann Arbor, Michigan

Carolyn P. Greenberg, M.D.

Associate Professor of Clinical Anesthesiology
Columbia University College of Physicians and Surgeons;
Medical Director
Ambulatory Surgery Unit
Presbyterian Hospital
New York, New York

Steven Hall, M.D.

Anesthesiologist-In-Chief
Children's Memorial Hospital
Evanston, Illinois

Raafat S. Hannallah, M.D.

Professor of Anesthesiology and Pediatrics
The George Washington University Medical Center;
Vice-Chairman of Anesthesiology
Children's National Medical Center
Washington, D.C.

Surinder K. Kallar, M.D.

Professor and Interim Chairman of Anesthesiology
Director of Ambulatory Anesthesia;
Medical Director
Ambulatory Surgery Center
Department of Anesthesiology
Medical College of Virginia/Virginia Commonwealth University
Richmond, Virginia

Patricia A. Kapur, M.D.

Associate Professor of Anesthesiology
Department of Anesthesiology;
Director
UCLA Surgery Center
UCLA Medical Center
Los Angeles, California

Jocelyn McClain, M.D.

Assistant Clinical Professor
College of Medicine at Peoria
University of Illinois
Peoria, Illinois

Sujit K. Pandit, M.D., Ph.D.

Professor of Anesthesiology
School of Medicine
University of Michigan
Ann Arbor, Michigan

Ramesh I. Patel, M.D.

Associate Professor of Anesthesiology and Pediatrics
The George Washington University Medical Center;
Medical Director
Ambulatory Surgery Unit
Children's National Medical Center
Washington, D.C.

D. Janet Pavlin, M.D.

Associate Professor
Department of Anesthesiology
University of Washington School of Medicine;
Head
Ambulatory Anesthesia
University of Washington Medical Center
Seattle, Washington

Beverly K. Philip, M.D.

Past President
Society for Ambulatory Surgery;
Associate Professor of Anesthesia
Harvard Medical School;
Director
Day Surgery Unit
Brigham and Women's Hospital
Boston, Massachusetts

Yung-Fong Sung, M.D.

Associate Professor of Anesthesiology
Emory University School of Medicine;
Chief of Anesthesiology
Ambulatory Surgery Center/The Emory Clinic
Wesley Woods Geriatric Hospital
Atlanta, Georgia

Rebecca S. *Twersky,* M.D.

Associate Professor of Anesthesiology
Director
Division of Ambulatory Anesthesia
SUNY Health Science Center at Brooklyn;
Medical Director
Ambulatory Surgery Unit
The Long Island College Hospital
Brooklyn, New York

To my loving, supportive, and understanding family

David,
Baila,
Yitzy,
and
Naomi

Preface

As we complete the last decade of the twentieth century, we witness the evolution of health care. The development of sophisticated medical and surgical technology, and advances in anesthesia, pharmacology, and drug delivery systems have contributed greatly to the explosive growth of ambulatory surgery that has occurred during the past two decades. By the year 2000, it is expected that nearly 70% of all elective procedures in the United States will be performed on an ambulatory surgical basis. Similar growth patterns are expected in Canada and abroad in Europe and Australia. Additionally, the growth of freestanding surgical centers will contribute to more ambulatory procedures than allowed in the past. These developments have placed a tremendous onus on physicians, nurses, and other health care professionals to meet the demands of a rapidly growing specialty.

It is no coincidence that *The Ambulatory Anesthesia Handbook* has been published. The intention of this handbook is to address the clinical and administrative concerns that have arisen from the daily practice of ambulatory surgery. The handbook is directed to anesthesiologists both in training and practice, as well as other physicians, health care professionals, administrators, and nurses involved in the care of ambulatory surgery patients. Practical approaches to the common problems encountered in this rapidly growing field have been addressed. The expansive role of physicians, nurses, health care extenders, ancillary health professionals, and administrators has led to questions about recommendations and guidelines for actual practice. This book is intended to guide these individuals through the steps of treating the ambulatory surgery patient.

The text contributors, who are acknowledged and respected authorities in the field of ambulatory surgery, provide succinct and comprehensive discussions of the basic areas involved in the preoperative management of outpatients, including modalities of preoperative assessment and laboratory testing, preoperative surgical and anesthesia considerations for a variety of procedures, protocols for managing the challenging pediatric and adult patients, techniques for administering general and regional anesthesia (including preoperative preparations and premedication), sedation techniques for adult and pediatric patients, anesthesia use outside the operating room, the process of discharging patients, and ways to assess quality of services rendered. Because of the current focus on health care reform and cost containment, one chapter is devoted to cost effectiveness—although ambulatory surgery is already a specialty that has been touted as cost savings containing to health care facilities.

How has ambulatory surgery changed, and how can we expect for it to change further? The development of various surgical procedures with the use of laser and laparoscopic techniques has resulted in the expansion of the list of procedures that can now be performed on an outpatient basis. Newer pharmacological agents that can be used for both general anesthesia and sedation have also contributed to short outpatient procedures and recovery time. Providing anesthesia and sedation outside the operating room both by anesthesiologists and nonanesthesiologists will continue. At the same time, the focus will remain on practicing cost-effective medicine. The future? An extension of the ambulatory surgery facility to accommodate more major procedures and extended periods of observation, the use of computerization in preoperative management, as well as quality assessment, and outcome evaluation will be integrated to the daily practice. What is needed now is aptly provided in this handbook.

I sincerely acknowledge the scholarly efforts of all the contributing authors and the members of my department who appreciated the importance of what I was doing and allowed me to complete the book. I would like to thank my secretary, Edna Morales, and research assistant Barbara McEwan for their devoted assistance; Bernard Wetchler, M.D., who has always been a source of inspiration to me in developing my interest in ambulatory surgery; and all of you who read this book and find its efforts worthwhile.

Rebecca S. Twersky

Contents

THE AMBULATORY ANESTHESIA HANDBOOK

1

Presurgical Evaluation and Laboratory Testing

Lucinda L. Everett and Surinder K. Kallar

Overview of the Preoperative Process

Preoperative evaluation is a fundamental part of the practice of anesthesiology, and it is particularly important in the ambulatory surgical population. Traditionally, inpatient anesthetic care included a preoperative visit by the anesthesiologist the night before the operation, which proved valuable in reducing patient anxiety and possibly in providing a better outcome.[1] With the proliferation of outpatient surgery and same day admit surgeries, this traditional visit is becoming less common. Very often, the patient and the anesthesiologist first meet just a few minutes before the patient is taken into the operating room. Understandably, these circumstances have changed the dynamics of the patient-anesthesiologist relationship, and, therefore, developing a good physician-patient relationship and effectively reducing patient anxiety has become a much greater challenge for the outpatient anesthesiologist.[2] In this new environment, it is imperative to use a screening mechanism that allows predetermination of the patient's fitness to undergo the proposed operation under some form of anesthesia. Failure to determine this in advance may cause last-minute postponement or cancellation of surgery, which gives rise both to resentment from the patient and to disruption of the operating room schedule. Ideally, the screening should take place a few days before the scheduled day of operation, so that additional laboratory tests or consultations can be obtained if necessary.

Appropriate preoperative evaluation allows the anesthesiologist to formulate an anesthetic plan for each patient, and also addresses whether that patient can be safely handled as an outpatient (Box 1-1). A mechanism to allow prearrival evaluation is critical for the smooth function of an ambulatory surgical center. This assessment should confirm that the patient's medical condition is adequately evaluated and treated, that the extent of the procedure is appropriate, and that the patient will have adequate social support during the postoperative period. Clear guidelines must be available to the health care personnel (e.g., surgeon, anesthesiologists, nurse-clinician, registered nurse, internist) who are to perform the preoperative screening. The person responsible for the screening should be able to distinguish patients who are suitable for outpatient operation from those who need further evaluation. Box 1-2 lists absolute and relative contraindications for outpatient operations. These criteria may vary from facility to facility, depending on local views, patient population mix, ease with which hospital admission is possible, and staff expertise.

Box 1-1 Goals of Preoperative Visit in Ambulatory Surgery

- Assess appropriateness of patient and of procedure for ambulatory facility
- Obtain medical information needed to plan anesthesia care
- Assess factors that affect risk of anesthesia
- Assess factors that might alter planned anesthetic technique
- Obtain informed consent
- Assess patient's social situation with respect to ambulatory surgery
- Provide preoperative education to patient (NPO and medication instructions)
- Acquaint patient with ambulatory surgical facility
- Provide patient with clear expectations for anesthetic care and postoperative course

Patient Selection

In general, the patient for ambulatory surgery should have no unevaluated medical problems, and no problems severe enough to require hospitalization after surgery. Chronic illnesses such as hypertension or diabetes should be well controlled. Ambulatory patients should be ASA physical status 1 or 2 (Table 1-1),[3] but status 3 and 4 patients are acceptable if their disease process is compensated. Preoperative screening would uncover any medical condition that might influence the anesthetic or surgical course, or that would preclude the performance of the procedure on an outpatient basis. A determination could be made if the existing medical condition requires further evaluation with laboratory tests or by consultation. Specific medical problems are discussed in Chapter 3.

Age

There is probably no upper age limit for ambulatory procedures if the medical condition is stable, and if the patient will have adequate care at home afterward. In the pediatric population,

---

Box 1-2 *Absolute or Relative Contraindications,*
Depending on the Type of Facility, for
Ambulatory Surgery

- Procedure associated with significant blood loss or severe postoperative pain
- Acute concurrent illness
- Poorly compensated or incompletely evaluated systemic disease (e.g., severe diabetes, asthma, coronary artery disease, morbid obesity)
- Severe systemic disease requiring invasive monitoring or intensive care follow-up (unstable ASA 3 or 4 patients)
- Sickle cell disease
- Coagulopathy
- Acute substance abuse
- Abnormal airway anatomy predisposing to difficult intubation
- Premature infants, infants with significant bronchopulmonary dysplasia, infants with a history of apnea, or infants requiring supplemental oxygen
- Susceptibility to malignant hyperthermia
- Children less than 1 year old with family history of sudden infant death syndrome
- Lack of social support or companion for patient during postoperative period
- Lack of understanding of postoperative requirements by patient or family

---

former premature infants with a risk of apnea are generally admitted for overnight monitoring at most centers.[4] Children less than 1 year old with a family history of sudden death syndrome are probably also best managed with overnight admission. Specific pediatric problems are detailed in Chapter 4.

Social History

It is important for the patient or family to adequately understand the plan for ambulatory surgery and the postoperative requirements. A responsible companion is necessary to accompany the

Table 1-1   American Society of Anesthesiologists Physical Status

Status	Description
1	A normal healthy patient
2	A patient with a mild systemic disease
3	A patient with a severe systemic disease that limits activity, but is not incapacitating
4	A patient with an incapacitating systemic disease that is a constant threat to life
5	A moribund patient not expected to survive 24 hours with or without operation

The designation *E* after the status refers to emergency operation, and generally would not apply to the ambulatory surgical patient.
American Society of Anesthesiologists: New classification of physical status. Anesthesiology 1963; 24:111.

patient home from surgery and be available for the first 24 hours. The patient must also have an adequate understanding of postoperative instructions, including the limitations on operating motor vehicles or machinery. The distance from home to the hospital and medical care alternatives in the patient's community may need to be considered for the patient who lives far from the ambulatory surgical center.

Procedure Selection

More and more types of procedures are being done on an ambulatory basis, particularly with the advent of laparoscopic technology. Procedures with significant intra- and postoperative physiologic consequences, such as open abdominal, thoracic, and intracranial procedures, as well as major vascular and orthopedic procedures, are not appropriate for ambulatory surgery. Surgery that does not involve significant fluid shifts or blood loss, that requires the patient to be able to ambulate and to tolerate oral intake after surgery, and that is not complicated by excessive pain or nausea and vomiting can be done on an ambulatory basis. A long duration of surgery itself is generally not a contraindication to ambulatory surgery if the capacity of the facility is not exceeded; however, staffing requirements for the recovery period, as well as the appropriateness of sending the patient home late in the day, must be considered. More specifics on procedure selection are found in Chapter 2.

Preoperative Evaluation

History

The cornerstone of evaluation of the patient before anesthesia is a thorough history (Box 1-3). Basic data should be collected, including age, height, weight, medications, allergies, and tobacco, alcohol, and drug use. The current state of health, recent acute illnesses, and status of known medical problems should also be

---

Box 1-3 The Preanesthetic Interview

- Age
- Scheduled procedure
- Medications
      Current medications and schedule; last dose
      Prior medications (steroids, chemotherapy)
- Allergies, including specific reaction
- Cigarette, alcohol, and drug history, including most recent use
- Anesthetic history, including specific details of any problems
- Prior surgical procedures and hospitalizations
- Family history, especially of any anesthetic problems
- Social history, especially with regard to postoperative caregiver
- Birth and developmental history (pediatrics)
- Obstetrical history; last menstrual period (females)
- Medical problems previously diagnosed; evaluation, treatment, and degree of control
- Review of systems, looking for signs or symptoms of undiagnosed medical problems, particularly cardiac, pulmonary, or neurologic disease, reflux, or bleeding tendency
- Exercise tolerance
- History of any airway problems (history of difficult intubation or airway disease, symptoms of temporomandibular joint disease, snoring or stridor, loose teeth)
- Patient concerns, preferences, or expectations regarding anesthesia

---

evaluated. Prior surgical and anesthetic experiences, as well as any family history of problems with anesthesia, are important. Reactions to medication, or problems with anesthesia experienced by the patient or the family, should be explored in detail and the specific reaction documented; prior records are helpful if there has been a problem. Box 1-4 lists typical preanesthetic questions that should be asked during the preoperative interview.

For each known medical problem, the duration, prior evaluation, and degree of control should be known. Questions should also be directed toward associated problems or end-organ damage, as appropriate. For a patient to be accepted for elective ambulatory surgery, the history should satisfy the anesthesiologist that the patient's medical problems have been adequately evaluated and that the problems are stable.

In addition to known problems, the review of systems may elicit signs or symptoms of other problems that could influence decision making about anesthetic care. Most important are previously undetected cardiac or pulmonary disease. Questions about exercise tolerance are a good starting point to detect cardiopulmonary problems; patients who are active without limitations or symptoms will rarely have significant disease.[5] In patients with risk factors for ischemic heart disease (age, sex, family history, hypercholesterolemia, diabetes, smoking, hypertension), the interviewer should be more persistent in questioning about chest pain, pressure, or tightness, and about exertional symptoms, including dyspnea.

Other undiagnosed disease states with anesthetic implications should also be sought in the review of systems. These include shortness of breath or wheezing, signs or symptoms of congestive heart failure, muscle weakness, gastrointestinal reflux, or unusual bruising or bleeding. The patient should be questioned about any range-of-motion limitations of the neck or jaw, loose teeth, history of snoring or sleep apnea, and problems with intubation. In the pediatric patient, the birth and developmental history are important. Females of childbearing age should be questioned closely about the possibility of pregnancy.

The preoperative interview provides an opportunity to assess whether the patient has adequate support (family or companion) for the ambulatory surgical process, to explore the patient's expectations and concerns about anesthesia, and to discuss options for anesthetic technique and for postoperative pain management.

Box 1-4 *Preanesthetic Questions*

- What operation are you having?
- Do you have any medical problems other than the condition for which you are having surgery?
- Do you feel sick at this time?
- Have you ever had a problem with your heart, such as chest pain, palpitation, or heart attack?
- How much physical activity can you endure?
- Do you get short of breath during normal activities?
- Do you have any problems with your blood pressure?
- Do you smoke or drink alcohol?
- Do you use any nonprescription drugs or other chemicals?
- Have you ever had bronchitis, pneumonia, or asthma?
- Do you wear dentures, eyeglasses, or contact lenses?
- Do you have any symptoms suggestive of obstructive sleep apnea, like snoring?
- Do you have any neurological problems, such as convulsions, severe headaches, or memory loss?
- Have you had a cough or cold recently?
- Have you ever had any jaundice or problem with your liver?
- Do you have reflux, hiatal hernia, or gastritis?
- Have you ever had a problem with your kidneys?
- Do you have any problems with your thyroid or adrenal glands?
- Do you bleed easily or have any problems with blood clotting?
- Do you have sickle cell disease or any other hemoglobin problems?
- Have you ever received a blood transfusion? Would you accept a blood transfusion if it were medically necessary?
- Do you take any medications on a regular basis? Have you taken any other medications in the last year?
- Have you ever had an operation?

Box 1-4 Preanesthetic Questions—cont'd

- Was there any problem with the anesthetic that you know of?
- Have you or anyone in your family ever had a problem with an anesthetic?
- Are you allergic to any medications?
- Is there anything else about your health that you think I should know?
- And to menstruating females ask:
  - When was your last menstrual period?
  - Could you possibly be pregnant?
  - Do you use any birth control?
    - For the parents of pediatric patients:
  - Was your child's delivery premature or at term?
  - Did your child experience any neonatal complications?
  - Does your child have a history of bradycardia or apnea?
  - Is there any history of sudden infant death syndrome (SIDS) in your family?

Instructions regarding NPO status, medications, and time of arrival to the facility should also be provided.

As will be discussed later, the preoperative evaluation process should be initiated before the patient's arrival for surgery to prevent delays and poor facility utilization, which may occur if the patient is not adequately evaluated or prepared. On the morning of surgery, the history should be confirmed, and any interim changes noted. The NPO status and last dose of medications should be ascertained. Patients should also be questioned about recent use of drugs or alcohol.

Physical Examination

The preanesthetic physical examination is tailored to obtain information pertinent to risk assessment and the development of an anesthetic plan (Box 1-5). Basic data includes height, weight, and general appearance. Baseline vital signs should include heart rate, respiratory rate, blood pressure (in both arms if indicated),

---

Box 1-5 Preoperative Physical Examination

- Height and weight
- Baseline mental status
- Vital signs (blood pressure, heart rate, respiratory rate, temperature, oxygen saturation)
- Airway evaluation
- Evaluation of heart and lungs
- Skin condition (e.g., turgor, jaundice, pallor).
- Landmarks for regional technique
- Neurologic function
- Vascular access
- Extremities (clubbing, edema, pulses)

---

and temperature. It is helpful to determine the oxygen saturation before any premedication. The baseline mental status should be noted, particularly in the elderly patient.

The chest examination should address any adventitious pulmonary sounds or restriction to airflow, and cardiac rhythm, murmurs, or gallops. The neck is examined for jugular venous distention or carotid bruits. Abdominal distention may alert the anesthesiologist to the potential for increased intraabdominal pressure or decreased respiratory reserve. Assessment of the adequacy of vascular access, skin integrity, peripheral neurologic deficits, clubbing of the extremities, edema, jaundice, or pallor complete the basic examination.

Airway Evaluation

The goal of preoperative evaluation of the airway is to detect patients with any abnormality that might predispose to difficult intubation or difficult mask ventilation. Unfortunately, no single method of evaluation has been shown to provide highly sensitive or specific prediction of the difficult patient.[6] Factors possibly predictive of difficult airway management are listed in Box 1-6. Condition of the teeth, gums, dentures, tonsils, and other intraoral structures should be noted. A general assessment of cervical spine movements, and functional status of the temporomandibular joint should be included as part of the routine airway assessment.

> ## Box 1-6 *Preoperative Evaluation of the Airway*
>
> - Mallampati classification (ability to view posterior pharynx)
> - Mentum-to-thyroid distance
> - Mandible-to-hyoid bone distance
> - Oral opening
> - Nares
> - Quality of dentition (teeth, gum, dentures)
> - Intraoral structures (tonsils, uvula, palates)
> - Mask fit (facial anatomy, beard, etc.)
> - Range of motion of neck
> - Obesity

***Table* 1-2**   Mallampati Classification for Airway Evaluation

The patient is asked to open his or her mouth and protrude the tongue maximally while in the sitting posture.

Class 1	Faucial pillars, soft palate, and uvula can be visualized.
Class 2	Faucial pillars and soft palate can be visualized, but uvula is masked by the base of the tongue.
Class 3	Only soft palate can be visualized.

Mallampati SR, Gatt SP, Gugino LD et al: A clinical sign to predict difficult tracheal intubation: a prospective study. Can Anaesth Soc J 1985; 32:429-34.

The Mallampati classification[7] correlates the view of the posterior pharynx with the view at laryngoscopy (Table 1-2). In the original study of 210 patients, all difficult laryngoscopy was either class 2 or class 3; however, subsequent studies have suggested a relatively poor predictive value, with both false-positive and false-negative results. The Mallampati classification remains the most commonly used test in airway evaluation; it should be used along with considerations of other factors. Frerk[8] suggests that a combination of the Mallampati classification and the thyromental distance improves predictive value.

Suspected difficult airway management may be a relative contraindication to ambulatory surgery; however, as anesthesiologists

1. Assess the likelihood and clinical impact of basic management problems:
   A. Difficult Intubation
   B. Difficult Ventilation
   C. Difficulty with Patient Cooperation or Consent

2. Consider the relative merits and feasibility of basic management choices:

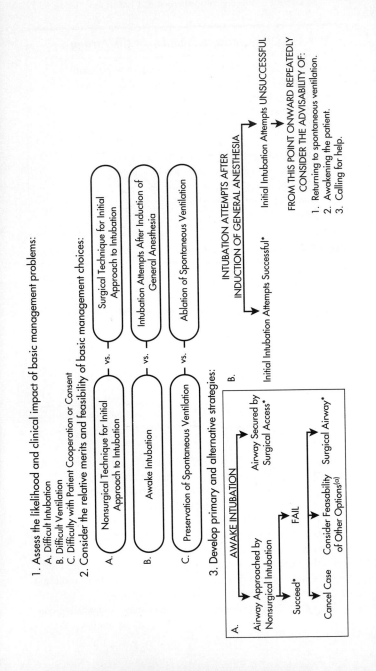

A. Nonsurgical Technique for Initial Approach to Intubation **vs.** Surgical Technique for Initial Approach to Intubation

B. Awake Intubation **vs.** Intubation Attempts After Induction of General Anesthesia

C. Preservation of Spontaneous Ventilation **vs.** Ablation of Spontaneous Ventilation

3. Develop primary and alternative strategies:

A. **AWAKE INTUBATION**

Airway Approached by Nonsurgical Intubation

Succeed* →

FAIL →

Cancel Case

Consider Feasability of Other Options[a]

Airway Secured by Surgical Access*

Surgical Airway*

B. **INTUBATION ATTEMPTS AFTER INDUCTION OF GENERAL ANESTHESIA**

Initial Intubation Attempts Successful*

Initial Intubation Attempts UNSUCCESSFUL

FROM THIS POINT ONWARD REPEATEDLY CONSIDER THE ADVISABILITY OF:
   1. Returning to spontaneous ventilation.
   2. Awakening the patient.
   3. Calling for help.

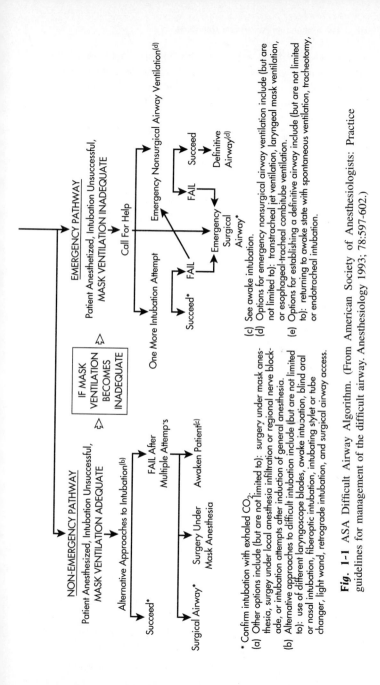

Fig. 1-1 ASA Difficult Airway Algorithm. (From American Society of Anesthesiologists: Practice guidelines for management of the difficult airway. Anesthesiology 1993; 78:597-602.)

NON-EMERGENCY PATHWAY
Patient Anesthesized, Intubation Unsuccessful,
MASK VENTILATION ADEQUATE

Alternative Approaches to Intubation[b]

Succeed*

FAIL After
Multiple Attempts

Surgical Airway*   Surgery Under   Awaken Patient[c]
                    Mask Anesthesia

⇨ IF MASK
VENTILATION
BECOMES
INADEQUATE ⇦

EMERGENCY PATHWAY
Patient Anesthezied, Intubation Unsuccessful,
MASK VENTILATION INADEQUATE

Call For Help

One More Intubation Attempt   Emergency Nonsurgical Airway Ventilation[d]

Succeed*   FAIL   FAIL   Succeed

                Emergency   Definitive
                Surgical   Airway[d]
                Airway*

* Confirm intubation with exhaled CO_2;

(a) Other options include (but are not limited to): surgery under mask anesthesia, surgery under local anesthesia infiltration or regional nerve blockade, or intubation attempts after induction of general anesthesia.

(b) Alternative approaches to difficult intubation include (but are not limited to): use of different laryngoscope blades, awake intubation, blind oral or nasal intubation, fiberoptic intubation, intubating stylet or tube changer, light wand, retrograde intubation, and surgical airway access.

(c) See awake intubation.

(d) Options for emergency nonsurgical airway ventilation include (but are not limited to): transtracheal jet ventilation, laryngeal mask ventilation, or esophageal-tracheal combitube ventilation.

(e) Options for establishing a definitive airway include (but are not limited to): returning to awake state with spontaneous ventilation, tracheotomy, or endotracheal intubation.

gain more widespread expertise with fiberoptic intubation, this may become an individual decision based on personnel, equipment availability, and time necessary to prepare and perform these techniques. Certainly, the equipment required to manage the difficult airway should be available on site in every facility where sedatives or general anesthetics are given, and personnel should have the expertise required to follow the American Society of Anesthesiologists Difficult Airway Algorithm (Fig. 1-1).[9]

Laboratory and Ancillary Testing

Blood tests, x-rays, and other diagnostic testing should only be ordered when specifically indicated by a thorough history and physical examination. This practice represents a radical departure from that of several decades ago, when laboratory screening panels were deemed necessary for all patients undergoing anesthesia or surgery. The practice of limiting tests to those indicated by the history and examination is well validated in the literature.[10] Overordering and blanket panel approaches generate high direct costs, and potentially place patients at risk from further tests done to evaluate abnormal (often false-positive) results. In several large studies, screening laboratory tests did not significantly contribute to patient care.[11,12]

The American Society of Anesthesiologists supports the concept that "no routine laboratory or diagnostic screening test is necessary for the preanesthetic evaluation of patients."[13] The Joint Commission on Accreditation of Healthcare Organization (JCAHO) and the Accreditation Association for Ambulatory Health Care (AAAHC) do not mandate specific preoperative laboratory testing, but let each facility determine an appropriate presurgical work-up. Departments and health care facilities are encouraged to develop appropriate guidelines for preoperative testing after considering its potential impact on outcome. State and hospital requirements may exist regarding preoperative testing; and although legal requirements must be observed, they may be obsolete. Practice groups may wish to request that obsolete rules be updated to reflect current practice. Laboratory tests, if indicated, are considered valid for up to 2 months before surgery if the initial results were normal.[14] Each facility must develop its own policy.

A given laboratory test should be ordered only if the incidence of abnormality in the patient population is such that there is a reasonable probability of demonstrating a finding that would alter patient management or risk assessment. For the healthy ambulatory patient having a minor surgical procedure, one can argue that no laboratory testing is required (Fig. 1-2). For patients with underlying medical conditions, and for patients in certain age groups, blood tests are ordered for specific indications, as listed in Table 1–3.

Hematologic and Biochemical Tests

A determination of the hemoglobin or hematocrit is indicated in patients at risk for anemia or polycythemia when the suspected abnormality would alter anesthetic management or the decision to proceed with surgery. Concern in recent years over blood-borne infections has led the medical community to reassess what is considered an acceptable degree of anemia in the normovolemic patient; the physiologic endpoint is related to oxygen-carrying capacity, and it differs depending on the underlying condition. Chronic anemia is generally well tolerated, and for procedures that do not involve significant blood loss, hemoglobin concentrations above 7 gm/dl are considered acceptable in patients without cardiac disease. In patients with more significant illnesses, a hemoglobin concentration of at least 10 gm/dl is considered desirable.

Preoperative determination of the hemoglobin is appropriate for menstruating females, for patients with a history of anemia, blood dyscrasia or malignancy, or chronic illness, and for patients with a history of polycythemia or congenital heart disease. In the pediatric population, however, it has not been shown to be useful for healthy children more than 1 year old,[12] although it should be performed for younger children and for those in whom sickle cell disease cannot be ruled out by history or prior testing.

The remaining components of the complete blood count, the white cell and platelet counts, are indicated only rarely in the ambulatory surgery patient. The white count may be useful in the overall evaluation of the patient with cancer, particularly after chemotherapy; it may also be ordered when there is suspicion of infection. The platelet count is only indicated when there are factors predisposing to or suggesting thrombocytopenia, such as a bone marrow abnormality, recent chemotherapy, history of liver disease or hypersplenism, or history of abnormal bruising or bleeding.

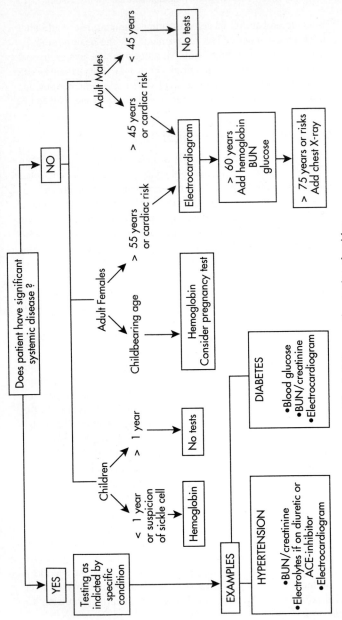

Fig. 1-2 Preoperative testing algorithm.

Table 1-3 Indications for Laboratory Testing

No laboratory test is indicated merely because the patient is undergoing anesthesia or surgery. Laboratory tests should be chosen according to specific indications based on a comprehensive history and physical examination. Some guidelines are listed below.

Test	Indications
Hemoglobin	Menstruating females, children less than 1 year old or with suspected sickle cell disease, history of anemia, blood dyscrasia or malignancy, congenital heart disease, chronic disease states, age greater than 60 years
WBC count	Suspected infection or immunosuppression
Platelet count	History of abnormal bleeding or bruising, liver disease, blood dyscrasias, chemotherapy, hypersplenism
Coagulation studies	History of abnormal bleeding, anticoagulant drug therapy, liver disease, malabsorption, poor nutritional status
Electrolytes, blood glucose, BUN/creatinine	Patients with hypertension, diabetes, heart disease, or disease states with the potential for fluid-electrolyte abnormalities. Patients taking digoxin, diuretics, steroids, or ACE-inhibitors
Liver function tests	Patients with liver disease, history of or exposure to hepatitis, history of alcohol or drug abuse, drug therapy with agents that may affect liver function
Pregnancy test	Patients in whom pregnancy cannot be reliably ruled out by history (some suggest all females of childbearing years)

Continued.

Table 1-3 Indications for Laboratory Testing—cont'd

Test	Indications
Urinalysis	No indication in preanesthetic evaluation; surgeon may request to rule out infection before certain surgical procedures, particularly those involving prosthetic implants
Electrocardiogram	Males more than 45 years old, females more than 55 years old, history or symptoms of cardiac disease, history of hypertension, diabetes, morbid obesity, significant pulmonary disease, cocaine abuse
Chest x-ray	Patients with symptoms of pulmonary disease, airway obstruction, cardiac disease, malignancy, history of heavy smoking, age greater than 75 years
Cervical spine flexion/extension	Patients with rheumatoid arthritis or Down's syndrome

Abnormal platelet function despite a normal platelet count can also occur in patients with a history of bruising or bleeding, particularly those on aspirin, and is best evaluated with a template bleeding time.

As with the platelet count, coagulation studies are not indicated unless there is a history of unusual bleeding, anticoagulant drug therapy, liver disease, or poor nutritional status. The prothrombin time (PT) measures the integrity of the extrinsic and common coagulation pathways, while the activated partial thromboplastin time (APTT) evaluates the intrinsic and common path. Spurious results may occur with polycythemia, hemolysis, or incomplete filling of the sample tube. Clinically significant changes in these clotting times are rarely an incidental finding; thus, preoperative screening for coagulopathy in the general population is not cost-effective or necessary.

Electrolyte concentrations and tests of renal function (blood urea nitrogen and creatinine concentrations) are indicated in patient populations with potential abnormalities, such as patients with hypertension, diabetes, or congestive heart failure. These tests should also be performed in patients taking diuretics, digoxin, angiotensin-converting enzyme (ACE) inhibitors, or steroids. The lowest acceptable level of serum potassium in the preoperative patient remains controversial; currently, it is not deemed necessary to replete the potassium to above 3.0 mg/dl, except perhaps in patients on digoxin. Blood glucose should be determined in patients with known or suspected diabetes, or those on steroids.

Liver function testing in the preoperative period is also somewhat controversial. Although a small percentage of the population may have asymptomatic viral hepatitis when presenting for surgery, most of these will acknowledge exposure, and the incidence is such that routine screening is not cost-effective. If a single test is desired, the AST (aspartate aminotransferase) is suggested.[15] In patients with liver disease, elevated transaminases reflect hepatocellular destruction; the prothrombin time and serum albumin are good indicators of synthetic function; and the conjugated bilirubin will be elevated in biliary obstruction.

Preoperative urinalysis has not been shown to be useful as a screening test, and should be replaced by specific blood chemistry tests indicated by the history or examination. In certain situations, the surgeon may request a urinalysis to rule out infection, particularly before insertion of prosthetic devices.

Pregnancy Testing

One study in ambulatory patients suggested that even a careful history did not pick up the possibility of pregnancy in all cases. Since testing is now easy and relatively inexpensive, and since the risk of drug exposure in an unsuspected pregnancy is significant, some clinicians recommend pregnancy tests in all women of childbearing age.[16] If the facility's policy is to perform routine pregnancy testing, patients should be informed of this before the test, and referrals for counseling and follow-up care should be made available if pregnancy is diagnosed.

HIV Screening

Screening for human immunodeficiency virus (HIV) has been suggested by some health care provider groups, but remains controversial because of confidentiality issues and because of the profound implications of the diagnosis. Although the disease has a relatively high prevalence, nearly all infected individuals have some known risk factor. Universal precautions in the operating room setting remain the recommended method for dealing with the possibility of HIV infection in the surgical patient.

Electrocardiogram and Chest X-Rays

Like blood tests, the electrocardiogram (ECG) and chest x-ray contribute little other than cost when ordered indiscriminately. Potential indications for a preoperative ECG include evaluation of cardiac rhythm and conduction, prior myocardial infarction, or ischemia. The resting ECG alone is not a sensitive or specific test for potential ischemia, or myocardium at risk. In patients with risk factors for coronary artery disease, a baseline ECG may be useful for comparison purposes if problems occur in the perioperative period. However, if there is clinical suspicion of ischemic heart disease, further evaluation may be appropriate (see Chapter 3). Current recommendations suggest that preoperative ECGs should be obtained in males more than 45 years old, females more than 55 years old, and other patients with history or risk factors suggesting cardiac disease, including cocaine abuse.[17-19]

Chest radiographs have not been shown to provide useful information that would not otherwise be suspected based on the history or physical examination.[20] Therefore, current recommendations are to require a chest x-ray only in patients with abnormal physical findings, history of cardiac or pulmonary disease, history of heavy smoking, or age greater than 75 years.[21] Examples of specific clinical questions to be answered by a chest x-ray would include presence or absence of a suspected infiltrate, of interstitial fluid in a patient with congestive heart failure, or of malignancy or pulmonary fibrosis in patients with other tumor or exposure to toxins or drugs. In general, if the clinical status is good, the radiograph will add little to clinical decision making. In patients with clinical abnormalities, it may assist in determining the etiology or reversibility of a disease process and help in assessing whether to proceed with surgery.

Pulmonary Function Tests

Pulmonary function tests (PFTs) are often overused in the preoperative setting. A basic question to be asked before ordering this examination is how it will augment the available clinical information. In patients with obstructive disease such as asthma or chronic obstructive pulmonary disease, PFTs will only serve to confirm the clinical impression. Areas in which they may be useful include patients with dyspnea or hypoxemia of undetermined etiology, assessment of the potential response to bronchodilators, or suspicion of disease severity sufficient to require postoperative ventilation or to preclude surgery.[22,23] Further cardiac or pulmonary evaluation is discussed along with the specific medical problems in Chapter 3.

Cervical Spine X-Ray

Evaluation of the cervical spine by radiograph is indicated in patients at risk for atlantoaxial subluxation.[24] The two main groups included here are patients with rheumatoid arthritis and those with Down's syndrome. Atlantoaxial instability occurs in significant numbers of these patients, and the condition may be asymptomatic; hence, preoperative evaluation of the spine is felt to be indicated unless it can be guaranteed that the neck will not be manipulated. An alternative approach would be to use the fiberoptic or Bullard laryngoscope during surgery in all of these patients.

Logistics of Preoperative Evaluation

The preoperative evaluation process may be conducted in several different ways, depending on the practice setting and patient population (Box 1-7). Ideally, the patient would be seen before

---

Box 1-7 Mechanisms for Preoperative Evaluation

- No evaluation until day of surgery
- Telephone screening
- Screening by registered nurse or nurse practitioner; referral to anesthesiologist, if needed
- Written health questionnaire (paper-and-pencil method)
- Computer-aided survey (e.g., Health Quiz Prescreen)
- Rely on surgeons to screen and refer
- Require visit to primary care physician
- Preoperative visit to anesthesiologist in ambulatory surgery center
- Preoperative visit to anesthesiologist in preoperative assessment clinic

---

Modified from Kallar SK, Everett LL: Controversies in ambulatory anesthesia: preoperative evaluation. Anesthesiology Rev 1992; 19:27-32.

the date of surgery by the clinician who is to be his or her anesthesiologist. However, a separate visit may be inconvenient for the patient, and impractical in some settings. Telephone screening is adequate for many patients,[25] and it provides an opportunity to obtain some baseline information and to give preoperative instructions to the patient. Patients with a complicated medical history should be seen in advance; these patients may be identified by the surgical provider using guidelines supplied by the anesthesiologist. The relative advantages and disadvantages of these methods are summarized in Box 1-8.

Although other physicians or physician extenders (nurse practitioners, CRNAs, or physician assistants) may participate in the preoperative assessment, the anesthesiologist is responsible for review of the information and final determination of the patient's condition. Preanesthesia assessment of all patients is a JCAHO requirement and an ASA standard. The ASA standards require an anesthesiologist to determine that the patient is fit for the planned anesthetic (see Box 1-9).[26] The JCAHO requires that "a licensed independent practitioner with appropriate clinical privileges" make a determination based on the preanesthesia assessment that the patient is an appropriate candidate to undergo the planned anesthesia.[27] It also requires that the patient be reevaluated immediately before the induction of anesthesia.

Box 1-8 *Advantages and Disadvantages of Methods of Preanesthetic Evaluation*

Preanesthesia Clinic

Advantages

Comprehensive evaluation is possible
Ready accessibility of consultation and laboratory tests
Patient's questions can be answered directly
Can obtain informed consent
Can give a prescription for preoperative medications

Disadvantages

Patient may still not meet anesthesiologist
Requires an extra trip to the hospital
Time-consuming for the patient
Usually not reimbursed by third-party payor
May not decrease patient anxiety

Telephone Interview

Advantages

Saves the patients an extra trip to the hospital
Patient has opportunity to speak to the anesthesiologist
Patient's questions can be answered directly

Disadvantages

Time-consuming, often frustrating for the health
    professional
Low contact rate
Physical examination is not possible

In patients who require a preoperative visit for evaluation, we prefer that the anesthesiologist initially see the patient, because other providers are not always attuned to specific anesthesia-related concerns. If further evaluation is required, consultation may be obtained from the patient's own physician or a specialist, and the particular question asked by the anesthesiologist rather than making a blanket request for "preoperative clearance." Box 1-10 lists situations when a consultation might be beneficial. The consultation should be directed toward expert assessment of existing organ dysfunction and whether the patient is fully optimized. Mechanisms for consultation at a convenient site, and in a timely manner,

Box 1-9 **Basic Standards for Preanesthesia Care**
(American Society of Anesthesiologists)

These standards apply to all patients who receive anesthesia or monitored anesthesia care. Under unusual circumstances (e.g., extreme emergencies), these standards may be modified. When this is the case, the circumstances shall be documented in the patient's record.

Standard I: An anesthesiologist shall be responsible for determining the medical status of the patient, developing a plan of anesthesia care, and acquainting the patient or the responsible adult with the proposed plan.

The development of an appropriate plan of anesthesia care is based upon

1. Reviewing the medical record
2. Interviewing and examining the patient to
   a. Discuss the medical history, previous anesthetic experiences, and drug therapy
   b. Assess those aspects of the physical condition that might affect decisions regarding perioperative risk and management
3. Obtaining and/or reviewing tests and consultations necessary to the conduct of anesthesia
4. Determining the appropriate prescription of preoperative medications as necessary to the conduct of anesthesia

The responsible anesthesiologist shall verify that the above has been properly performed and documented in the patient's record.

American Society of Anesthesiologists, Approved by House of Delegates on October 14, 1987.

are helpful in providing comprehensive patient care. There must be a procedure for quick procurement of any necessary records and the result of consultations; surgeons should be aware of the need to send any pertinent records with the patient.

Since the anesthesiologist who meets the patient at the preoperative visit may not be the person who provides anesthesia care during surgery, some consensus on patient acceptability is required within each practice. We suggest that departments agree on guidelines for acceptable patients so that frustrating last-minute cancellations can be prevented.

Box 1-10 Indications for Cardiologist or Internist Consultation

- Recent myocardial infarction (less than 6 months)
- Unstable angina
- Uncontrolled severe hypertension, diabetes, chronic obstructive pulmonary disease, significant renal or liver disease
- Significant and symptomatic cardiac arrhythmia
- Exercise intolerance without an obvious cause
- Recent abnormal ECG changes suggestive of coronary artery disease
- Congestive cardiac failure
- Bleeding disorders (e.g., hemophilia)
- Hemoglobinopathies (e.g., sickle cell anemia)

The preoperative visit to the anesthesiologist may occur at the site of ambulatory surgery or, in a larger medical center, in an integrated preoperative assessment clinic.[28] Visits to the ambulatory surgery center offer the patient the opportunity to become acquainted with the specific facility and personnel he or she will see on the day of surgery, while a preoperative assessment clinic may have more comprehensive facilities for preadmission registration, laboratory evaluation, and radiology. Ideally, for patient convenience and staffing flexibility for anesthesia and nursing personnel, all of these facilities would be located together and adjacent to the ambulatory surgery center.

A written questionnaire may be helpful in obtaining baseline information from patients (Fig. 1-3). This may be given to the patient at the surgeon's office and returned before surgery, or it may be completed as the first step of a preoperative assessment visit. A handheld computer developed by Roizen asks patients a series of questions, then provides a summary of problems with anesthetic implications and a list of recommended laboratory tests (Fig. 1-4).[29]

The preoperative visit or initial screening call should be made far enough in advance to allow intervention, if needed, before surgery. By doing this, there is sufficient time for further evaluation,

The Methodist Medical Center of Illinois
Ambulatory SurgiCare

Patient Preanesthesia/Surgery Questionnaire

Name _____ Age _____ Weight _____ Height _____
Date/Time of Operation _____ Arrival Time _____
Person to drive you home _____ Phone# _____

1. Please tell us if you have or have had any of the following;
   if you check yes, please explain.
   Blood pressure problems: ☐Yes ☐No _____
   Heart problems/chest pain: ☐Yes ☐No _____
   Hepatitis/jaundice: ☐Yes ☐No _____
   Bleeding problems: ☐Yes ☐No _____
   Diabetes: ☐Yes ☐No _____
   Epilepsy/seizures/severe headache: ☐Yes ☐No _____
   Asthma/breathing problem: ☐Yes ☐No _____
   Loose, false, or capped teeth: ☐Yes ☐No _____

2. List any major illnesses other than usual childhood illnesses:
   _____
   _____

3. List any operations you have had: _____
   _____

4. List any medicines, steroids, inhalers, or drugs you take now or have taken
   in the past year. _____

	Yes	No
5. Have you or a blood relative ever had a problem with an anesthetic? _____	☐	☐
6. Are you allergic to local anesthesia, any medicines, idodine, or tape? _____	☐	☐
7. Date of last period: ____ Could you possibly be pregnant?	☐	☐
8. Do you smoke? _____	☐	☐

(Please check if you take any medicine, injections, or pills for:)
☐Heart ☐Lungs ☐Diabetes ☐Kidney ☐Blood pressure

**Patients, please do not write below the double line —
for use of Anesthesia Department**
═══

Anesthesia Note

☐ NPO   ☐ Chart reviewed   ☐Lab data reviewed
☐ Anesthesia management and risk explained to patient/responsible party
☐ Patient's condition satisfactory to proceed with anesthesia as planned
☐ General   ☐ Regional   ☐Local with sedation

Date _____ Time _____ Signature _____

Fig. 1-3 Preoperative questionnaire for the Methodist Medical Center of Illinois. (From Wetchler BV, editor: Anesthesia for ambulatory surgery, ed 2, Philadelphia, 1991, JB Lippincott.)

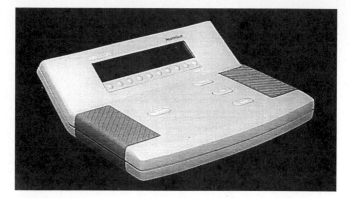

Fig. 1-4 Health Quiz Prescreen. (Courtesy of Nellcor Incorporated, Pleasanton, Calif.)

or if postponement is required, the surgical time can be used for another patient without wasting valuable resources. A follow-up telephone contact the day before surgery is useful to ask about any interim illness, and to reinforce preoperative instructions.

A mechanism must exist for obtaining, reviewing, and following up results of any laboratory tests ordered. The ambulatory surgery center or preoperative assessment clinic must maintain good communication with the referring surgeon and ensure that the surgeon is made aware of any problems or potential delay of the scheduled procedure. Finally, documentation of the preoperative visit or telephone call, along with any laboratory results, surgical consent, and surgeon's note, should be maintained in a single patient file, which should be available for final review on the day before scheduled surgery. The particular paper flow pattern that best suits the needs of the practice setting must be determined on an individual basis; some considerations are summarized in Table 1-4.

Preoperative evaluation by the anesthesiologist may be reimbursed by third-party payors as a consultation. It is hoped that the efforts of the anesthesiologist in this area will help to curtail medical costs by limiting unnecessary laboratory tests, by contributing to appropriate patient selection, and, ultimately, by limiting postoperative complications.

Table 1-4 Logistical Issues in Preoperative Evaluation

Issue	Ideal	Considerations
Whether to see all patients	Have adequate medical information available on all patients for surgery Avoid last-minute cancellations	Ability to determine which patients should be seen Patient convenience Preoperative teaching
Timing of preoperative visit, if required	Allow adequate time for further evaluation Coordinate with visit to surgeon if possible	
Who sees patient	Anesthesiologist who will do case (Responsible anesthesiologist must review/confirm preoperative evaluation at the time of surgery)	Difficult logistically Adequacy of screening of healthy patients by registered nurse Possibility of using nurse practitioner, physician assistant, CRNA, under anesthesiologist's direction; internist or family practitioner is an alternative

Guidelines for preoperative evaluation	Consensus exists within the practice that allows consistency between anesthesiologists Patient seen preoperatively would be acceptable to any anesthesiologist in the group	Recognize need for case-by-case evaluation
Mechanism for review of laboratory tests, if any are required	Any needed test is reviewed, with appropriate follow-up of abnormal values	Need rapid turnaround; routing of results to ambulatory surgical center or preoperative evaluation clinic Preexisting agreement with consultants (internist, cardiologist) may be useful Fax capability useful for records
Mechanism to obtain records or consultation from other physicians	On-site consultation available Needed records are obtained Surgeons are aware of need to send pertinent records when patients are referred	
Mechanism to communicate with referring surgeon when cancellation or further evaluation is necessary	Surgeon is kept aware of patient's status and any potential delay	
Matching preoperative paperwork with ambulatory surgery center record	Documentation of preoperative evaluation is available for anesthesiologist review before scheduled surgery	Find optimal paper flow pattern for practice setting

Preoperative Instructions and Psychological Preparation

The preoperative visit should be a time for exchange of information: The personnel in the ambulatory surgery center learn about the patient, and the patient should in turn learn what to expect from ambulatory anesthesia and surgery. Any particular implications of the patient's underlying medical condition or planned procedure should be discussed, and the recommendations or options for anesthesia presented to the patient. Preoperative instructions should include specific fasting instructions, medications to take or withhold before surgery, and time and place to arrive on the day of surgery. The patient should be given a summary of what to expect upon arrival at the ambulatory surgery center, the anticipated duration of stay, and the need for a companion when discharged.

Specific concerns of the patient should be addressed; assurances that the patient's needs will be met may help to minimize anxiety on the morning of surgery. A brief discussion of management of postoperative pain and other potential complications is also reassuring to the patient. Similarly, contact with some of the personnel in the ambulatory surgery center before the day of surgery will help make the experience more comfortable for the patient.

Written instructions and information, perhaps in the form of a brochure, can provide the patient with a resource to review in the days before surgery (Box 1-11). This information should include an overview of the concept of ambulatory surgery; preoperative procedures, including testing; instructions regarding fasting and medications; and instructions for arrival and discharge, including parking. A single-page summary of the most important information, including patient-specific information, should be provided (Box 1-12). The patient should be encouraged to call the ambulatory surgery center with any questions or concerns before or after surgery.

Box 1-11 *Topics for Ambulatory Surgery Brochure*

Overview of concept of ambulatory surgery
Preoperative procedures
        Scheduling
        Preregistration
        Testing
Expectations for the day before surgery
        Preoperative phone call
        Eating and drinking
        Sleep
Expectations for the morning of surgery
        Fasting instructions
        Instructions on clothing, make-up, valuables
        Arrival—time and place, transportation, and parking
        Necessity of a caretaker for patient's children or
            other children in the family of a child having
            surgery
        Necessity of a companion to accompany patient
            home
Registration
        Financial materials required
        Proof of guardianship, if legal guardian is not parent
            (for children)
Preoperative preparation
        Nursing check-in
        Preoperative evaluation by anesthesiologist
        Intravenous line placement
        Options for premedication
        Options for anesthesia
Expectations for the recovery period
        Duration of stay in postanesthesia care unit
        Potential for and management of pain, nausea, and
            vomiting
Expectations for the remainder of the 24 hours after surgery
        Residual anesthetic effects
        Acceptable options for travel home (private car,
            van, or taxi with a companion. Bus, subway,
            walking are unacceptable.)
        Limitations on driving, operating equipment, mak-
            ing important decisions, and caring for children
        Need for companion
Mechanism for postoperative instructions and follow-up

Box 1-12 *Sample Checklist for Ambulatory Surgery (Instructions for Adult Patient)*

Have you

_____ had nothing to eat or drink since midnight the night before your surgery?

_____ had no alcohol or tobacco products since midnight the night before your surgery?

_____ made arrangements for child care for the day of your surgery and for 36 hours after surgery?

_____ arranged for a responsible adult to take you to the center, stay with you, and take you home after surgery?

_____ taken your regular medication as directed by the anesthesiologist?

_____ brought with you the names of your medications, a list of any allergies, and your insurance card or other necessary financial information?

_____ worn loose-fitting clothes and left all of your valuables at home?

Date of surgery _____

Type of surgery _____

Arrival time _____

Special instructions _____

From Ambulatory Surgery Center, Medical College of Virginia Hospitals, Richmond, Va.

Summary

Preoperative evaluation serves to provide the anesthesiologist with information needed to assess risk and to plan anesthetic care. The most important components of the preoperative assessment are a careful history and physical examination. Laboratory and ancillary tests should be ordered only when indicated by the results of the history and physical examination, and not used as screening panels. Careful communication between surgeon and anesthesiologist, and a uniformly organized preoperative process, are essential to the smooth functioning of an ambulatory surgery center. Contact with the ambulatory surgery center before scheduled surgery provides the patient with necessary instructions and information, and should serve to reduce anxiety and provide a more patient-focused experience.

References

1. Egbert LD, Battit GE, Turndorf H, Beecher HK: The value of the preoperative visit by an anesthetist: a study of doctor-patient rapport. JAMA 1963; 185:553-5.

2. Twersky RS, Lebovits AH, Lewis M, Frank D: Early anesthesia evaluation of the ambulatory surgical patient: does it really help? J Clin Anesth 1992; 4:204-7.

3. American Society of Anesthesiologists: New classification of physical status. Anesthesiology 1963; 24:111.

4. Welborn LG: Perioperative apnea in the premature infant. Anesthesiol Clin North Am 1991; 9:885-97.

5. Fleisher LA, Barash PG: Preoperative cardiac evaluation for noncardiac surgery: a functional approach. Anesth Analg 1992; 74:586-98.

6. Wilson ME: Predicting difficult intubation. Br J Anaesth 1993; 71:333-4.

7. Mallampati SR, Gatt SP, Gugino LD et al: A clinical sign to predict difficult tracheal intubation: a prospective study. Can Anaesth Soc J 1985; 32:429-34.

8. Frerk CM: Predicting difficult intubation. Anaesthesia 1991; 46:1005-8.

9. American Society of Anesthesiologists: Practice guidelines for management of the difficult airway. Anesthesiology 1993; 78:597-602.

10. Macario A, Roizen MF, Thisted RA et al: Reassessment of preoperative laboratory testing has changed the test-ordering patterns of physicians. Surg Gynecol Obstet 1992; 175:539-47.

11. Narr, BJ, Hansen TR, Warner M: Preoperative laboratory screening in healthy Mayo patients: cost-effective elimination of tests and unchanged outcomes. Mayo Clin Proc 1991; 66:155-9.

12. Roy WL, Lerman J, McIntyre BG: Is preoperative hemoglobin testing justified in children undergoing minor elective surgery? Can J Anaesth 1991; 38:700-3.

13. American Society of Anesthesiologists: Statement on routine preoperative laboratory and diagnostic screening. Approved by House of Delegates on October 14, 1987, and last amended on October 13, 1993. American Society of Anesthesiologists, 1994 Directory of Members, Park Ridge, Ill, p. 775.

14. Macpherson DS, Snow R, Lofgren RP: Preoperative screening: value of previous tests. Ann Int Med 1990; 113: 969-73.

15. Roizen MF, Cohn S: Preoperative evaluation for elective surgery—what laboratory tests are needed? Adv Anesthesia 1993; 10:25-47.

16. Manley S, Dekelaita G, Feldman L et al: Is routine preoperative pregnancy testing necessary? Anesthesiology 1992; 77:A41.

17. Goldberger AL, O'Konski M: Utility of the routine electrocardiogram before surgery and on general hospital admission: critical review and new guidelines. Ann Intern Med 1986; 105:552-7.

18. Gold BS, Young ML, Kinman JL et al: The utility of preoperative electrocardiogram in the ambulatory surgery patient. Arch Intern Med 1992; 152:301-5.

19. Parosokos JA: Who needs a preoperative electrocardiogram? Arch Intern Med 1992: 152:261-3.

20. Tape TG, Mushlin Al: How useful are routine chest x-rays of preoperative patients at risk for postoperative chest disease? J Gen Int Med 1988; 3:15-20.

21. Archer C, Levy AR, McGregor M: Value of routine preoperative chest x-rays: a meta-analysis. Can J Anaesth 1993; 40:1022-7.

22. Zibrak JD, O'Donnell CR, Marton K: Indications for pulmonary function testing. Ann Int Med 1990; 112:763-71.

23. Zibrak JD, O'Donnell CR, Marton K: Preoperative pulmonary function testing. Ann Int Med 1990; 112:793-4.

24. Crosby ET, Lui A: The adult cervical spine: implications for airway management. Can J Anaesth 1990; 37:77-93.

25. Patel RI, Hannallah RS: Preoperative screening for pediatric ambulatory surgery: evaluation of a telephone questionnaire method. Anesth Analg 1992; 75:258-61.

26. American Society of Anesthesiologists: Basic standards for preanesthesia care. Approved by House of Delegates on October 14, 1987. American Society of Anesthesiologists, 1994 Directory of Members, Park Ridge, Ill, p. 734.

27. Joint Commission on the Accreditation of Healthcare Organizations: Accreditation manual for hospitals, Chicago, 1994, JCAHO, p. 6.

28. Conway JB, Goldberg J, Chung F: Preadmission anaesthesia consultation clinic. Can J Anaesth 1992; 39:1051-7.

29. Lutner RE, Roizen MF, Stocking CB et al: The automated interview versus the personal interview. Do patient responses to preoperative questions differ? Anesthesiology 1991; 75:394-400.

Common and Special Ambulatory Procedures 2

Jocelyn R. McClain and Rebecca S. Twersky

Ambulatory facilities
**Perioperative considerations for
   common ambulatory procedures**
   Gynecology
   General surgery
   Ophthalmology
   Otolaryngology
   Dental extractions
   Plastic procedures
   Podiatry
   Orthopedics
   Urology
   Pain
   Medical
Special ambulatory procedures
Summary

Ambulatory Facilities

As predicted, ambulatory surgery has grown phenomenally. There are more surgical centers, more procedures, as well as a higher percentage of patients receiving outpatient surgery (Fig. 2-1 and Table 2-1). It is no longer a promising concept, but a reality with

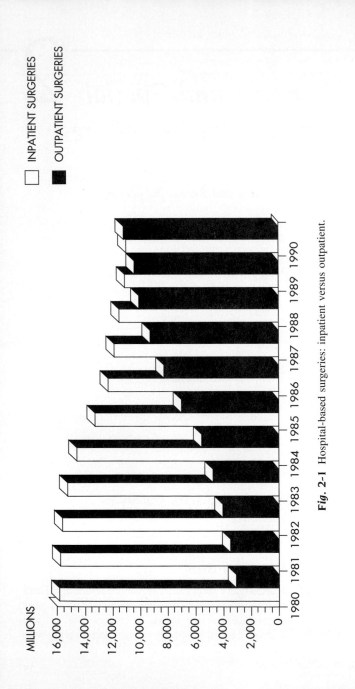

Fig. 2-1 Hospital-based surgeries: inpatient versus outpatient.

Table 2-1   Growth Projections for Surgery Centers

Year	Number of facilities	Total number of surgeries	Number of surgeries per facility
1983	239	377,266	1578
1984	330	517,851	1569
1985	459	783,864	1708
1986	592	1,033,604	1746
1987	865	1,383,540	1712
1988	964	1,722,367	1787
1989	1221	2,162,391	1771
1990	1381	2,618,739	1896
1991	1510	3,016,000	1997
1992	1643	3,456,000	2103
1993	1708	3,817,000	2235

Source: SMG Marketing Group.

seemingly endless bounds. The changes in health care finances support this growth.

Rapid advances in surgical technology and improvements in anesthetic care have made outpatient surgery desirable and safe. Ambulatory surgery is marketed in a variety of settings, each with its own advantages and disadvantages. Hospital-based facilities, freestanding facilities, and physician office–based facilities are the major categories (Table 2-2).[1]

In the hospital-based facility, outpatient surgery may be performed on the same campus or removed from the hospital yet retain its affiliation. The hospital unit may be integrated in the main operating room, or it may have separate operating room suites, separate postanesthesia care units, and even separate

Table 2-2   Surgery Center Facilities by Type of Ownership

Type	Number of facilities	Percentage of total
Corporate chain	158	11.4
Independent	1129	81.8
Hospital owned	94	6.8
Total	1381	100.0

Based on 1990 figures. Source: SMG Marketing Group.

staffing. Freestanding ambulatory centers maintain no hospital affiliation and are often physician-owned. These facilities have flourished as a constant shift from inpatient to outpatient services has occurred. Expansion is predicted to occur driven by four forces: (1) improved construction and operation of surgical centers; (2) new surgical techniques; (3) improved anesthetic agents; and (4) regulations influencing ambulatory surgery.[2]

Physician office–based surgery has also grown with more procedures being offered, thus allowing lower costs to both patients and third-party payors. However, other facilities investing more in high-tech equipment—often capturing specialty niches—are likely to remain for the more minor procedures. The growth of this market segment and success in financial management have brought about another layer of outpatient care. These patients, although suitable for ambulatory surgery, require prolonged observation in excess of the average 2- to 3-hour ambulatory stay. Minimal stay status offers the physician and hospital added flexibility in managing more procedures for a wider range of patients. Recovery care centers is the next level of care, offering postoperative supervision for up to 72 hours.

Perioperative Considerations for Common Ambulatory Procedures (See Table 2-3)

Gynecology

Laparoscopy

Laparoscopy in gynecologic surgery has allowed for significant advances in outpatient surgery. Laparoscopy can be used diagnostically for infertility and pelvic pain, as well as therapeutically for ovarian cystectomies, laser ablation of endometriosis, removal of ectopic pregnancies, and myomectomies.

Laparoscopy is the endoscopic examination of the intraabdominal cavity. The incisions are small and, therefore, cause little patient discomfort. A periumbilical incision is made, through which a Verres needle is inserted (Figs. 2-2 and 2-3). Carbon dioxide (CO_2) is insufflated through this needle to obtain the pneumoperitoneum; therefore, it is important that this needle pass through the fascial planes and the peritoneum. This pneumoperitoneum allows better visualization of the intraabdominal and pelvic cavities. When the needle is inserted correctly and when CO_2 insufflation has begun, the intraabdominal pressure stays well

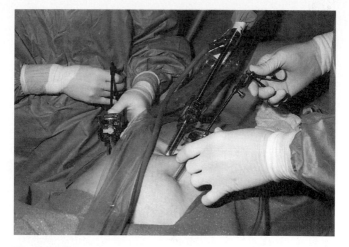

Fig. 2-2 *Center,* 10 mm trocar with camera inserted; *left,* 12 mm trocars with operating instruments.

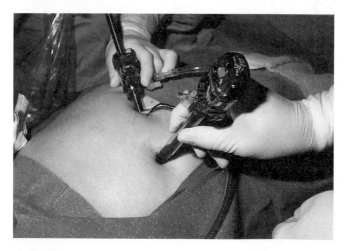

Fig. 2-3 *Center,* Umbilical 10 mm trocar; *left,* 12 mm trocar placement.

below 19 mm Hg. Should the pressure gauge rise abruptly and CO_2 flow cease, the surgeon must recheck the needle positioning. After obtaining an adequate pneumoperitoneum (usually with

Text continued on p. 44.

Table 2-3 Perioperative Considerations for Common Ambulatory Procedures

Procedure	Risks	Postoperative considerations	Common anesthesia techniques
Gynecology			
Laparoscopy (diagnostic, LTS, laser)	Bowel perforation Ventilatory impairment due to CO_2 insufflation Aspiration Bleeding CO_2 laser burns, corneal injury	Bleeding Pain Nausea/vomiting	General Spinal Epidural
Dilatation and curettage	Uterine perforation Bleeding	Bleeding Nausea/vomiting	General Spinal Epidural
Hysteroscopy	Pulmonary edema	Hyponatremia Urinary retention	General Spinal Epidural
General Surgery			
Breast biopsy	Minimal bleeding	Nonspecific	Local anesthesia MAC General

Procedure			
Inguinal herniorrhaphy	Bleeding Laser surgery—bowel perforation, CO_2 insufflation complications	Pain Urinary retention	General Ilioinguinal field block Spinal Epidural Caudal (pediatrics) Local anesthesia, MAC
Hemorrhoidectomy	Airway control Bleeding Patient positioning	Pain Urinary retention	Spinal Epidural General
Ophthalmology Cataract extraction	Minimal	Nonspecific	MAC Retrobulbar or peribulbar block
Strabismus correction	Oculocardiac reflex	Nausea/vomiting Pain	General (pediatrics) MAC, general (adults)
Otolaryngology Tonsillectomy and adenoidectomy	Aspiration Bleeding Endotracheal tube displacement	Nausea/vomiting Pain	General
Myringotomy and tube insertion	Minimal	Nonspecific	General MAC (adults)

Continued.

Table 2-3 Perioperative Considerations for Common Ambulatory Procedures—cont'd

Procedure	Risks	Postoperative considerations	Common anesthesia techniques
Otolaryngology—cont'd			
Sinus surgery	Blood loss	Bleeding	General
	Local anesthesia toxicity	Nausea/vomiting	MAC
Laryngoscopy	Vocal cord edema	Respiratory difficulty	General
	Laryngospasm	Bleeding	General with insufflation
	Laser injury and airway fires		
Panendoscopy	Tracheal or bronchial tears		
Dental			
Oral rehabilitation/extractions	Aspiration	Bleeding	Local/sedation
	Bleeding	Nausea/vomiting	General
Plastics and Reconstructive			
Miscellaneous procedures	Local anesthesia toxicity	Nausea/vomiting	General
Aesthetic surgery	Prolonged surgery	Hematoma	MAC
		Nerve injuries	
		Drowsiness	

Procedure			
Liposuction	Fluid loss Fat embolus	Hypotension Blood and fluid replacement	General MAC
Podiatry			
Bunionectomy	Tourniquet	Nonspecific	MAC Regional block
Orthopedics			
Arthroscopy: knee and shoulder	Tourniquet Prolonged surgery	Pain	Regional, general
Carpal tunnel	Minimal	Nonspecific	Regional MAC
Urology			
Cystoscopy	Bleeding	Hematuria Bladder spasm Urinary retention	General Spinal/epidural MAC
Lithotripsy	Arrhythmias	Hematuria Pain from fragmented calculi	General MAC Spinal/epidural

approximately 3 L), the Verres needle is removed and a trocar inserted. The size of the trocar will vary depending on what procedure is to be done. The laparoscope is then passed through the self-sealing opening in the hollow trocar. In order to maintain a pneumoperitoneum, the laparoscope is connected to the insufflator and set to deliver a constant flow of 200 ml per minute. A second puncture site for cannula insertion is made for manipulation of the uterus. This second puncture is often made near the bladder.[3]

Laparoscopic tubal sterilization

Laparoscopic tubal sterilization has become the most common operation performed in the United States.[3] The fallopian tubes may be electrocauterized or silastic rings or clips may be placed, depending on surgeon preference. Electrocautery is a safe, popular method that is permanent, which may not be attractive to certain patients who later seek microvascularization and reanastomosis of the tubes. A current delivered between a positive and a negative electrode destroys the tissue. The surgeon views the procedure to ensure destruction and to measure the degree of current passing through. The placement of silastic rings or clips only occludes the tube; therefore, the potential for reanastomosis is greater. Clips and silastic rings are associated with a greater degree of postoperative pain. It should be noted that many surgeons use multiple methods of sterilization (cutting, cautery, and clips) to decrease the failure rate. Box 2-1 illustrates the important features for laparoscopic

---

Box 2-1 *Important Features of Laparoscopic Tubal Sterilization*

CO_2 pneumoperitoneum
Relaxed abdomen for trocar insertion
Risk of bowel puncture and vessel gas embolus
Empty bladder
Empty stomach
Ventilation concerns regarding CO_2 absorption
Trendelenburg position
Use of silastic rings or clips versus electrocauterization of tubes
Risk of aspiration

tubal sterilization. Intraoperative morphine and local anesthetic infiltration of the mesosalpinx have been recently evaluated for their analgesic effects.[4, 5] General anesthesia is utilized most frequently; however, spinal or epidural anesthesia can be administered in patients undergoing brief procedures and whose body habitus can tolerate pneumoperitoneum without significant respiratory embarrassment.

Diagnostic laparoscopy

Diagnostic laparoscopy may be performed in the work-up of pelvic pain and infertility. Laser ablation of endometriosis is often involved. The same major concerns of laparoscopy apply. In addition, one must consider the impact of the use of laser in the operating room: *LASER* (light amplification by stimulated emission of radiation) is used for surgical cutting, vaporization, coagulation, and cauterization. In particular, the CO_2 laser with a wavelength of 10,600 amperes is often used in gynecologic surgery. The characteristics of the laser are determined by the wavelength of light emitted by the medium used. Carbon dioxide laser does not penetrate deeply into tissue layers. Therefore, safety precautions must specifically prevent absorption of laser energy by superficial tissue in undesired locations. Corneal injury is a possible danger of CO_2 laser. Protective eyewear must be used by all hospital personnel in the room in which laser is being used. The patient's eyes must be protected by the same eyewear. In addition, after the patient's eyes have been taped shut, moist gauze should be used to cover the eyes, because water is an effective absorber of CO_2 laser. Moist towels are also used to shield the surgical drapes from the laser to prevent potential fires.

Postlaparoscopic pain is the main factor that requires intervention during the recovery period both in the hospital and after discharge. Oral or parenteral nonsteroidal antiinflammatory drugs (NSAIDs) have particular usefulness in managing postlaparoscopy pain.[6, 7]

Dilatation and curettage

Dilatation and curettage is performed to obtain endometrial sampling and to evaluate abnormal uterine bleeding. The patient is placed in the Trendelenburg position with the legs in stirrups. The surgeon must initially clamp and then dilate the cervix. This is the time of greatest stimulation. Following this, the uterus is sounded to determine the depth of the cavity. During the curettage stage, there is risk of uterine perforation. At this time, the patient must not move. Perforation and hemorrhage would require further exploratory surgery. Intraoperative bleeding is minimal, and recovery is rapid.

Dilatation and curettage for incomplete abortion or termination of pregnancy

Dilatation and curettage for incomplete abortion or termination of pregnancy has several important features. After incomplete abortion, the cervix is usually dilated as a result of partial passage of the products of conception, whereas nulliparous patients who present for termination of pregnancy may have laminaria tents in the endocervix. These are placed in the firm, undilated cervix of the nulliparous patient 12 to 24 hours before the procedure to allow the cervix to dilate slowly. The use of the laminaria reduces the incidence of cervical laceration and uterine perforation. Instead of sharp curettage as is used in diagnostic D&C, suction curettage is used. Suction curettage causes less trauma to the uterine wall and is associated with less blood loss. Blood loss may be related to the length of the gestation, anesthetic technique, or possible development of coagulopathy as a result of released tissue thromboplastins. Uterine contractility aids in decreasing blood loss, and is prompted by the complete evacuation of all products of conception. In addition, oxytocin infusion or intramuscular methylergonovine is often administered to increase uterine tone. Anesthetics that relax uterine tone should be avoided. Postoperative bleeding, cramping from continued oxytocin infusion, as well as nausea and vomiting can occur. Appropriate intervention should be instituted, and the patient observed until bleeding is minimal.

Hysteroscopy

In diagnostic hysteroscopy the endocervical canal and uterine cavity are examined to determine the distribution and characteristics of lesions and to perform selected biopsies. Hysteroscopy is usually performed with a 4 mm hysteroscope and a 5 mm diagnostic hysteroscopic sheath. This sheath is passed through the end of the cervix, and because of the scope's small size, the procedure usually requires little or no cervical dilatation. The gynecologist must decide which method will be used for distention of the uterine cavity: CO_2 insufflation, low-molecular-weight dextran, or glycine. There are differences in costs as well as in the cleaning procedure of the instruments. When CO_2 is used, bubbles, mucus, and blood will easily obscure the view. This is not the case when dextran 70 (Hyskon) is used.[8] When endometrial ablation or resection is performed, CO_2 or dextran may enter the systemic circulation, allowing the possibility of gas embolization or fluid overload. In addition, dextran 70 may cause anaphylaxis or coagulopathy. The risk of anaphylaxis is reduced by the routine use of dextran 1 (Promit). Dextran 70 is a polyvalent hapten that may form antibody complexes as any antigen does. Dextran 1, however, is a monovalent hapten that can only bind individual sites of antibodies. Without the formation of an immune complex, anaphylaxis does not occur. Administration of a molar excess of monovalent hapten just before intravenous administration of dextran 70 competitively prevents formation of immune complexes.[9]

A solution of dextran 70 or glycine is the preferred distending and irrigating agent. The procedure is performed with the patient in the Trendelenburg position with the legs in stirrups. If significant irrigation fluid is used, patients are at risk for developing dilutional hyponatremia or pulmonary edema. Diuretic therapy with furosemide may be used postoperatively.

Cervical cone biopsy

Cervical cone biopsy is performed in patients who have abnormal cervical cytology. The goal of the procedure is to obtain a plug of tissue incorporating two thirds of the depth of the endocervix and the entire transformation zone. The plug may be cone-shaped or cylindrical.[10] In addition, cervical conization may be used for the treatment of chronic intraepithelial neoplasia. The procedure may be performed with a scalpel or with a CO_2 laser. In the latter instance, the precautions for laser use in the operating room should be instituted. Conization is reserved for patients in whom the diagnosis could not be made by colposcopy-directed biopsies. The cervix is well vascularized; therefore, the risk of bleeding is significant. Hemostatic sutures may be placed in the cervix before conization, or dilute solutions of epinephrine may be injected to induce local vasospasm and thereby reduce blood loss. If epinephrine is used, one must be cautious for possible intravascular injection with resultant vasospasm of coronary as well as systemic vessels leading to myocardial ischemia and significant hypertension. As with many gynecological procedures, cervical and intrauterine manipulation may result in prostaglandin release, which can result in continued postoperative pain. Nonsteroidal antiinflammatory agents have been found useful to combat pain.

General Surgery

Breast biopsy

Breast biopsy is a surgical procedure commonly performed on an outpatient basis. Cancer prevention education has increased women's awareness and readiness to perform self-breast examinations, undergo mammography, and seek medical attention earlier rather than later. Simple procedures, such as needle aspiration of cysts, may be performed in the physician's office. Palpable masses, depending on their location, may be biopsied under local anesthesia, local anesthesia with sedation, or general anesthesia. Nonpalpable masses detected on mammography require needle localization by x-ray technique to assist surgical biopsy. The method for needle localization requires no preoperative sedation. The patient is taken to the radiology department, where localizing needles are placed. The patient is returned to the operating room, where the biopsy procedure is performed. Special care is taken not to disrupt needle placement while positioning the patient. Breast biopsies may be incisional or excisional in type. Incisional breast biopsy involves incision and partial removal to obtain a specimen. Excisional biopsy involves removal of the entire mass. In most instances, a circumareolar incision can be used, even when the lesion is at some distance from the nipple. When this is not possible, a curved incision is used. After removal of the mass, the specimen is sent to the pathology laboratory for frozen section. If needle localization is required, the specimen will be sent for examination by xeroradiography, and the radiologist informs the surgeon if the suspicious area has been removed. After removal of the lesion, careful hemostasis is achieved. The patient is fit for discharge on the same day.

Special concerns for the patient undergoing breast biopsy include anxiety due to fear of malignancy, fear of disfigurement, and embarrassment of body exposure. In addition, although they are sedated, these patients may still be aware of conversation in the operating room, particularly when pathologists inform the surgeon of the diagnosis. Postoperatively serosanguinous drainage may be expected. Minimal to mild pain can usually be controlled with oral analgesics (e.g., acetaminophen with codeine, with oxycodone, or related compounds).

Inguinal herniorrhaphy

Inguinal herniorrhaphy is a common procedure performed on patients of all ages and both sexes. Repair of inguinal hernia is strongly recommended in all patients so that strangulation of bowel can be prevented. All but very large hernias can be repaired on an outpatient basis. There are numerous surgical techniques that are performed using various general, regional, and local anesthetic techniques. A long-acting local anesthetic can be intra-operatively injected at the surgical site to make the patient more comfortable during the postoperative period and to promote early ambulation. Again, several options are available for the adminis-tration of local anesthetic, including field block, direct bathing of the nerve as it is visualized during the surgical procedure, ilioinguinal and iliohypogastric nerve block, and wound margin infiltration (see Chapter 8). Bilateral hernia repair is more com-monly performed in pediatric outpatients than in adult outpatients. Various combinations of general, caudal, and ilioinguinal block have been successfully reported in this population.[11, 12]

Laparoscopic inguinal herniorrhaphy, a relatively new proce-dure performed on an outpatient basis, may represent an advance in laparoscopic technique that enables improved repair. The most important concerns in this procedure are carbon dioxide, pneumo-peritoneum development and respiratory effects, necessity of placing the patient in the Trendelenburg position, and the possi-bility for bleeding and bowel perforation on trocar insertion. A CO_2 pneumoperitoneum is induced, and a 10 mm trocar is placed at the umbilicus. At the level of the umbilicus, two trocars are placed laterally to the rectus muscle in the left and right mid-lower abdomen. A 10 mm trocar is placed on the site of the hernia, and a 5 mm trocar is placed on the contralateral side. A straight or 30-degree angle diagnostic laparoscope, video equipment, and dis-posable trocars are used (Figs. 2-4 and 2-5). The patient should be in the Trendelenburg position to displace intraabdominal contents cephalad. After identifying the hernia defect, the peritoneum over the defect is opened using a combination of blunt dissection and cautery, separating the hernia sack from the myofascial layers. Propylene mesh and endoclips are used for surgical repair. In a

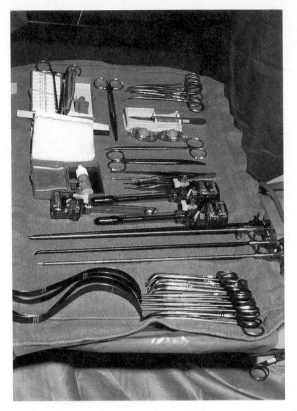

Fig. 2-4 Laparoscopy equipment. *From top to bottom:* Scissors, antifog solution for camera lens, trocars, and right-angle dissector.

series of 63 procedures performed by Sailors et al.,[13] the myofascial defect was loosely packed with rolled propylene mesh; however, this technique is not universal. An additional sheet of propylene mesh is used to cover the hernia defect; it is placed over the transverse abdominus arch, Cooper's ligament, and ileopubic tract. Then the peritoneum is approximated over the mesh sheet with standard laparoscopic clips.

A small number of patients have received inguinal herniorrhaphy with this repair; however, laparoscopic herniorrhaphy is still under evaluation for safety and efficacy. Preliminary results show

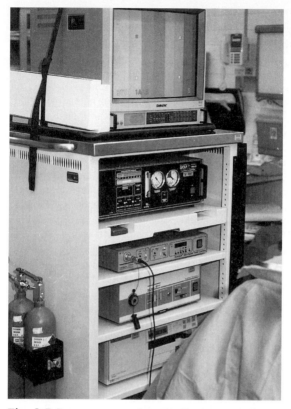

Fig. 2-5 Laparoscopy equipment. *From top to bottom:* Viewer, insufflator and gauges, camera source, light source, recorder, CO_2 tanks on side.

fast recovery and return to work, little postoperative pain, and high patient satisfaction. The selection of patients and surgical skill are important. Continued experience with laparoscopic operative techniques should reduce potential problems.

Common postoperative problems that follow conventional herniorrhaphy include urinary retention, which may delay discharge from the facility, and pain management. It has been reported that the incidence of urinary retention following herniorrhaphy was higher in patients older than 53 years of age who receive general anesthesia and greater than 1200 ml of fluid. Spinal anesthesia and minimal fluid administration appear to lessen the incidence of urinary retention.[14]

Hemorrhoidectomy

Hemorrhoids are classified as external or internal based on their site of origin. External hemorrhoids occur in the lower third of the anal canal, and internal hemorrhoids occur in the upper two thirds of the canal. Patients presenting for hemorrhoidectomy are those who have failed conservative management and treatment by injection of sclerosing solution, and those who initially present with very large hemorrhoids. Therefore, extensive repair, with its higher risk of postoperative bleeding and a prolonged observation period, is often necessary. Pain management is another reason for prolonged observation of these patients.

The important concerns with this procedure are the amount of blood loss, the positioning of the patient, and airway control, which includes appropriately placed bolsters for ventilation for the patient in the prone position. The surgical procedure may be a formal or a limited hemorrhoidectomy. The limited hemorrhoidectomy is usually compatible with the ambulatory time frame. It is wise to ascertain the proposed position of the patient, which is determined by surgeon preference, before anesthetizing the patient: Improper positioning will make visualization difficult for the surgeon and may lead to increased patient morbidity. Lateral, jackknife, prone, or lithotomy positions may be chosen. The buttock is spread apart, exposing the hemorrhoid. Local anesthetic (lidocaine or bupivacaine) *with* epinephrine is often used to decrease the amount of bleeding.[15] In the limited method, the hemorrhoid is excised, after which no attempt is made to close the mucosa. White petrolatum gauze and a simple dry dressing are placed on the wound. In the formal approach, the hemorrhoid is excised by removing the mucosal and submucosal tissue. Initial anal dilatation may be very painful for an inadequately anesthetized patient. The mucosa is closed in this procedure. Local anesthetic may be injected to provide postoperative pain relief, and white petrolatum gauze is placed in the anal canal between the internal and external sphincters.

Postoperative pain control and urinary retention are common problems. The incidence of postoperative urinary retention in patients who have undergone surgery for benign anorectal disease ranges from 0% to 70%, and is significantly increased when a long-acting local anesthetic agent is used and when more than 1000 ml of intravenous fluid is administered perioperatively.[16] To reduce the incidence of postoperative urinary retention, perioperative fluid restriction, use of shorter-acting local anesthetics, and delayed catheterization (until a palpable bladder is detected) are suggested.

Circumcision

Circumcisions are ideal outpatient procedures, because postoperative pain can easily be managed with local blocks, which allow for early ambulation. The removal of foreskin requires careful hemostasis. Postoperative pain can be managed with a series of penile blocks or the application of lidocaine jelly or spray. Application of topical lidocaine has been found highly effective with the same duration of analgesia as morphine and nerve block.[17]

Ophthalmology

Cataract extraction

A cataract is an opacity of the crystalline lens that may impair vision and interfere with the lifestyle of otherwise functional older adults. Cataract extraction has become an extremely common procedure performed in freestanding and hospital-affiliated ambulatory surgery units, many of which devote a large percentage of patient care and procedure time to cataract extraction. These patients are generally geriatric patients with multiple medical problems on multiple medications. Therefore, preoperative assessment is of paramount importance to ensure safe and uncomplicated surgery. Outpatient cataract surgery has been highly successful, and it is a procedure that is well accepted by the general population. However, to maintain this trend we must continue to consider the multiple medical problems these patients can have, as well as the occasional need to admit them to the hospital. These patients are older, they may live alone, and they may not have a home environment suitable for postoperative recovery.

There are different methods of removing the cataract. The method selected by the surgeon will depend on the ophthalmic examination.

Intracapsular cataract extraction

In intracapsular cataract extraction (ICCE), the opaque lens with the lens capsule is completely removed, and the intraocular lens is placed in the anterior chamber. This procedure is performed in selected cases of subluxation, dislocation, and lens-induced glaucoma.

Extracapsular cataract extraction

In extracapsular cataract extraction (ECCE), the lens is removed while the zonules and posterior lens capsule remain intact and clear. A rim of anterior lens capsule also remains to support a posterior chamber intraocular lens. Extracapsular cataract extraction has largely supplanted ICCE. Newer forms of ECCE include phacoemulsification and phacofragmentation. Phacoemulsification is a popular technique that is quick and simple for well-skilled hands. The lens is fragmented by ultrasonic vibrations, irrigated, and aspirated simultaneously. An intraocular lens is then placed.[18] Regional eye block (peribulbar or retrobulbar) is routinely performed with or without additional sedation. Use of long-acting local anesthetics minimizes the need for intraoperative analgesics. Occasionally carbonic anhydrase inhibitors (e.g., acetazolamide, methazolamide) or mannitol may be administered to reduce intraocular pressure. When these agents are used, appropriate assessment of electrolyte and metabolic homeostasis should be made.

Strabismus repair

In pediatric practice, the most common ocular surgery is strabismus repair. This procedure corrects involuntary gaze preference by strengthening or lengthening the appropriate muscle. Pediatric patients undergo the procedure under general anesthesia; however, regional block is an option for the cooperative adult. The patient should be placed in the supine position with the head stabilized and the neck extended. Use of an oral RAE tube allows the surgeon to operate with relative ease. A fornix or limbal approach may be used to access the rectus muscle. After separating the eyelids with an eyelid speculum, the surgeon grasps the globe with forceps and gently elevates it from the orbit. The conjunctiva is grasped with forceps, and Wescott scissors are used to penetrate the scleral surface of the eye. A tenotomy hook can then be passed into the incision and slid underneath to secure the rectus muscle.[19]

At this point, anesthetic concerns include oculocardiac reflex, postoperative nausea and vomiting, postoperative pain control, and (controversial) use of succinylcholine. Muscle manipulation may stimulate the oculocardiac reflex, which involves a trigeminal and vagal nerve pathway. The response is most commonly bradycardia, which may be resolved by cessation of muscle manipulation, and may be attenuated by atropine. The reflex may also decrease in intensity with continued stimulation. The incidence of nausea and vomiting after strabismus repair ranges from 30% to 85%, which is higher than that seen after other procedures with similar anesthetic technique. Decreasing its incidence and severity would improve postoperative comfort and shorten patients' stay at the facility. Droperidol has been shown to decrease nausea and vomiting. The ideal pediatric dose is not clear. The suggested dose ranges from 20 to 75 µg/kg. Lerman et al. suggest that droperidol be given at the time of induction, anticipating approximately 10 minutes until eye manipulation.[20] The perioperative use of intravenous droperidol is not without disadvantages. Even in small doses, it may produce profound and protracted somnolence, as well as hypotension, restlessness, and extrapyramidal effects. Metoclopramide may have some advantage over droperidol, as it enables effective antiemesis without excessive somnolence.[21] The incidence of vomiting warrants further studies with comparisons to newer agents such as the 5-HT_3 antagonists (e.g., granisteron, ondansetron, and dolasetron). Other methods aimed at control of postoperative nausea and vomiting include intraoperative gastric suctioning, replacement of preoperative fluid deficits, and the avoidance of opioids. Postoperative analgesia is often adequately treated with acetaminophen. The reversal of skeletal muscle relaxation has also been incriminated in increasing the incidence of nausea and vomiting. With new short-acting muscle relaxants (such as mivacurium), this may be prevented. Routine pediatric use of succinylcholine is no longer advised. With implications for forced duction testing and malignant hyperthermia, viable alternatives are available. In the age-appropriate patient, the author prefers propofol induction with propofol maintenance infusion. Propofol infusion alone is associated with a lower incidence of emesis in the 24 hours following surgery as compared with propofol/N_2O or halothane/N_2O/droperidol technique.[22, 23]

Otolaryngology

Tonsillectomy and adenoidectomy

Although adenotonsillectomy is a common otolaryngologic procedure, it is still not performed as frequently as it was in the past. It is indicated in carcinoma, abscess, sleep apnea, and recurrent tonsillitis.[24] As an ambulatory procedure, it is controversial because of the potential for severe consequences of postoperative bleeding.[25, 26] Typically, serious posttonsillectomy bleeding does not occur immediately after surgery; there are two peak times, one at 12 to 24 hours, the second at 5 to 10 days postoperative. It is commonly caused by premature separation of the formed granulation tissue from the pharyngeal surfaces. Clot evacuation and control of bleeding may require surgical intervention if application of topical caustic solutions is unsuccessful. Delayed hemorrhage may also be due to inadvertent placement of suture through a major vessel. Bleeding occurs when the suture dissolves.[27] These patients are most often observed under some type of minimal stay admission. The choice of discharge status may be guided somewhat on an individual basis. Box 2-2 lists the inappropriate patients for tonsillectomy and adenoidectomy. The preoperative medical evaluation becomes crucial in patient selection. Patients with a history of blood dyscrasia of any form; chronic aspirin users; and those with a recent history of upper respiratory infection, allergic disorders, or episodes of acute tonsillitis are not candidates for ambulatory surgery.[28] Children less than 3 years old reportedly have higher episodes of

---

Box 2-2 Exclusion Criteria for Ambulatory Surgical Tonsillectomy and Adenoidectomy

Lingual tonsillectomy
History of blood dyscrasia
Sickle cell disease
Leukemia
Chronic aspirin ingestion
Recent history of allergic disorder
Recent acute tonsillitis or upper respiratory infection
Sleep apnea
Inappropriate social factors
Children less than 3 years old

postoperative respiratory difficulty and should not have this surgery as outpatients.[29] In addition, blood loss in the very young patient may significantly alter circulating blood volume. One must also carefully search for a history of sleep apnea. The progression of this state involves episodes of hypoxia that may lead to increased pulmonary artery pressure, cor pulmonale, and heart failure. Adult patients who undergo tonsillectomy often have redundant pharyngeal tissue and should be observed postoperatively for episodes of hypoxia. Patients with congenital airway abnormalities are also at risk and should be observed for longer durations. One must also consider social factors, such as responsibility of caregivers and distance from hospital. Lingual tonsillectomy in the adult is often performed on an inpatient basis because it is a technically more difficult procedure with increased risk of bleeding.

The procedure is performed in the supine position after induction of general anesthesia and insertion of an endotracheal tube, commonly a RAE tube. The surgeon places a Crowe-Davis mouth gag, which holds the mouth open for the surgeon, and holds the endotracheal tube in place. Alternatively, a Jennings mouth gag may be used, but its placement requires temporary disconnection of the anesthesia circuit from the endotracheal tube. Proper attention must be paid to the airway at this time because the endotracheal tube may easily become kinked by the mouth gag. It is important to observe for breath sounds and peak airway pressure to ensure adequate ventilation at this step. Also as the surgeon opens the mouth and directs his or her attention to the surgical procedure, inadvertent extubation may occur.

The tonsil is then grasped with a tenaculum, and the mucosal membrane over the superior pole of the tonsil is incised. Dissection of the superior pole is done with an elevator, and a snare is used to encircle and dissect the tonsil from its inferior attachments. Hemostasis is then obtained using packing, cautery, or ligature, as determined by the surgeon.[30] The other tonsil is then removed. Often the stomach will be emptied before extubation, because ingested blood contributes to postoperative nausea and vomiting. The tonsil or capsule may be infiltrated with a local anesthetic mixture; however, the effectiveness of bupivacaine infiltration in reducing pain and analgesic requirements has been questioned in both children and adults.[31, 32] The procedure of adenoidectomy is often combined with tonsillectomy. It is also performed using a mouth gag. Two red Robinson catheters are placed through the mouth to act as a palate retractor. The adenoid tissue is then removed using curettes, and the base of the adenoid is coagulated using electrocautery. Common immediate postoperative concerns are postoperative nausea, vomiting, and bleeding. The overall incidence of bleeding from tonsillar or adenoid surgery has been estimated to be less than 1% of cases. Immediate post-adenoidectomy bleeding (within the first 24 hours) is usually controlled easily with pressure hemostasis. Occasionally nasopharyngeal packing may be required. Pack strings are tied extranasally to prevent pack movement and subsequent airway obstruction.[27] The pack should be removed before discharge. Evaluation for discharge should be after a reasonable period of observation (4 to 6 hours) or at least until there is no evidence of bleeding, minimal nausea and vomiting, and adequate hydration.

Myringotomy

Bilateral myringotomy and tube placement is a very common otolaryngologic procedure performed as ambulatory surgery in children with unresolved serous otitis media. The procedure is brief, and the child undergoes general anesthesia typically by mask only. Young children usually do not tolerate the procedure under local anesthesia in the office setting. General anesthesia is induced with the patient's head turned for surgical positioning, and then the area is prepped. The surgeon, with the use of a microscope, makes a small (2 mm) incision in the anterior inferior quadrant of the tympanic membrane and inspects the middle ear. A polyethylene ventilating tube is then inserted. Antibiotic solution is then instilled into the ear, and a small piece of cotton placed in the canal. The procedure is repeated on the other ear, and the child is awakened. Because these procedures are short and generally performed in children with mask induction, intravenous lines are not necessary. Resumption of oral intake can be initiated as soon as the child is alert and the gag reflex is intact.

Sinus surgery

Nasal and sinus procedures performed by the otolaryngologist on an outpatient or minimal stay basis include nasal septal reconstruction, submucous resection of the nasal septum or inferior turbinates, intranasal ethmoidectomy, antromental windows, Caldwell Luc, and nasal polypectomy. Endoscopic techniques have become popular in performing many of these procedures. The choice of local anesthesia with sedation or general anesthesia is determined by the extent of the procedure required, surgeon skill, and patient acceptance. Major surgical concerns are blood loss, use of cocaine, and posterior pharyngeal packing. The septal area is very vascular, because of the capillary network that branches from the anterior and posterior ethmoidal arteries, the superior labial artery, and the spinal palatine artery.[30] Injury to the ethmoidal artery, particularly the anterior ethmoidal artery, can cause temporary bleeding with risk of intraorbital hematoma. Continued bleeding will lead to increased intraorbital pressure and irreversible optic nerve damage. For this reason the surgeon may not want the eyes taped shut for the procedure. Lubricating gel may be used to facilitate orbit exposure and direct visualization. The surgeon will use an agent to promote local vasoconstriction of this vascular area before any manipulation. Cocaine and lidocaine with epinephrine (1:100,000 or 1:200,000) are most often selected.[33-35] Epinephrine-associated dysrhythmias can occur during inhalation anesthesia (Table 2-4). Factors for arrhythmia include perfusion of the site injected, the speed of injection, presence of lidocaine and other concomitant anesthetic drugs, and age. It has been found that children are less susceptible than adults to the arrhythmogenicity of epinephrine. The dosage of cocaine must be limited to less than 3 mg/kg to avoid toxic sequelae. Cocaine-related hypertension and arrhythmia may require intraoperative treatment. Posterior pharyngeal packing, when used, may be a source of airway obstruction, which must be kept in mind during the postoperative period.

There are many endoscopic sinus techniques. Clinicians using the Messerklinger technique or the Wigand technique report

Table 2-4   Arrhythmogenic Doses of Epinephrine with Inhalation Anesthesia

Agent	ED_{50} (µg/kg)
Desflurane	7.0
Enflurane	10.9
Halothane	2.1 (children, 10 µg/kg)
Isoflurane	6.7

A positive response is defined as three or more premature ventricular contractions in the 5 minutes after starting the injection.

excellent results.[36] Antrostomy, or antral window, is performed for chronic sinusitis unresponsive to conservative measures. In this procedure, debris can be removed through a small perforation made in the inferior meatus. Antrostomy is performed when more aggressive investigation of the sinuses is not required. The initial perforation is carefully enlarged by fracturing the turbinate bone. Petrolatum gauze is placed in the nasal cavity and removed after 24 hours. An accompanying procedure is often nasal and sinus polypectomy, because polyp formation is one cause of chronic sinusitis. Nasal polyp snares and Takahashi forceps are used. Septoplasty procedures involve the removal of destroyed cartilage. The septum is then refashioned and sutured back in place. After satisfactory repair of the deviated septum, petrolatum gauze packing is placed in the finger of a surgical glove and inserted using hemostats for proper positioning. This may or may not be sutured in place, and is usually removed within the next 24 hours. These procedures are performed in the supine position with a 15- to 20-degree head elevation. Nausea compounded by continued mouth breathing due to nasal packing are causes of prolonged stay and possible hospital admission.

Laryngoscopy, esophagoscopy, and bronchoscopy

Panendoscopy may be performed to evaluate cancer staging or to treat vocal cord polyps. Appropriate airway evaluation is crucial. Discussion with the surgeon and evaluation of films will aid in developing an airway management plan. Throughout the procedure, the airway is shared between surgeon and anesthesiologist, who must maintain good communication. The anesthetic must provide profound block of laryngeal reflexes, muscle relaxation, attenuation of cardiovascular responses, adequate ventilation, and quick return of laryngeal response at the conclusion of the procedure. The duration of these procedures is unpredictable, but ranges from minutes to an hour or longer. Again, this emphasizes the need for effective communication with the surgeon. Total intravenous anesthetic with propofol, alfentanil, and mivacurium is the author's preference, because these agents obviate the need for delivery of inhaled agents through a commonly shared airway.

After induction of general anesthesia, the laryngoscope is positioned and a suspension apparatus is placed to free the surgeon's hands for the procedure. A ventilation mode should be selected before induction of anesthesia; ventilation options include a small endotracheal tube, which allows room for the surgeon to maneuver instruments; repeated intubations and extubations; or jet ventilation. The advantages and disadvantages must be considered for each patient and each procedure. If CO_2 or neodymium YAG laser is used in the procedure, it will also influence the choice of ventilation mode. The use of laser offers precision in coagulation, incision, and vaporization of tissue; minimal tissue damage due to edema; and less postoperative pain. However, there are hazards associated with laser that cannot be ignored (see next section). Laser-aided microlaryngoscopy may be used to remove small polyps or nodules. Performance of bronchoscopy allows biopsy, brushing, and washing samples to be taken and sent for pathological evaluation. Bronchoscopy with esophagoscopy allows complete examination of the neck area in search of a primary cancer. When the yield from this procedure is negative, cervical lymph node biopsy is required.

Postoperative airway complications may be heralded by edema, laryngospasm, or hemorrhage.

Laser airway surgery

The most feared hazard of laser airway surgery is airway fire. Surgical personnel participating in these procedures should be familiar with the protocol for management of airway fire (Box 2-3). The high-intensity beam can directly ignite combustible

---

Box 2-3 Appropriate Management of Airway Fire

1. Immediately stop ventilation.
2. Disconnect breathing circuit from endotracheal tube.*
3. Remove endotracheal tube.
4. Extinguish fire with water.†
5. Ventilate the patient with mask.
6. Examine extent of damage by laryngoscopy/ bronchoscopy.
7. Ventilate with humidified oxygen.
8. Continue management in ICU setting.

* It is of paramount importance that one disconnect the endotracheal tube from the breathing circuit *before removing it* to prevent a blow-torch effect. Oxygen supports combustion.
† It is probable that the surgeon or nurse has already extinguished the fire.

objects in the surgical field, and it may reflect off shiny objects and ignite objects not in the surgical field. The endotracheal tube sits precariously close to the laser beam and emits gases that will readily support combustion. For this reason, a different type of endotracheal tube and gas are selected. Several types of endotracheal tubes are used with CO_2 laser, each of which has inherent shortcomings. The choices of material include polyvinyl chloride (PVC), silicone, red rubber, and metal. The only noncombustible endotracheal tube is the uncuffed metal tube; however, it is noncompliant and may damage the airway. The shiny surface could also deflect the laser beam. Polyvinyl chloride tubes ignite and burn readily, producing molten, toxic debris. The resultant tissue damage is secondary to direct thermal injury as well as chemical injury. The PVC cuff is not protected from ignition by the laser beam, nor is the tubing below the cuff. The cuff may be filled with saline to serve as a heat sink, because water as well as tissue readily absorbs laser energy. Silicone tubes crumble when ignited, while red rubber tubes tend to char. Red rubber tubes are more resistant to ignition and do not disintegrate.[37] Red rubber tubes may be wrapped with metallic tape to lessen the area of flammable material likely to contact the laser beam. Of course, this too has its disadvantages. Sosis has shown that the 3M tape No. 425 wrapped red rubber tube offers the most protection from CO_2 laser.[38] The endotracheal tube must be taped smoothly and without any gaps that would result in a rough surface that could damage the mucosa. Also pieces of tape must not be left hanging free; they may be aspirated, or they may obstruct the airway. There are several endotracheal tubes designed specifically for use with CO_2 laser; however, studies have shown that the ideal cuffed CO_2 laser–proof tube is not yet available.[39]

Neodymium (Nd) YAG laser is used for debulking bronchial tumors. It penetrates deeper into layers of tissue than does CO_2 laser. With YAG laser, airway fire prevention is even more difficult, because no specially designed tube material exists for its use. Though its beam passes through PVC tubing, any debris on the tube can absorb the beam and ignite the endotracheal tube. It has been suggested that ventilation modes other than endotracheal tube be selected for use with YAG laser.[40] The ventilating bronchoscope serves this purpose. Complications of YAG airway surgery include perforation of the trachea or bronchi, perforated great vessels, and often fatal hemorrhage and bronchospasm.

The selection of gas mixture is an important consideration for laser airway surgery. Oxygen and nitrous oxide support combustion; therefore, when they are used, ignition is more likely when the beam contacts combustible material. These agents should be used in the lowest possible concentration to maintain adequate oxygenation. Room air, nitrogen, or helium may be used for this purpose. In particular, helium diffuses heat well, which may decrease laser-induced endotracheal tube ignition.

Dental Extractions

The primary dental procedure performed in the ambulatory surgery unit is tooth extraction. This procedure may not be done in an office setting for many reasons: full-mouth and multiple extractions often require general anesthesia; the patient's medical condition may necessitate close monitoring; or the patient may be mentally retarded and require deep sedation or general anesthesia. The procedure may be performed with local anesthesia and sedation or with general anesthesia. Nasotracheal intubation allows a clear operating field. In this procedure, the teeth are removed using forceps clamps. A local anesthetic with epinephrine is used when cardiovascular status is stable. After complete removal of all tooth fragments, the gum is sutured and hemostasis is obtained. Gauze may be placed between the gums at case completion. Postoperative bleeding and emesis are frequent occurrences.

Plastic Procedures

Rhytidectomy

Plastic surgery is among the growing list of procedures now primarily performed in the physician's office. Patients seeking rhytidectomy, or face-lift, hold high expectations for good results. In general, patients undergoing plastic procedures have varying motivations and expectations that should be explored before surgery. The procedure is usually performed under local anesthesia with sedation. Lidocaine 0.5% with epinephrine 1:200,000 or 1:400,000, or 0.5% bupivacaine, is used. If general anesthesia is also used, the arrhythmogenicity of epinephrine in the presence of inhalation agents must be recognized (Table 2-4). The total amounts of local anesthetic delivered must be considered so that symptoms of toxicity can be prevented. Major concerns of rhytidectomy are the long duration of the procedure and the inaccessibility of the airway. Even a nasal cannula can be obtrusive in the surgical field. Deep conscious sedation is required.

The major complications are hematoma and facial nerve paralysis. The procedure is individualized for each patient's appearance. In general, an incision is made from the horizontal hairline of the forehead behind the hairline to the crus of the ear helix. The incision continues anterior to the ear, around the lobe, then toward the occiput, and it then crosses the superior mastoid area. The skin flap thus created is then raised, meticulous hemostasis is obtained, and the flap is drawn upward and backward. Care must be taken not to pull the flap too aggressively and compromise blood supply to the area.

Blepharoplasty

Blepharoplasty may be performed with local anesthesia, with local anesthesia and sedation, or with general anesthesia. In this procedure, excess skin or herniated fat is removed from the eyelid. Local anesthetic is used, usually 1% lidocaine with epinephrine 1:100,000. The incision is made in the upper lid, from the medial canthal ligament to the lateral canthal ligament, such that the scar will fall in the natural crease of the lid. Fat is removed gently with careful and meticulous care for hemostasis. Fat may also be removed from the lower lid in a similar manner. The skin is closed, and no dressing is applied. The patient should be instructed to apply ice compresses continuously for 48 hours.

Rhinoplasty

For rhinoplasty, the anesthetic choices are general anesthesia, local anesthesia, or intravenous sedation. Cocaine 4% and lidocaine with epinephrine are used. Each surgeon's technique may be different, and the surgery is individualized for desired patient results. In this procedure, an intercartilaginous incision is made between the upper and lower lateral cartilages and skin of the dorsum of the nose is elevated. Any bony deformity is removed and the cartilaginous portion of the deformity is made congruous with the new level of bone. The nasolabial angle is then altered, and the caudal edge of the septum is trimmed to the desired angle. At the conclusion of the procedure, petrolatum gauze packs are inserted in the nasal cavity. Steri-Strips and a plaster splint are applied. Postoperative care may require more prolonged recovery in a 24-hour observation unit or recovery care center. Postoperative pain, nausea, and vomiting are common.

Podiatry

Many different podiatry procedures can be performed in ambulatory surgery units under local anesthesia with sedation. A tourniquet is used to reduce bleeding in the surgical field. In longer procedures, it is often the tourniquet that becomes unbearable and sedation becomes directed at decreasing the awareness of the tourniquet.

Bunionectomy

Repair of the hallux valgus, or bunion, is a common podiatry procedure. Hallux valgus is a prominence of the distal medial aspect of the great toe and the varus deformity of the first metatarsal. The valgus deformity occurs at the metatarsal phalangeal joint. The primary patient complaint is of pain at the bunion site. There are many procedures to correct it: bunionectomies, osteotomies, metatarsal fusions, and tendon transfers. Two commonly performed procedures are the McBride and Keller bunionectomies. The procedure is selected by the surgeon based on the age of the patient and the extent of the deformity. The McBride procedure involves a lateral sesamoidectomy, bunionectomy, and adductor tenotomy with reattachment of the adductor to the neck of the metatarsal. The Keller procedure involves a proximal phalangectomy of the great toe. The foot is placed in Elastoplast dressing, and the patient is given a stiff shoe for limited ambulation. Postoperative pain is managed with oral narcotic combinations and nonsteroidal antiinflammatory drugs.

Orthopedics

There are several anesthetic concerns associated with the use of the pneumatic tourniquet in orthopedic surgery, which is used to provide a bloodless field of operation for the surgeon. The tourniquet size should be appropriate for the patient. The cuff's width should be greater than half the limb diameter. Smooth padding should be placed under the tourniquet to protect the patient's skin. The tourniquet should inflate uniformly, and the tourniquet pressure should be frequently checked. Maintenance of tourniquet pressure is particularly important when an intravenous regional block is performed. The tourniquet is usually inflated to 100 mm Hg above systemic blood pressure in the lower extremity, and approximately 50 mm Hg above systemic blood pressure in the upper extremity. Hemodynamic changes occur when the tourniquet is in place and when it is released. The changes are of little concern in the young, healthy patient, but hemodynamics must be considered in the management of patients with coexisting medical problems. These changes include increases in blood pressure and central venous pressure that are probably secondary to shift of total blood volume. On release of the tourniquet, blood pressure will fall. In addition, metabolic acidosis may develop in the ischemic limb. The occurrence of these changes and their physiologic effect is impacted by the duration of tourniquet inflation. Suggested time limits are subject to controversy. Recommendations vary from 30 minutes to 4 hours.[41] When considering length of tourniquet inflation, one must consider the cardiopulmonary status of the patient and the size of the limb involved, including possible use of bilateral tourniquets. Tourniquet pain occurs with regional anesthesia and with sedation techniques after approximately 30 to 45 minutes of inflation, despite adequate block. In fact, the patient is usually quite comfortable for the procedure, but unable to bear the tourniquet pain. Its etiology and treatment are unclear. An attempt may be made to decrease the patient's awareness of the pain with narcotic administration or further sedation. If pain persists and the procedure is lengthy, general anesthesia may be necessary for patient comfort.

Carpal tunnel release

Carpal tunnel syndrome is caused by compression of the median nerve by the fibrous ligament at the wrist. The symptoms are numbness, paresthesia, and pain in the fingers and hand. Its repair gives relief to these patients. The procedure may be performed with local infiltration or with regional anesthesia, in particular, Bier block. This block offers the surgeon a clear operating field: The arm is exsanguinated and a tourniquet is used.

In this procedure, a palmar skin incision is made, and the transverse carpal and volar carpal ligaments are exposed. Another incision is made through the ligament to expose the carpal canal. The median nerve must be identified so that it is not inadvertently severed. The nerve and the injured area are examined and further repair is made as necessary. Long-acting local anesthetics may be infiltrated for postoperative analgesia. The incision is closed, dressed, and wrapped for wrist immobilization. The procedure is usually short, and tourniquet pain is rarely a concern. It should be noted that some centers are performing these procedures using an endoscopic technique. In endoscopic median nerve decompression, a transverse skin incision is made and the transverse carpal ligament is surgically released using special instruments.[42] A general or regional anesthetic is recommended, although a skilled surgeon may perform the procedure on a patient under local anesthesia. The injected local anesthetic increases the amount of tissue fluid, which can obscure endoscopic viewing. The use of small amounts of local anesthetic prevents this. Postoperatively, the wrist is splinted.

Arthroscopy

Knee arthroscopy is a procedure that allows the internal knee capsule to be examined. It may be used therapeutically, as well as diagnostically for patients with chronic symptoms; during the procedure, removal of loose bodies, synovial biopsy, resection of adhesions, or repair of torn menisci may be performed. Local anesthesia with sedation, general anesthesia, or regional anesthesia may be used. The regional techniques include spinal, epidural, and three-in-one femoral sciatic block, although the latter is rarely appropriate, given the delayed recovery of motor function and the requirements for ambulatory discharge. The major concern with arthroscopic knee surgery is the use of the tourniquet. The local anesthetic approach to knee arthroscopy is somewhat unique. In addition to local skin infiltration for trocar insertion, the internal knee capsule can be bathed with the anesthetic, by one injection or by continuous irrigation. This method is most successful when extensive movement of the joint is not necessary, as muscle relaxation is often inadequate. Addition of intraarticular opioids in conjunction with local anesthesia has shown mixed results, but intraarticular morphine and bupivacaine combined have provided prolonged postoperative pain relief.[43, 44] Drug dose and presence of tourniquet may influence effectiveness.

General anesthesia may be offered, depending on patient, surgeon, and anesthesiologist preference. The newer anesthetic agents are decreasing discharge time and undesirable side effects. Propofol maintenance infusion is advantageous for short procedures, and it is associated with a lower incidence of postoperative emesis. The choice of regional anesthesia also offers decreased discharge time and may be most suited for orthopedic procedures, which are generally performed on young, healthy, active patients. They will appreciate as rapid a return to normal activity as possible. The choice of spinal anesthesia in the outpatient has its advantages and disadvantages. Given consideration to points of patient selection, choice of short-acting local agent, small gauge tip and adequate postoperative hydration, this method offers excellent operating conditions. Procedures on the knee require anesthesia of the femoral obturator and lateral femoral cutaneous nerves. A three-in-one block (lumbar plexus block, a block of the lateral femoral cutaneous nerve, femoral nerve, and obturator nerve) may be used by those proficient in this technique. It involves a single injection of a large quantity of local anesthetic into the fascial envelope of the femoral nerve. This large quantity spreads upward into the pelvis, where the obturator and lateral femoral cutaneous nerves travel in conjunction with the femoral nerve.[45] If work on the posterior aspect of the knee is anticipated, a femoral sciatic nerve block will also be necessary; however, its appropriateness for outpatient anesthesia has been questioned because it is associated with prolonged recovery from block. Epidural block offers the advantages of a regional technique, less likelihood of postdural puncture headache, excellent operating conditions, and, with proper selection of a local agent, faster recovery times than those seen with spinal and general anesthesia.[46]

Arthroscopy is performed on the patient in the supine position with the knee extended and elevated. A trocar is inserted into the superior and medial aspect of the knee to enable saline irrigation. A second incision for the arthroscope is made, and it is connected to drainage tubes. A continuous flow of saline enables clear visualization of structures, as well as removal of debris. Operative instruments can be inserted as needed through separate incision sites to perform various procedures. The arthroscope can be attached to a camera for simultaneous viewing and for later viewing.

Shoulder arthroscopy may be performed with regional inter-scalene blockade, with general anesthesia, or with interscalene anesthesia and light general anesthesia. In performing the inter-scalene block, the selection should be guided by anesthesiologist skill. Potential complications include pneumothorax and intravas-cular injection. Airway management and proximity of operating site should also be considered. Neurologic assessment in the early postoperative period is required by many surgeons. The procedure is performed with the patient in the lateral or beach chair position.[47]

Postoperative pain following arthroscopy can be treated initially with intravenous opioids. Parenteral or oral nonsteroidal antiinflammatory drugs can provide longer postoperative relief. Additionally, cold-pack treatments can provide good pain relief, be initiated in the PACU, and continued at home.

Urology

Cystoscopy

Cystoscopy is a procedure used for evaluation of prostatic hypertrophy, resection of bladder tumor, ureteral stent placement, and treatment of urethral strictures. The procedure involves the placement of a cystoscope through the urethral meatus. With the aid of irrigating fluid, the bladder is distended, and then its structure may be visualized. This is usually a brief procedure that can be performed under any form of anesthesia. Topical local anesthetic (Urojet) may be adequate for simple follow-up cancer monitoring; for other indications, regional anesthesia or general anesthesia may be required. Urinary retention or hematuria can occur postoperatively. Some patients may be discharged with an indwelling catheter.

Extracorporeal shock wave lithotripsy

Extracorporeal shock wave lithotripsy (ESWL) is a procedure utilized for the disintegration of ureteral and renal stones. It has replaced open nephrolithotomy and offers faster recovery with decreased morbidity. In addition, with second-generation lithotriptors, patients do not need to be submersed in a water bath. Second-generation lithotriptors use biplanar fluoroscopy to target the stone and then apply shock waves specifically. After successful stone disintegration, the resulting particles may be passed in the urine, or, if necessary, a ureteral stent may be placed to maintain ureter patency. The anesthetic requirement is for a still patient, so that frequent repositioning of the focused shock waves can be minimized. Application of EMLA (eutectic mixture of local anesthetics) at least 45 minutes before the procedure has been successful.[48] In most circumstances, sedation is adequate. Short-acting intravenous sedatives and analgesics (specifically propofol and alfentanil) are ideal for the outpatient because during the procedure, the stimulus is intense but short-lived. These agents provide an adequate plane of sedation that is not prolonged. Infusion techniques are discussed in Chapter 9. Complications of ESWL include cardiac arrhythmias, which can be minimized by use of lithotriptors that link the shock wave to the R-wave of the electrocardiogram. This delays the shock wave so that it does not occur during the vulnerable period. Postoperative concerns include pain from fragmented urinary calculi and bleeding.

Pain

Trigger point injection

In the pain clinic, one of the most common procedures is trigger point injection to treat myofascial pain. The technique is simple and effective, especially when combined with the spray-and-stretch method. A trigger point is an area of tenderness in a muscle or supporting structures, and it may be surrounded by an extended area of referred pain. Clinically the patient will exhibit a hyperirritable site within a taut band of skeletal muscle. Pain may be elicited by palpating this point. In addition to pain, there is weakness and decreased range of motion of the affected muscle. Exacerbations can be caused by overuse, cold weather, stress, fatigue, and direct pressure. Use of direct pressure aids in locating the trigger point. On palpation, the muscle will feel ropey or bandlike. A local twitch response may be elicited and, when present, is thought to be confirmation of the myofascial syndrome. The trigger point is the most sensitive point with the ropey band. It is at this point that a small 22- to 25-gauge needle is placed perpendicular to the muscle plane. Local anesthetic with or without corticosteroid is then injected into the muscle. Injection of local anesthetic is preferred over saline injection or no injection (termed *dry needling*). After trigger point injections, patients benefit from muscle stretch techniques. With the spray-and-stretch technique, a vapocoolant spray (e.g., ethyl chloride or fluoromethane) is used to enhance the ability of muscle fibers to stretch to their full range of motion. Other modalities include use of moist deep-heat massage and TENS. A physical therapist working with these patients postinjection is beneficial.

Epidural steroid injection

Epidural steroid injections are commonly and easily performed on an outpatient basis. Epidural steroids are indicated in the treatment of nerve root irritation and resulting inflammation. They have also been used in treatment of radicular pain secondary to herniated disc; back pain secondary to degenerative spine with disc narrowing, spondylolysis, or spondylolisthesis; trauma; and postlaminectomy.[49] The technique may be performed with the patient sitting or in the lateral decubitus position. Placement of the patient with the painful side down is thought to promote contact of the steroid solution with the affected nerve roots. Every attempt to perform the block at the affected nerve root level should be made. After sterile prep and drape, the epidural space is localized with a standard Touhy needle by a loss-of-resistance method. Aspiration is performed to rule out subdural puncture. If a mixture of local anesthetics is to be used, a test dose should first be injected. Most commonly, methylprednisolone 80 mg, or triamcinolone 50 to 75 mg, with 6 to 10 ml of saline or local anesthetic is used. Following injection, a period of monitoring and observation to ensure adequate recovery of blockade is prudent. The patient may be discharged, usually within 1 hour. The total number of injections that may be performed is somewhat controversial, but is usually dependent on the patient's response. If complete relief is obtained after one injection, no further treatment is necessary. If there is no improvement after the first injection, the procedure may be repeated once or twice, or not repeated at all. Repeat injections for pain that recur after initial relief are controversial. If there is a partial response to the first injection, the procedure may be repeated twice. A maximum of three injections is recommended, more than this brings no further pain relief. Complications from epidural steroid injections are rare, and the incidence of inadvertent subdural puncture is 1%.

Stellate ganglion block

The list of clinical conditions that have been treated with stellate ganglion block is long. The more common conditions include reflex sympathetic dystrophy, herpes zoster, postherpetic neuralgia, phantom limb pain, and pain associated with vascular insufficiency. The technique may be performed in an ambulatory setting; however, proper monitoring must be accomplished, and resuscitative drugs, suction, oxygen, cardiac defibrillator, and airway management equipment must be readily available, because of the risk of life-threatening complications. Intraspinal or intravascular injection may result in seizures or respiratory compromise. Pneumothorax is also a risk when C-7 is the chosen landmark. All patients should be informed of the possibility of disturbing side effects, such as hoarseness, subjective shortness of breath, partial sensory and motor block of the arm, ptosis, myosis, and nasal congestion. The more common approach to stellate ganglion block is performed with the patient in the supine position at the level of C-6 or Chaussignac's tubercle. A small roll of towels placed behind the patient's shoulders will enhance neck extension and facilitate palpation. After localizing the cricoid cartilage and sliding the palpating finger to the medial border of the sternocleidomastoid muscle, the clinician may feel the tubercle using gentle but firm pressure (Fig. 2-6). The site is swabbed with alcohol and punctured with a posteriorly directed 23-gauge needle. This needle should enter in a plane perpendicular to the table on which the patient rests. The needle will usually contact Chaussignac's tubercle at 2 to 2.5 cm, and it should then be withdrawn slightly from the periosteum before injection. To prevent cerebrospinal fluid or intravascular injection, the needle must be carefully aspirated. A test dose of 0.5 ml to 1 ml of 1% lidocaine is then given, and if there are no sequelae, a total of 5 ml to 10 ml of anesthetic solution (composed of equal amounts of 0.75% bupivacaine and 2% lidocaine) is usually adequate to obtain a sympathetic block.[50]

Medical

Gastrointestinal endoscopy

Gastrointestinal endoscopies are not routinely performed in the operating room, but are common outpatient procedures in the office or in gastrointestinal suites. Esophagogastroduodenoscopy, sigmoidoscopy, and colonoscopy can be used to diagnose suspected cancer, esophagitis, polyps, and ulcers. Flexible endoscopes are more comfortable for the patient. Various instruments designed for use with endoscopes allow for biopsy, foreign body removal, and polypectomy. When polypectomy is performed, bleeding may be controlled by applying pressure, fulguration, or electrocautery. In addition to bleeding, there is a risk of bowel perforation. Endoscopy is performed with the patient in the lateral position, with sedation.

Other medical procedures performed on an ambulatory basis include chemotherapy, bronchoscopy, and cardiac catheterization.

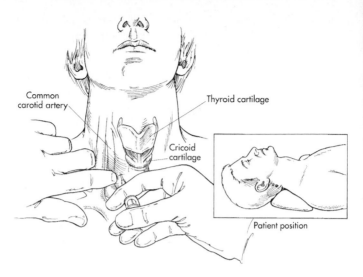

Fig. 2-6 Stellate ganglion block. C-6 anterior tubercle is directly beneath the operator's index finger. The carotid artery is retracted laterally when necessary. The needle is perpendicular to all skin planes and is inserted directed posteriorly. *Inset:* Patient positioned for stellate ganglion block. Pillow or roll should be between the shoulders to extend the neck, to bring the esophagus toward the midline, and to facilitate palpation of Chaussignac's tubercle. (From Williams MR: Subdural/central nerve blocks. In Raj PP, editor: Practical management of pain, ed 2, St Louis, 1992, Mosby, pp. 758-65.)

Only the latter two may require sedation or anesthesia, and general considerations are discussed in Chapters 9 and 10.

Special Ambulatory Procedures

The list of procedures performed on an outpatient basis is constantly increasing. What is considered today a procedure requiring a 24-hour observation period may soon be considered a strictly ambulatory procedure. The increase in the number of procedures performed in the outpatient arena reflects improvement in anesthetic pharmacology, anesthetic techniques, surgical equipment, and surgical techniques. The most important feature, however, is our choice of patients for any particular procedure. It should be emphasized that we must use our increasing knowledge of outcome analysis to tailor each patient's surgical experience to his or her needs. Varying levels of skill among surgeons would determine appropriate setting. A surgeon well skilled in a certain procedure will feel confident in discharging a patient the same day. We will need to change our mind set from procedure-oriented definitions of what is ambulatory surgery to patient/surgeon/procedure-oriented considerations. The uncommon ambulatory procedures presented here illustrate this point. The procedures in all instances are not suited for early discharge; however, with a skilled surgeon and an appropriate patient, same day discharge or 24-hour observation is possible (Box 2-4).

Laparoscopic cholecystectomy has been performed in the United States since 1988. The procedure does not result in a large debilitating scar, which reduces inpatient stay. Gynecological laparoscopies have long been performed as outpatient procedures. Now the laparoscopic technology is advancing in other specialties as well. In a series of laparoscopic cholecystectomies performed by Riddick, it was found that almost 50% of the patients could have the procedure done on an outpatient basis.[51] As one would suspect, younger patients without previous surgery were more likely to have the procedure performed with same evening discharge. They further found that nonseptic patients with acute cholecystitis tolerated the outpatient experience well. However, it was felt that patients with more severe disease (i.e.,

---

Box 2-4 Procedures Considered for Short-Stay or Extended Observation Admission

Tonsillectomy
Cholecystectomy
Thyroidectomy
Submandibular gland excision
Parotidectomy
Scleral buckle
Vitreoretinal surgery
Transurethral resection of the prostate (TURP)
Bone marrow harvest

showing signs of infection and inflammation) required hospital admission. There are reports of outpatient open cholecystectomies as well. Saltzstein et al. performed a series of 94 consecutive cholecystectomies and reported that 68% of eligible patients were discharged on the same day.[52] Those patients best tolerating the procedure exhibited no significant comorbidity, did not undergo common bile duct expiration, and were less than 55 years old. They also attributed part of the success of early recovery to the use of a midline incision that did not violate abdominal muscles, and to the routine use of subfascial injection of long-acting local anesthetic.

The scope of same-day otolaryngology procedures is increasing. Ambulatory parotidectomies, submandibular gland resections, and thyroidectomies have been reported.[53, 54] Helmus's review of selected head and neck surgeries make several key points that undoubtedly contribute to an 80% same-day discharge rate.[55] Major resections with airway and deglutition implications were avoided. Proper patient selection is stressed, as is the need for proper and complete preoperative assessment. When an extended period of observation is necessary, the surgery should be scheduled for early morning. Finally the point is made that physicians, nurses, anesthesia team, and hospital administrators must work cohesively to obtain any degree of success. These procedures can be done safely within the general guidelines outlined. It is evident that these procedures may be suitable for select patients, some surgeons, and certain centers.

Vitreoretinal surgery has moved into the arena of outpatient and short-stay surgery. Many of these patients can be managed safely and effectively, in part because of newer retinal reattachment procedures, such as balloon buckling and pneumatic retinoplexy, which is performed quickly and simply. Wilson[56] reviewed 255 consecutive scleral buckling and vitrectomy operations. Patients were divided into two groups: (1) Patients undergoing procedures under general anesthesia with postoperative hospitalization for several days; and (2) patients undergoing procedures under local anesthesia whenever appropriate, and managed on an outpatient or short-stay basis. Patients in group 2 whose status necessitated a change from ambulatory to inpatient admission were children or were people having lengthy or difficult procedures, poor health, decreased vision in other eye, inadequate home care, or general anesthesia. The technical success rate in both groups showed no difference.

Postoperative hospitalization after vitreoretinal surgery has continued, despite the newer, faster techniques and the evidence that unrestricted postoperative physical activity has little or no effect on the outcome.[56] Although many surgeons still prescribe bed rest postoperatively and prefer patients to remain in the hospital, selected patients for vitreoretinal surgery may be candidates for same-day or short-stay surgery.

Transurethral resection of the prostate (TURP) has been performed on an outpatient basis. The introduction of the laparoscopic technique has facilitated outpatient prostate surgery. Considerations in patient selection include health of the patient, ability of family to care for him, the home environment, and the motivation of the patient for outpatient surgery. Interestingly, the volume of the resection did not influence the decision. Postoperatively the patient is assessed for patient stability, cessation of bleeding, return of neurologic function, and absence of discomfort.[57]

The list of uncommon ambulatory procedures further includes autologous bone marrow harvesting,[58] mediastinoscopy and anterior mediastinotomy,[59] vascular access surgery,[60] radiofrequency catheter ablation of accessory atrioventricular pathways,[61] vaginal hysterectomy,[62] orthopedic procedures such as anterior cruciate ligament repair, and shoulder reconstruction. The list will continue to grow as surgical equipment, surgical skill, and anesthetic drugs continue to improve. Success will depend on our ability to design the appropriate experience for the appropriate patient.

Summary

Advances in surgical techniques have contributed to the increased growth of ambulatory surgery. Both freestanding and hospital-based ambulatory surgery facilities are now performing a wide variety of procedures for the various specialties, including ophthalmology, gynecology, otolaryngology, orthopedics, plastic surgery, general surgery, podiatry, urology, gastroenterology, dentistry, and pain management. Familiarity with the commonly performed ambulatory surgical procedures enables the anesthesiologist to plan accordingly for an appropriately tailored anesthetic administration. A review of the common perioperative considerations for common ambulatory procedures has been presented. Anesthetic techniques are factors in the surgical considerations, as much as patient characteristics.

Office-based surgery is also experiencing growth as many procedures are being shifted into the office practice. As the financial demand for ambulatory surgery increases, so does the list of surgical procedures. What is now being performed on a 24-hour observation admission may soon shift in to the ambulatory arena. Laparoscopic cholecystectomy, vaginal hysterectomy, thyroidectomy, and vitreoretinal surgery are being performed in a few centers on an outpatient basis. With further improvements in techniques and pain management, this list will continue to grow.

References

1. Henderson J: Ambulatory surgery: past, present and future. In Wetchler BV, editor: Anesthesia for ambulatory surgery, 1991, Philadelphia, JB Lippincott, p. 6.
2. Davis J: Ambulatory surgery: how far can we go? Med Clin North Am 1993; 77(2):365-75.
3. Garfield J: Anesthesia for gynecologic surgery. In Rogers M, editor: Principles and practice of anesthesiology, St Louis, 1993, Mosby, pp. 2105-36.
4. Snyder D, Dorin A, van Amerongen D et al: Low dose morphine injected into the mesosalpinx may provide analgesia for outpatient laparoscopic tubal occlusion. Anesthesiology 1993; 79(3A):A27.
5. Snyder D, Dorin A, van Amerongen D et al: Topical versus mesosalpinx injected bupivacaine for outpatient laparoscopic yoon ring tubal occlusion. Anesthesiology 1993; 79(3A):A11.
6. Rosenblum M, Weller RS, Conrad PL et al: Ibuprofen provides longer lasting analgesia than fentanyl after laparoscopic surgery. Anesth Analg 1991; 73:255-9.
7. Edwards ND, Barclay K, Catling SJ et al: Day case laparoscopy: a survey of postoperative pain and an assessment of the value of diclofenac. Anaesthesia 1991; 46:1077-80.
8. Hurt WG: Outpatient gynecologic procedures. Surg Clin North Am 1991; 71(5):1099-110.
9. Renck H, Ljungströem KG, Hedin H et al: Prevention of dextran induced anaphylactic reactions by hapten inhibition. A Scandinavian multicenter study of the effects of 20 ml dextran 1, 15% administered before dextran 70 or dextran 40. Acta Chir Scand 1983; 149:355-60.

10. Rogers M, editor: Principles and practice of anesthesiology, St Louis, 1993, Mosby, pp. 2105-36.

11. Langer JC, Shandling B, Rosenberg M: Intraoperative bupivacaine during outpatient hernia repair in children: a randomized double blind trial. J Pediatr Surg 1987; 22:267-70.

12. Hannallah RS, Broadman LM, Belman AB et al: Comparison of caudal and ilioinguinal/iliohypogastric nerve blocks for control of post-orchiopexy pain in pediatric ambulatory surgery. Anesthesiology 1987; 66:832-4.

13. Sailors DM, Layman TS, Burns RP et al: Laparoscopic hernia repair: a preliminary report. Am Surg 1993; 59(2):85-9.

14. Petros JG, Rimm EB, Robillard R et al: Factors influencing postoperative urinary retention in patients undergoing elective inguinal herniorrhaphy. Am J Surg 1991; 161:431-3.

15. Davis JE: General surgery of the major ambulatory surgical patient. In Davis JE: Major ambulatory surgery, Baltimore, 1986, Williams & Wilkins, pp. 274-82.

16. Petros J, Bradley T: Factors influencing postoperative urinary retention in patients undergoing surgery for benign anorectal disease. Am J Surg 1990; 159:374-6.

17. Tree-Trakarn T, Pirayavaraporn S: Postoperative pain relief for circumcision in children: comparison among morphine, nerve block and topical analgesia. Anesthesiology 1985; 62:519-22.

18. Feldman M, Albert S: Anesthesia for ophthalmologic surgery. In Rogers M, Tinker J, Covino B et al, editors: Principles and practice of anesthesiology, St Louis, 1993, Mosby, pp. 2241-56.

19. Tasman W, editor: Duane's clinical ophthalmology, vol 6, Philadelphia, 1993, JB Lippincott, pp. 2-25.

20. Lerman J, Eustis S, Smith DR: Effect of droperidol pretreatment on postanesthetic vomiting in children undergoing strabismus surgery. Anesthesiology 1986; 65:322-5.

21. Broadman L, Ceruzzi W, Patane P et al: Metoclopramide reduces the incidence of vomiting following strabismus surgery in children. Anesthesiology 1990; 72(2):245-8.

22. Watcha M, Simeon R, White P et al: Effect of propofol on the incidence of postoperative vomiting after strabismus surgery in pediatric outpatients. Anesthesiology 1991; 75:204-9.

23. Weir PM, Munro HM, Reynolds PI et al: Propofol infusion and the incidence of emesis in pediatric outpatient strabismus surgery. Anesth Analg 1993; 76:760-4.

24. Kirk G: Anesthesia for ear, nose and throat surgery. In Rogers M, Tinker J, Covino B et al, editors: Principles and practice of anesthesiology, St Louis, 1993, Mosby, pp. 2257-74.

25. Colclasure JB, Graham SS: Complications of outpatient tonsillectomy and adenoidectomy: a review of 3,340 cases. Ear, Nose Throat J 1990; 69:155-60.

26. Reiner SA, Sawyer WP, Clark KF, Wood MW: Safety of outpatient tonsillectomy and adenoidectomy. Otolaryngol Head Neck Surg 1990; 102:161-8.

27. Kornblat A, Kornblat A: Tonsillectomy and adenoidectomy. In Paparella M, Shumrick DA, Gluckman JL, Meyerhoff WL, editors: Otolaryngology, vol 3, Philadelphia, 1991, WB Saunders, pp. 2149-65.

28. Orkin FK, Gold B: Selection. In Wetchler BV, editor: Anesthesia for ambulatory surgery, Philadelphia, 1991, JB Lippincott, pp. 85-125.

29. Tom LW, DeDio RM, Cohen DE et al: Is outpatient tonsillectomy appropriate for young children? Laryngoscope 1992; 102:277-80.

30. Busby D: Otorhinolaryngological surgery. In Kassity K, McKittrick JE, Preston FW, editors: Manual of ambulatory surgery, New York, 1982, Springer-Verlag, pp. 26-50.

31. Schoem SR, Watkins GL, Kuhn JJ, Thompson DH: Control of early postoperative pain with bupivacaine in pediatric tonsillectomy. Ear, Nose Throat J 1993; 72(8):560-3.

32. Schoem SR, Watkins GL, Kuhn JJ et al: Control of early postoperative pain with bupivacaine in adult local tonsillectomy. Arch Otolaryngol Head Neck Surg 1993; 119(3):292-3.

33. Karl HW, Swedlow DB, Lee KW, Downes JJ: Epinephrine-halothane interactions in children. Anesthesiology 1983; 58:142-5.

34. Moore M, Weiskopf R, Eger E et al: Arrhythmogenic doses of epinephrine are similar during desflurane or isoflurane anesthesia in humans. Anesthesiology 1993; 79:943-7.

35. Johnston R, Eger E, Wilson C: A comparative interaction of epinephrine with enflurane, isoflurane and halothane in man. Anesth Analg 1976; 55(5):709-12.

36. Danielson A: Functional endoscopic sinus surgery on a day case outpatient basis. Clin Otolaryngol 1992; 17:473-7.

37. Keon T: Anesthetic management during laser surgery. Intl Anesthes Clin 1992; 30(4):99-107.

38. Sosis, MB: What is the safest endotracheal tube for Nd-YAG laser surgery? A comparative study. Anesth Analg 1989; 69:802-4.

39. Kirk G: Anesthesia for ear, nose, and throat surgery. In Rogers M, Tinker J, Covino B et al, editors: Principles and practice of anesthesiology, St Louis, 1993, Mosby, pp. 2257-4.

40. Keon T: Anesthetic management during laser surgery. Intl Anesthes Clin 1992; 30(4):99-107.

41. Concepcion M: Anesthesia for orthopedic surgery. In Rogers M, Tinker J, Covino B et al, editors: Principles and practice of anesthesiology, St Louis, 1993, Mosby, pp. 2187-214.

42. Agee JM, McCarroll HR, Tortosa RD et al: Endoscopic release of the carpal tunnel: a randomized prospective multicenter study. J Hand Surg 1992; 17(6):987-95.

43. Joshi GP, McCarroll SM, O'Brien TM et al: Intraarticular analgesia following knee arthroscopy. Anesth Analg 1993; 76:333-6.

44. Stein C, Comisel K, Haimerl E et al: Analgesic effect of intraarticular morphine after arthroscopic knee surgery. N Engl J Med 1991; 325(16):1123-6.

45. Mulroy M: Peripheral nerve blockade. In Barash P, Cullen B, Stoelting R, editors: Clinical anesthesia, ed 2, Philadelphia, 1992, JB Lippincott, p. 868.

46. Wetchler BV, editor: Anesthesia for ambulatory surgery, Philadelphia, 1991, JB Lippincott, pp. 366-74.

47. Bernstein R, Rosenberg A, editors: Manual of orthopedic anesthesia and related pain syndromes, New York, 1993, Churchill Livingstone, p. 282.

48. Gajraj NM, Pennant JH, Watcha MF: Eutectic mixture of local anesthetics (EMLA) cream. Anesth Analg 1994; 78:574-83.

49. Benzon H: Epidural steroids. In Raj PP, editor: Practical management of pain, ed 2, St Louis, 1992, Mosby, pp. 818-28.

50. Raj PP: Chronic pain. In Raj PP, editor: Clinical practice of regional anesthesia, New York, 1991, Churchill Livingstone, pp. 489-98.

51. Riddick EJ, Olsen DO: Outpatient laparoscopic laser cholecystectomy. Am J Surg 1990; 160:485-7.

52. Saltzstein E, Mercer L, Peacock J et al: Outpatient open cholecystectomy. Surg Gynecol Obstet 1992; 174(3):173-5.

53. LoGerfo P, Gates R, Gazetas P: Outpatient and short-stay thyroid surgery. Head Neck (March/April) 1991; 97-101.

54. Steckler RM: Outpatient parotidectomy. Am J Surg 1991; 162:303-5.

55. Helmus C, Grin M, Westfall R: Same-day-stay head and neck surgery. Laryngoscope 1992; 102:1331-4.

56. Wilson D, Barr C: Outpatient and abbreviated hospitalization for vitreoretinal surgery. Ophth Surg 1990; 21(2):119-22.

57. McLoughlin M, Kinahan T: Transurethral resection of the prostate in the outpatient setting. J Urol 1990; 143:951-2.

58. Thorne AC, Stewart M, Gulati S: Harvesting bone marrow in an outpatient setting using newer anesthetic agents. J Clin Oncol 1993; 11(2):320-3.

59. Vallieres E, Page A, Verdant A: Ambulatory mediastinoscopy and anterior mediastinotomy. Ann Thorac Surg 1991; 52:1122-6.

60. Didlake R, Curry E, Rigdon E et al: Outpatient vascular access surgery: impact of a dialysis unit–based surgical facility. Am J Kid Dis 1992; 19(1):39-44.

61. Kalbfleisch SJ, El-Atassi R, Calkins H et al: Safety, feasibility and cost of outpatient radiofrequency catheter ablation of accessory atrioventricular connections. J Am Coll Cardiol 1993; 21(3):567-70.

62. Stovall T, Summitt RL, Bran D et al: Outpatient vaginal hysterectomy: a pilot study. Obstet Gynecol 1992; 1:145-9.

3

Management Dilemmas of Adult Patients

Rebecca S. Twersky

The success of ambulatory surgery lies in the proper selection and screening of patients. Previous chapters have discussed preoperative evaluation utilizing preanesthesia clinics, health questionnaires, consultative services of other physician specialties (e.g., cardiologists, internists, endocrinologists, pediatricians), and of other health care professionals involved in the patient's overall care. Appropriate preoperative testing has also been addressed. This information will allow the anesthesiologist to assess the patient properly and to identify those patients at particular risk for complications if they undergo the outpatient procedure. The next two chapters deal with management options for relatively common dilemmas encountered in ambulatory surgery. This chapter focuses on the adult patient.

Geriatric Patient

Age alone is not a significant risk factor for perioperative complications in ambulatory surgery and should not exclude a patient. Americans more than 65 years old constitute the fastest growing segment of the population and will continue to account for a significant portion of ambulatory surgery cases. It is predicted that by the year 2000, over 15% of the U.S. population will be more than 65 years old.[1] It is not uncommon for patients in their eighties and occasionally in their nineties to be scheduled for cataract extraction, cystoscopy, and other minor ambulatory procedures. Evaluation of the geriatric patient should proceed as it would for any patient. Researchers have found only a weak correlation between age and complication rate following ambulatory surgery.[2-4] The preoperative evaluation of older adults is often challenging, because of multiple concurrent medical problems (Box 3-1). Each disorder must be evaluated for the degree of

---

Box 3-1 Considerations in the Geriatric Patient

Multiple medical problems
Polypharmacy, chronic medications
Cognitive impairment
Sensory deficits (hearing or visual loss)
Limited mobility
Social situation

Box 3-2 *Physiologic Changes of Aging*

Cardiovascular
   Increased blood pressure
   Decreased baroreceptor sensitivity
   Increased incidence of arrythmias, heart block, bradycardia
   Increased stroke volume
Pulmonary
   Decreased vital capacity, forced expiratory volume in 1 second (FEV_1), PaO_2
   Increased closing capacity, FRC
Central Nervous System
   Decreased CBF, cerebral oxygen consumption ($CMRO_2$)
   Increased incidence of cerebrovascular disease
   Increased incidence of Alzheimer's dementia
   Decreased amounts of neuronal substance, neurotransmitters
   Impaired thermoregulation
Renal and Liver Function
   Decreased glomerluar filtration rate (GFR), creatinine clearance less than 1 ml/min/year >40 years
   Decreased hepatic blood flow
   Decreased levels of serum proteins
Musculoskeletal
   Decreased amounts of muscle mass, lean body mass
   Increased amounts of adipose tissue
Miscellaneous
   Depressed airway reflexes
   Impaired glucose tolerance
   Impaired homeostasis and fluid and electrolytes

compensation and its potential impact in the context of the planned procedure. Preoperative approaches to several of these medical problems are discussed in this chapter.

The normal physiologic changes of aging have an effect on perioperative management (Box 3-2). Blood pressure changes may be more exaggerated; older adults show less of a heart rate response to hypotension and may be at risk for orthostatic hypotension. In addition, patients may be on long-term drug therapy, which can further compound changes in systemic circulation. There is also an increased incidence of silent myocardial infarction (MI) and of coronary artery disease (CAD); therefore,

Box 3-3 *Pharmacologic Differences in the Elderly*

Decreased protein binding, resulting in
    Exaggerated pharmacologic effect
    Rapid rise concentration of drug in brain
Decreased renal and liver function resulting in
    Reduced drug clearance
    Smaller induction doses of intravenous agents
    Reduced maintenance dose requirements
Decreased neuronal mass, resulting in
    Decreased minimum alveolar concentration (MAC)
    Increased sensitivity to drug

preoperative electrocardiograms (ECGs) should be carefully evaluated.[5] Further investigation is warranted if there is evidence of an old MI, left bundle branch block, left anterior hemiblock, or intraventricular conduction defects that have not been previously noted.[1] Geriatric patients are more at risk for hypoxemia, aspiration, and hypothermia. The pharmacologic effects of intravenous and inhalation agents are influenced by the physiologic changes that have occurred in the elderly (Box 3-3). This is manifested as increased drug sensitivity, a reduction in dosage necessary for intravenous induction and maintenance, decreased minimum alveolar concentration (MAC), and prolonged anesthetic effect. Patients who receive general anesthesia may have prolonged recovery and postoperative confusion. Chung et al. reported that cognitive changes occurred in the elderly even after cataract extraction with a retrobulbar block and supplemented intravenous sedation.[6-7] Ventilatory response to hypoxemia and hypercarbia is reduced, and proper recovery period with supplemental oxygen should be administered. A longer postoperative period of observation may be needed. A busy ambulatory surgery facility must respect the slow pace of many of the geriatric outpatients, and sufficient time must be provided for their adequate preoperative preparation and for their recovery.

The geriatric patient is also challenging in terms of pre- and postoperative teaching. The patient must understand instructions clearly, or assistance must be sought for the patient. With the preoperative assessment, a plan for administering the patient's regular medications during the perioperative period must be formulated. The social situation should also be carefully assessed. The advantages of ambulatory surgery for geriatric patients centers around the brief hospital stay, which allows them an earlier return to their own familiar environment, and a resumption of their daily activities, diet, and medication schedule. Ensuring that the patient is discharged to a *responsible* home setting will further minimize complications. If necessary, home care support should be sought.

Cardiovascular Disease

With coronary artery disease (CAD), cerebrovascular disease, and hypertension occurring in approximately 68 million Americans,[8] it is quite common to be evaluating elective ambulatory surgery patients with some degree of cardiovascular disease. As cardiovascular disease continues to be a significant factor in perioperative morbidity and mortality, it is critical during preoperative assessment to obtain an accurate medical history and physical examination in order to determine the patient's fitness for outpatient surgery (Box 3-4). The physical examination and cardiac status have been clinically correlated (Box 3-5). It is clear that recent MI (within 6 months) and congestive heart failure (CHF) are significant risk factors for perioperative morbidity. Associated risks for cardiovascular disease include hypertension, diabetes mellitus, obesity, smoking, hyperlipidemia, and increased age; however, their risks for perioperative ischemia remain controversial. Many patients undergoing noncardiac surgery remain in a less well-defined risk group. To what extent should these patients undergo further preoperative testing, particularly if they are scheduled for outpatient surgery? Recommendations with regard to specific cardiovascular diseases are discussed below.

Hypertension

Hypertension affects about 25% of adults and 50% of the elderly in the United States. Additionally, half the cases are never diagnosed, and two thirds of patients with diagnosed hypertension receive inadequate therapy.[9] Often, during the preoperative anesthesia visit, the clinician will discover the poorly treated and the newly diagnosed hypertensive patient. At what blood pressure can a patient undergo ambulatory surgery? First, going beyond the

Box 3-4 *Evaluation of Cardiovascular Disease*

History

Coronary artery disease
Chest pain at rest and with exercise
Stable vs. unstable angina
Previous MI and associated complications
CABG surgery or angioplasty

Valvular heart disease or congestive heart failure
Dyspnea, angina, cyanosis, edema, nocturia, fatigue
MI, rheumatic fever, congenital heart disease
Recurrent pneumonia or bronchitis

Arrhythmias
Syncope, dizziness, palpitations

Hypertension and vascular disease
Stroke, claudication, renal disease, diabetes

Miscellaneous
Chronic medication
Other diseases affecting cardiovascular function

Physical Examination

Level of orientation
Blood pressure, heart rate and rhythm
Cyanosis, capillary filling
Peripheral edema
Hepatomegaly
Jugular venous distension, pulsation
Precordial pulsations, cardiomegaly
Auscultation of heart and lungs
Ventilatory rate and pattern
Body weight, height, temperature
Evidence of peripheral vascular disease

numerical blood pressure, the degree of cardiac disease should be evaluated. Preoperative evaluation should involve a search for associated cardiovascular disease—ischemic heart disease, arrythymias, cardiomyopathy, evidence of CHF, and end-organ disease, including cerebrovascular or renal impairment. Appropri-

Box 3-5 *Clinical Correlation with Cardiac Examination*

Left ventricular dysfunction, myocardial infarction, ischemia
Cardiomegaly, rales, dyspnea, peripheral edema, jugular venous distension, S_4 gallop, apical systolic murmur
Left ventricular regional wall motion abnormalities
Abnormal precordial systolic bulge
Increased left ventricular end diastolic pressure
S_3 gallop
Mitral regurgitation, papillary muscle dysfunction
Apical systolic murmur
Aortic stenosis
Pansystolic murmur with radiation
Mitral stenosis
Diastolic murmur at base
Aortic regurgitation
Diastolic murmur at apex

ate laboratory testing should be based on presence of end-organ disease. Preoperative ECGs are frequently abnormal. Further cardiac testing—such as echocardiogram, stress test, or dipyridamole-thallium scan—would only be necessary if there is evidence of impaired myocardial performance.

Outpatient surgery should be deferred and therapy instituted in patients with newly discovered hypertension and in those with treated, uncontrolled hypertension with confirmed diastolic blood pressure greater than 110 mm Hg. Patients with poorly controlled hypertension have greater intraoperative fluctuations in blood pressure, which increase the risk for increased perioperative cardiac morbidity.[10-12] Extreme swings in blood pressure may occur on induction of anesthesia, endotracheal intubation, and extubation. Additionally, altered baroreceptor reflexes and intravascular volume depletion make these patients more prone to hypotension and exaggerated pressor response. The ultimate goal is to maintain the patient's blood pressure close to the value of chronic control. In general, perioperative blood pressure should be maintained within 20% of baseline chronic values. Tachycardia is a greater determinant of perioperative MI in hypertensive patients, and treatment with esmolol or longer-acting beta blockers is recommended.[13] Knowledge of the patient's antihypertensive medication is important, as some medications interact with anesthesia (Table 3-1). Patients must be instructed to continue all their antihypertensive medication (except diuretics) to improve perioperative hemodynamic control.

Coronary Artery Disease

Preoperative evaluation of the patient with known coronary artery disease (CAD) or ischemic heart disease should include a detailed cardiac history and examination (Box 3-4). Evidence of ventricular dysfunction, limited exercise tolerance, or change in anginal pattern may place the patient at high risk for what is a relatively low-risk procedure.[14] An algorithm for preoperative cardiac evaluation and testing uses exercise tolerance to determine the need for further cardiac work-up (Fig. 3-1).[15] Resting 12-lead ECGs are recommended for patients aged 40 to 50 years and older; this can serve as a baseline, but rarely does it show anything new in patients with known CAD. The anesthesiologist may need to consult with the patient's internist or cardiologist to obtain a better history, and to gather information about previous ECGs and noninvasive and invasive cardiac work-ups. Specialized cardiac testing is directed toward assessing the amount of functional myocardium, the vulnerability to ischemia, and the global cardiac activity (Table 3-2). The accuracy, specificity, and cost-effectiveness vary,[16] and tests should be selected when abnormal results would affect patient management. The patient with unstable angina may benefit from coronary artery bypass or percutaneous transluminar coronary angioplasty before undergoing elective outpatient surgery. Patients with stable cardiac status do not need additional preoperative therapy, provided that the cardiologist, internist, or family physician examines the patient and indicates that the patient's management has been optimized.

Should patients wait 6 months following a recent MI before undergoing elective ambulatory surgery? Within 6 months of an MI, the risk of reinfarction postoperatively may be no different than that after a 6-month waiting period.[17,18] Shah et al.[18] reported no perioperative MI in noncardiac surgery patients who had had an MI in the past 6 months and who received monitored anesthesia care, but found similar rates of reinfarction *following* general and regional anesthesia. Although prospective data are lacking for ambulatory patients, select patients who have had an MI 4 to 6

Table 3-1   Antihypertensive Drugs

Drug	Perioperative considerations
Diuretics	Hypovolemia, electrolyte abnormalities
Beta blockers (e.g., propanolol, labetelol, atenolol)	Rebound hypertension and tachycardia on withdrawal, additive myocardial and chronotropic depressant effects with anesthesia, bronchospasm
Alpha$_1$ blockers (e.g., prazosin)	Decrease minimum aveolar concentration (MAC), additive hypotension with anesthesia, rebound hypertension and tachycardia on withdrawal
Alpha$_2$ agonists (e.g., clonidine)	Decrease MAC, additive hypotension with anesthesia
Arteriolar vasodilators (hydralazine)	Postural hypotension
Calcium channel blockers (e.g., nifedipine, verapamil, diltiazem)	Decreased contractility and conduction delays, additive hypotension with anesthesia, decrease MAC, potentiate neuromuscular blocking agents
Angiotensin-converting enzyme (ACE) inhibitors (e.g., lisinopril, enalapril, captopril)	Hypotension with anesthesia, hyponatremia
False neurotransmitters (methyldopa)	Decrease MAC, bradycardia, orthostatic hypotension, poor response to indirect-acting vasopressors

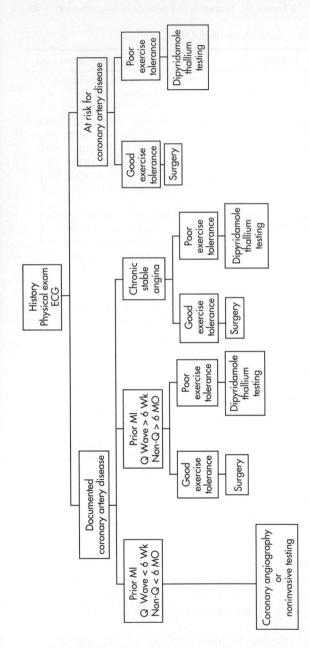

Fig. 3-1 Preoperative cardiac evaluation. Algorithm for patients undergoing surgical procedures associated with a low-to-moderate risk of perioperative myocardial ischemia. (From Fleisher LA, Bararsh PG. Anesth Analg 1992; 74:586-98.)

Table 3-2   Specialized Cardiac Testing

Procedure	Function
Exercise stress testing	Can detect ST-segment changes; identify heart rate and blood pressures associated with ischemia; positive test may not correlate with likelihood of cardiac complication
Echocardiography	Evaluates global and regional ventricular function; valvular function; estimate of ejection fraction; noninvasive; questionable predictive value
Technetium pyrophosphate	Extremely sensitive and specific for acute MI
Dipyridamole thallium-201	Provides information regarding myocardial perfusion; Extremely sensitive for acute MI; may induce coronary steal; not useful as screening tool; used in patients who cannot undergo exercise stress testing
Ambulatory monitoring	Arrhythmia and ischemia detection

months previously may undergo ambulatory procedures, if their preoperative cardiac status and the proposed procedure are carefully evaluated.

Preoperative medications, particularly beta blockers, should be continued. Nitrates should not be withheld; calcium channel blocker administration appears to make little difference in the incidence of ischemia during surgery,[19] and antihypertensives should be continued. Antiplatelet drugs (e.g., aspirin, dipyridmole) may need to be discontinued if significant intraoperative bleeding is anticipated.

The incidence of ischemia is greater in the postoperative period, and strategies to decrease postoperative ischemia include prevention of tachycardia and hypertension, preservation of coronary artery blood flow, and aggressive pain management.[20-24] Choice of anesthetic may not affect outcome. However, the incidence of perioperative infarction following ambulatory surgery is rare. Warner et al.[25] reported an incidence of perioperative MI following outpatient surgery of 1:3220. Only 2 out of 14 MIs occurred within 8 hours of surgery; one patient succumbed 7 days later. Gold et al. reported that the likelihood of hospital admission following ambulatory surgery was greater in patients with CAD than in those with other medical diseases.[3] Surgery on ASA physical status 3 and 4 patients can be done on an outpatient basis if their medical conditions are well controlled.

Valvular Heart Disease

Patients with valvular disease may undergo ambulatory surgery if there is no evidence of congestive heart failure, if there is no significant impairment in myocardial performance, and if compensatory mechanisms for maintaining cardiac output are intact. Valvular disease can cause dysrhythmias, alterations in pulmonary and peripheral vascular resistance, and changes in preload and myocardial oxygenation. Although the prevalence of rheumatic valvular disease is declining, congenital bicuspid aortic stenosis, mitral valve prolapse, IHSS, and calcific mitral insufficiency are encountered more frequently.[9] Valvular lesions can be classified as stenotic lesions that produce pressure overload on the ventricles, or regurgitant lesions resulting in volume overload. Only aortic stenosis is considered a significant risk factor in noncardiac surgery.[26,27] The preoperative evaluation should assess the severity of cardiac disease (Table 3-3). Exercise tolerance is useful in classifying the patient. Patients in New York Heart Association (NYHA) class 1 and 2 can undergo outpatient surgery, and those in class 3 may be considered as outpatient candidates for minor procedures. The patient must be able to lie flat, even during a regional or local anesthetic procedure. Congestive heart failure, manifesting as dyspnea, orthopnea, and fatigue, should be treated, and myocardial contractility optimized, before elective surgery.

Table 3-3   New York Heart Association Classification of
                Patients with Heart Disease

Class	Description
1	Asymptomatic
2	Symptoms with ordinary activity but comfortable at rest
3	Symptoms with minimal activity but comfortable at rest
4	Symptoms at rest

Anxiety, diaphoresis, and resting tachycardia may be evidence of
a compensatory increase in sympathetic nervous system activity.
Cardiac dysrhythmias, especially atrial fibrillation, are common.
Symptoms of angina, even when coronary arteries are normal,
may occur when valvular stenosis impinges on outflow or when
ventricular hypertrophy impedes diastolic coronary perfusion. In
the physical examination, identification of the location, intensity,
and radiation of the heart murmur assists in characterizing the
valvular lesion. Medical management commonly includes digitalis
therapy, which increases myocardial contractility and slows ventricular heart rate, particularly in the presence of atrial fibrillation.
Control of heart rate is adequate if the resting ventricular rate is
less than 80 beats per minute. Prolongation of P-R interval,
significant bradycardia, or premature ventricular beats on the ECG
may suggest digitalis toxicity. Diuretic therapy may also be used
to treat fluid overload. Laboratory testing for serum drug levels
and potassium levels should be measured, because hypokalemia
further exacerbates digitalis toxicity. Many patients may be taking
anticoagulants, and the decision to stop oral anticoagulant therapy
or to convert to heparin for the perioperative period should be
discussed among the physicians involved in the perioperative
management. Echocardiography is the best noninvasive diagnostic
tool for characterizing the valvular lesion. Should all adult patients
with evidence of heart murmur undergo an echocardiogram?
Clinical history and physical examination should clarify the need;
if necessary, consultation with a cardiologist should be sought.
Antibiotic prophylaxis should be followed according to the American Heart Association guidelines and are addressed further in
Chapter 6.

Anesthesia management is based on maintaining a cardiac
rhythm, blood pressure, and systemic vascular resistance that will

---

Box 3-6 Anesthetic Considerations for Patients with Valvular Heart Disease

---

Mitral Stenosis

Heart rate: normal to slow
Central blood volume: rapid increases should be avoided
SVR: normal to high
Other: avoid hypoxemia or increase in PVR that may induce CHF

Aortic Stenosis

Heart rate: normal sinus rhythm
SVR: normal
Central blood volume: keep full

Mitral Regurgitation

Heart rate: normal to fast
SVR: normal to low
Other: avoid drug-induced myocardial depression

Aortic Regurgitation

Heart rate: normal to high
SVR: normal to low
Other: avoid drug-induced myocardial depression

---

minimize the pathophysiology. Valvular stenotic lesions require strict maintenance of preload, contractility, rate, and rhythm (preferably sinus rhythm) within a narrow range. Valvular insufficiency or regurgitant lesions benefit from maintaining lower pulmonary or peripheral vascular resistance, which promotes forward flow. Often combined lesions are present, and management should be geared toward the more hemodynamically significant impairment (Box 3-6).

Mitral Valve Prolapse

Mitral valve prolapse (MVP) (see Box 3-7) is a fairly common condition, occurring in approximately 4% of the population, with a slightly higher prevalence in women.[28] These patients may have already undergone echocardiographic studies because of the incidental finding of a murmur or click on physical examination, or because of symptoms of chest pain, palpitations, anxiety, or

---

Box 3-7 Considerations in the Patient with Mitral Valve Prolapse

- Documentation of the diagnosis
- Clinical manifestations
    Chest pain
    Dysrhythmia or palpitations
    Valvular insufficiency or ventricular dysfunction
    Neurologic manifestations
    Anxiety
- Need for endocarditis prophylaxis

Box 3-8 Complications Associated with Mitral Valve Prolapse

- Cardiac arrhythmias (junctional rhythm, PVCs)
- A-V heart block
- ST-segment and T-wave changes
- Mitral regurgitation
- Infective endocarditis
- Ruptured chordae tendineae
- Transient ischemic attack
- Sudden death (rare)
    Keep heart slow and full

---

embolic phenomena. Patients with prolapse of a structurally abnormal valve have a higher incidence of complications than those with prolapse of a structurally normal valve. Potential complications include valvular regurgitation, endocarditis, and stroke (Box 3-8). There may be associated dysrhythmias even in asymptomatic patients.[29] It has been suggested that anxiety disorders result from mitral valve prolapse, and that valvular disorder is associated with adrenergic hyperactivity; however, neither of these have been shown to have a causal relationship.[30] In the absence of significant valvular regurgitation, the perioperative risk is probably not increased; patients with a structurally abnormal valve and regurgitation should receive antibiotic prophylaxis for bacterial endocarditis according to AHA recommendations (see Chapter 6).

Pacemaker

The presence of a well-embedded, functioning pacemaker should not exclude a patient from undergoing ambulatory surgery. The patient should be evaluated for the presence of other associated cardiovascular disease, i.e., ischemic or valvular heart disease, and the approach would be similar to that previously discussed for these disorders. Preoperative evaluation should involve determining the reason for the pacemaker, the patient's underlying rhythm, the drug therapy, and exact type of pacemaker (chamber sensed, chamber paced, sensing pattern, and default rhythm). Most modern pacemakers can convert to a fixed-rate asynchronous pacemaker in the presence of electrocautery interruptions without the need for reprogramming. However, the clinician must plan appropriately and be capable of reprogramming a pacemaker if necessary. Pacemaker battery changes on an ambulatory surgery basis is not universally accepted. Most patients should remain in a monitored setting until adequate pacemaker function has been established.

Pulmonary Disease

Asthma

Asthma is a common disease estimated to affect 5% to 10% of the U.S. population, or approximately 10 million patients, more than 3 million of whom are children. Despite a better understanding of its pathogenesis and improvements in treatment, asthma-associated morbidity and mortality have recently increased.[31] The National Institute of Heart, Blood, and Lung has issued new guidelines for the management of asthma, which emphasize inflammation as a vital factor in pathogenesis and therapy.[32] During preoperative evaluation, the clinician should ascertain the severity and control of the asthma, stimuli that trigger asthma attacks (allergy, respiratory infection, cold, exercise), and drug therapy that the patient uses for treatment (Box 3-9).

Treatment is related to asthma severity (Box 3-10). Mild asthma (symptoms less than three times a week, pulmonary function usually normal) can be managed by bronchodilators as needed, while moderate to severe asthma with more persistent symptoms may necessitate maintenance antiinflammatory steroid

---

Box 3-9 The Patient with Asthma or Chronic Obstructive Pulmonary Disease

---

- Baseline status (functional status and lung examination)
- Medication use (scheduled and demand medications)
- History of exacerbations: frequency, severity, triggers, intubation
- History of recent exacerbation or respiratory infection
- History of severe bronchospasm may contraindicate ambulatory surgery
- Use of corticosteroids
- Pulmonary function testing not indicated preoperatively in most patients

---

Box 3-10 Current Treatment of Asthma

- Steroids: used to reduce inflammation; bronchiolar relaxation
- Cromolyn sodium: mast cell stabilizer; preferred first-line treatment in children
- Beta$_2$ agonists: for acute bronchospasm
- Aminophylline: second-line treatment; least effective; good for nocturnal asthma

---

therapy. Whether mild cases require steroid administration is controversial.[33,34] Beta$_2$-specific adrenergic agonists are first-line treatment for emergency asthma and for prophylaxis of exercise-induced asthma. The administration route of choice is inhalation or nebulization; with oral administration, these agents have a slower onset of action, are less effective, and are more toxic. Theophylline was used for many years for acute and chronic asthma, but recent studies suggest that it is not effective in the acute setting in patients already optimized with beta-adrenergic drugs and steriods.[35] However, like beta-adrenergic drugs, long-acting, sustained-release oral preparations are helpful for controlling nocturnal asthma and for maintenance therapy. Serum concentrations should be maintained between 5 and 15 µg/ml to minimize side effects such as nausea, vomiting, irritability, insomnia, and arrhythmias. Anticholinergics such as ipratopium bromide (Atrovent) are not used in asthma; these are more helpful for patients with chronic bronchitis. Cromolyn sodium, administered in the inhaled form, is a mast-cell stabilizer and is considered first-line therapy in patients with allergic asthma. It has a very good safety profile. It is probably less effective than inhaled steroids, and its maximal effect may take up to 6 weeks to appear. Antiinflammatory steroid agents are being used more regularly in patients with moderate to severe asthma, and more aggressively and earlier than before. Patients may be instructed by their pulmonologists to take a short preoperative course of prednisone. Patients may also be taking inhaled steroids, which decrease the frequency of acute asthma episodes and lessen the need for concurrent medications, including oral steroids. They are effective in decreasing bronchial hyperreactivity. At higher doses, systemic effects may be seen, including adrenal suppression, cataracts, osteopenia (bone loss), and growth stunting.[33,34]

Whether all outpatients who have been receiving steroids should receive perioperative high-dose steroid replacement therapy is unclear. Steroids should be replaced in those patients with deficiencies. In low levels of stress, such as outpatient procedures, maintaining physiologic steroid levels seems sufficient. Patients who take their prednisone with milk or antacids to minimize gastric irritation may require parenteral steroids perioperatively. This, however, does not warrant high-dose replacement, unless there is evidence of impaired glucocorticoid response to surgical stress.[36] The potential harm from glucocorticoid excess is in patients with preexisting hypertension, diabetes, fluid retention, and gastric ulcers. Familiarity with the available steroid preparations is important when determining which to provide the outpatient (Table 3-4).

The physical examination should include an evaluation of the upper airway for rhinitis, otitis, nasal polyps, and infectious precipitants of asthma; chest examination for evidence of obstruction such as hyperexpanded chest, increased expiratory phase, wheezing, and rhonchi; and extremities for clubbing (almost never found in asthma, but rather in COPD). Peak flow is a parameter that can be followed in asthmatics during treatment, and it may validate clinical impression of patients with chronic illness.

Table 3-4 Exogenous Glucocorticoids

Compound	Trade name	Relative glucocorticoid potency	Equivalent dose (mg)
Short-acting			
Cortisone (as acetate)		1	25
Hydrocortisone (cortisol)	Solu-Cortef, A-HydroCort	0.8	20
Prednisone	Deltasone	3.5–4.5	5
Prednisolone	Hydeltrasol	4	5
Methylprednisolone	Solu-Medrol	5	4
Intermediate-acting			
Triamcinolone	Aristocort, Aristospan, Cinalone, Kenalog	5	4
Long-acting			
Dexamethasone	Decadron, Hexadrol	30	0.75

From Deutschmann CS: Anesthetic considerations in the use of corticosteroids and antibiotics. In Rogers MC, editor: Principles and practice of anesthesiology, 1993, St Louis, Mosby, p. 1595.

Simple observation of a forced expiratory maneuver can also provide important clinical insight. Pulmonary function, arterial blood gases, and chest x-rays are not needed for the stable asthmatic undergoing ambulatory surgery.

Chronic Obstructive Pulmonary Disease

The outpatient with chronic obstructive pulmonary disease (COPD), chronic bronchitis, or emphysema presents a great challenge. The pathophysiology of COPD is characterized by an obstruction to air flow with reversible and irreversible components. The degree to which each component is present determines the severity of the illness. The reversible component usually consists of bronchospasm, infection, secretion, and atelectasis, and should be treated with bronchodilators, antibiotics, and respiratory therapy before outpatient surgery. Preoperative evaluation should involve the same approach as that used for the asthmatic: current clinical status, determination of baseline pulmonary function, and drugs used in long-term therapy. The patient with COPD may have baseline wheezing and functional limitation. Additionally, these patients may be elderly or obese, or have concomitant cardiovascular and other systemic diseases that further compound their evaluation. Smoking history is frequently positive, and stopping smoking is helpful if done 6 to 8 weeks before surgery. This time period is required for mucus production to decrease, and for tracheal and bronchial cilia to return to normal function. Recovery of alveolar macrophages, immune response, and hepatic enzyme activity occurs after 6 to 8 weeks of smoking cessation. Abrupt cessation may increase the risk for mucus secretion and plugging; however, lower blood levels of bound carboxyhemoglobin and improvement in blood oxygen-carrying capacity can be achieved within 24 hours of smoking cessation.[37] Routine pulmonary function testing is not recommended, but may be helpful in determining the etiology of dyspnea, or, in severe COPD, in predicting need for continued ventilatory support after general anesthesia.[38] Similarly, baseline arterial blood gas determination or use of pulse oximetry may influence choice of anesthetic or need for further evaluation; resting hypercarbia or hypoxemia suggest increased perioperative risk.

A history of frequent exacerbations, steroid dependence, or need for intubation for respiratory support should prompt particular caution in evaluation and planning for outpatient surgery

(Box 3-9). Patients should be at their baseline or optimal status when presenting for surgery; wheezing, decline in functional status, or increase in sputum production suggest that the patient's condition is not optimized. Patients with pulmonary disease may be candidates for ambulatory surgery if they are well compensated at the time. All medications should be continued through the morning of surgery. Choice of anesthetic technique should be geared toward minimizing complications. If general anesthesia is required, airway manipulation should be avoided to decrease bronchospasm. The laryngeal mask airway (LMA) may be a reasonable alternative to laryngoscopy and intubation. Regional anesthesia may be preferred, when appropriate, with two caveats: A high level of spinal or epidural anesthesia may not be tolerated by patients with significant COPD, and caution should be used when administering upper extremity blocks (particularly the supraclavicular or interscalene approach to the brachial plexus) because pneumothorax or phrenic nerve block could have catastrophic results in these patients. Postoperatively, notwithstanding any respiratory embarrassment, these patients can be discharged.

Endocrine Disorders

Diabetes Mellitus

Diabetes mellitus, occurring in approximately 1% to 2% of the U.S. population, is the most frequently encountered endocrine disorder in ambulatory surgery. The pathophysiology of the disease includes a relative or absolute deficiency in insulin that leads to hyperglycemia and the inability to utilize glucose at the cellular level; disorders of lipid and protein metabolism are also involved. There are two types of primary diabetes: type 1, or insulin-dependent diabetes mellitus (IDDM), and type 2, or non-insulin-dependent diabetes mellitus (NIDDM). They differ in their age distribution, actual level of insulin production, cellular response to insulin, and treatment (Table 3-5).[39]

Evaluation for ambulatory surgery and anesthesia should include an assessment not only for diabetic control but also for comorbid disease (Box 3-11). Associated diseases may include renal insufficiency, CAD, silent ischemia, cardiomyopathy, arrhythmias, peripheral vascular disease, peripheral neuropathy, orthostatic hypotension, and gastroparesis, all of which have implications for the anesthesiologist. The "stiff joint syndrome" may be associated with unanticipated difficult intubation. These

Table 3-5 Characteristics of IDDM and NIDDM

	IDDM (Type 1)	NIDDM (Type 2)
Age of onset (years)	Less than 40	Greater than 40
Family history of diabetes	Uncommon	Common
Body habitus	Normal to wasted	Obese
Pathogenesis	Autoimmune mediated	Non-immune mediated
Physiologic state	Ketoacidosis prone	Hyperosmolar prone
Plasma insulin	Low to absent	Normal to high
Insulin therapy	Responsive	Responsive to resistant
Oral hypoglycemic therapy	Unresponsive	Responsive

patients may be identified by the "prayer sign" (inability to appose the palms of the hands with no space in between). At minimum, an ECG, and blood glucose and electrolyte levels should be performed. Additional testing would be determined by associated end-organ disease and their therapies. Patients at risk for aspiration may warrant pretreatment with gastrokinetics (metoclopramide 10 mg intravenously or orally), H_2 antagonists, or prophylactic antiemetics. General anesthetic agents have little effect on blood glucose and should be selected based on presence of other systemic diseases. Regional anesthesia causes relatively little metabolic disturbance, but patients with peripheral neuropathy warrant prior assessment of baseline function. Brittle diabetics are not appropriate candidates for outpatient surgery.

Treatment of diabetes is aimed at maintaining glucose homeostasis and preventing increased protein catabolism and electrolyte disturbances. Presence of cardiovascular disease, susceptibility to infection, and poor wound healing are factors that affect perioperative outcome. Ideally, blood glucose should remain adequately controlled, and acid-base chemistry and volume status should remain within normal limits throughout the perioperative period.[40] Perioperatively, it is preferred to maintain blood glucose at levels where resistance to infection and phagocyte function are not impaired, allowing normal wound healing to take place. The threshold for these effects is probably around 200 mg/dl, but the goal for glycemia control ranges between 120 and 180 mg/dl.[41] The determination of "how high is too high?" should be based on knowledge of the patient's usual blood glucose control, length and extent of the planned procedure, and the patient's ability to return to normal oral intake.

Preoperative instructions for the diabetic should include guidelines for insulin and medication administration and for preoperative fasting (NPO). Familiarity with the different treatments is important (Table 3-6). For the insulin-dependent diabetic, several

---

Box 3-11 *Considerations in the Diabetic Patient*

Degree of control
End-organ diseases
      Coronary artery disease
      Stiff ventricle (cardiac diastolic dysfunction)
      Renal insufficiency
      "Stiff joint syndrome," with potential difficult
          intubation
      Visual impairment (may affect discharge
          planning)
      Autonomic neuropathy (gastroparesis with
          nausea and vomiting)
      Peripheral neuropathy
Options for perioperative management
      Administer no insulin until after procedure
      Administer portion of long-acting insulin
      Administer insulin by sliding scale based on blood
          sugar
      Administer insulin by infusion
Goal in ambulatory surgery is rapid return to preoperative
    control
Patient's/family's ability to assess and manage glucose
    postoperatively

perioperative regimens have been described, and their selection depends on the preoperative glycemic control, reliability of the patient, and patient ability to self-monitor blood glucose. Insulin infusions, which have gained popularity in recent years,[40,42,43] may be impractical for brief outpatient procedures; an insulin infusion might be chosen for a longer procedure, but such a patient would require careful evaluation before discharge. Other options in managing the patient with IDDM include administering a portion (one third to one half) of the usual morning dose of long-acting insulin, or withholding the insulin until after surgery, when a reduced dose is given (Fig. 3-2). Insulin should be withheld from the fasting patient until the patient is in a monitored setting where an intravenous line can be started and dextrose administered. An effort should be made to schedule the surgery for diabetic patients early in the morning so as not to disrupt their usual routine. When this is not feasible, the patients should not eat solids for 8 hours, and should arrive to the ambulatory surgery facility early enough to determine whether clear liquids can be given, to check the fasting blood glucose level, and to follow one of the prescribed perioperative insulin regimens.

Most patients with NIDDM on oral antihyperglycemic drug therapy may safely omit their medication while fasting, and may resume taking the usual dose when they resume oral intake. Caution should be used in patients on long-acting drugs (e.g.,

Table 3-6   Treatment of Diabetes

	Onset of action (hours)	Duration of action (hours)
Insulin		
Regular	0.5-1	6-8
Semilente	1-2	12-16
NPH	1-2	18-26
Lente	2-4	18-26
70% NPH + 30% regular insulin	0.5	Up to 24
Oral Hypoglycemics		
Tolbutamide (Orinase)	Rapid	6-10
Chlorpropramide (Diabinese)	Slow	24-72
Glyburide (Micronase, Diabeta)	Intermediate	18-24
Glipizide (Glucotrol)	Very rapid	16-24

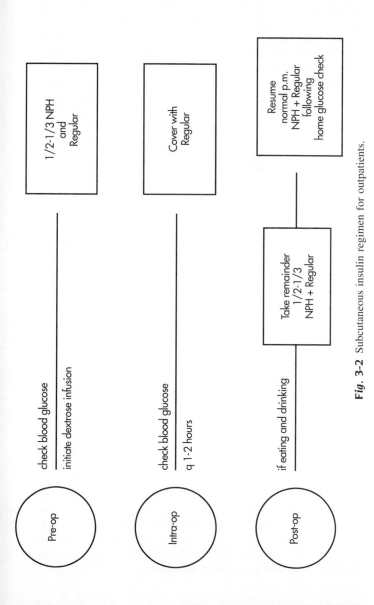

Fig. 3-2 Subcutaneous insulin regimen for outpatients.

chlorpropamide) that may cause residual hypoglycemia during the fasting period. The fasting blood glucose level should be determined preoperatively; if it is less than 250 mg/dl, no insulin need be given and intravenous fluids should not contain glucose. If the level is greater than 250 mg/dl, recommendations as presented for IDDM should be followed, and intravenous fluids containing dextrose should be administered.

For many diabetics, ambulatory surgery may be ideal to allow an early return to a near-normal regimen. However, because of autonomic nervous system dysfunction diabetics frequently have, postoperative nausea and vomiting and aggressive treatment with antiemetics and adequate hydration should be instituted. Also associated with diabetic autonomic dysfunction is bladder dysfunction, which may pose a problem if voiding criteria must be met for discharge. Blood glucose should be checked before discharge in patients who receive insulin perioperatively. Patients must be carefully evaluated to ensure that they can monitor their blood sugar, adjust their insulin dosage after discharge, and tolerate oral intake. Judicious perioperative glycemia control helps maintain the homeostatic balance so vital to the patient with diabetes.

Morbid Obesity

Preoperative evaluation of the morbidly obese patient (Box 3-12) should include a careful evaluation of the airway, as well as a search for coexisting diseases such as hypertension, restrictive lung disease, sleep apnea, and CHF.[44] Airway management as well as venous access may be challenging. Choice of an anesthetic technique should take into account potential difficulties with intubation and mask ventilation, as well as increased aspiration risk due to slower gastric emptying and increased intraabdominal pressure. If lipid-soluble anesthetics are used, emergence times may be longer, and postoperative ventilatory support may be required. However, with the new short-acting anesthetic agents, morbidly obese patients with an adequate airway and without significant cardiopulmonary pathology may be safely anesthetized on an outpatient basis. Patients with sleep apnea, daytime somnolence, resting hypoxemia, or evidence of Pickwickian syndrome are not suitable candidates for ambulatory surgery, except perhaps for brief procedures under local anesthesia.

Box 3-12 *Considerations in the Morbidly Obese*
           Patient

- Potential for difficult mask airway or intubation
- Potential for increased gastric residual and/or increased intragastric pressure
- Difficult venous access
- Altered volume of distribution and drug metabolism
- Potential end-organ manifestations:
    Ventricular failure
    Pulmonary hypertension
    Liver dysfunction
    Thromboembolic disease

End-stage Renal Disease

Only selected patients with chronic renal failure scheduled for the minor outpatient procedures are appropriate candidates.[45] The patient with chronic renal failure on dialysis (Box 3-13) may have one or several of the previously described diseases, including CAD, hypertension, CHF, and diabetes. Concerns specific to the dialysis patient include fluid volume and electrolyte status. During the history, signs and symptoms of volume overload and angina should be specifically addressed. Ideally, surgery should be planned for a day following dialysis, when the patient reaches his or her "ideal" weight. Immediately after dialysis, the patient has a relative intravascular volume depletion; while after more than one day, the patient begins to return to a volume overloaded state. Similarly, electrolyte shifts continue to occur for at least several hours after dialysis. It is also prudent to recheck the serum level of potassium (and glucose, if the patient is a diabetic) on the morning of surgery.

Local or regional anesthesia, when appropriate, may be best for the dialysis patient; general anesthesia, if chosen, should be accomplished with agents that minimize cardiovascular depression. The altered pharmacokinetics of renal failure should also be remembered, and alternatives to succinylcholine considered if the preoperative serum potassium level is borderline. A final consideration in the dialysis patient is a careful evaluation of the

---

Box 3-13 *Considerations in the Dialysis Patient*

- Associated diseases (hypertension, diabetes, coronary disease)
- Electrolyte and acid-base status
- Volume status
- Coagulation status and platelet function
- Timing of dialysis in the perioperative period
- Cognitive impairment common

Box 3-14 *Considerations in the Patient with Rheumatoid Arthritis*

- Potential for difficult airway
- Cervical spine instability or fixation
- Mandibular hypoplasia, particularly in juvenile onset rheumatoid arthritis
- Cricoarytenoid arthritis
- Pulmonary involvement
- Implications of medications
  Aspirin
  Steroids
  NSAIDS

---

functional status and need for postoperative supervision; mild neuropsychiatric impairment is relatively common in this population, and particular caution must be taken in discharge planning.

Rheumatoid Arthritis

Rheumatoid arthritis has several important anesthetic implications (Box 3-14). The cervical spine may have limited mobility or have instability. Because of the high incidence of asymptomatic instability, flexion and extension neck radiographs are suggested before elective surgery. The rheumatoid arthritis patient may also have cricoarytenoid arthritis, which may predispose to difficult intubation and to postoperative laryngeal edema. Cricoarytenoid arthritis is frequently asymptomatic and should be anticipated; a smaller endotracheal tube should be considered. Preoperative fiberoptic evaluation may be appropriate in patients with history of hoarseness or jaw pain. Medication history is also important in this population, as chronic aspirin, NSAIDs, or steroid use are common. If possible, aspirin should be discontinued a week before surgery; in patients who must remain on aspirin therapy, it may be appropriate to determine the bleeding time before a regional anesthetic technique is used.

Alcohol and Drug Abuse

Recent or chronic substance abuse may be a significant problem in patients presenting for ambulatory surgery. A careful history and high index of suspicion are needed. Ambulatory surgery for patients who have signs of acute intoxication should be postponed; for the chronic abuser, evaluation of the medical sequelae will help determine the patient's suitability for surgery. Intravenous drug abusers (Box 3-15) may have difficult venous access, and may place health care providers at risk of exposure to human immunodeficiency virus (HIV). In addition, intravenous drug users and cocaine users frequently have a low pain threshold and cooperate poorly with procedures such as intravenous catheter placement or regional anesthetic techniques. There have also been

---

Box 3-15 *General Considerations in the Intravenous Drug and Cocaine Abuse Patient*

- Difficult intravenous access
- Low pain threshold
- May be poorly cooperative
- HIV transmission risk
- Cardiomyopathy
- Myocardial ischemia
- Pulmonary changes: decreased compliance, chronic granulomatosis
- Nasal septal atrophy
- Altered sympathetic nervous system responses
- Drug withdrawal

anecdotal reports of substance injection into intravenous lines started in a medical setting, which prompts careful supervision of this patient population and awareness of this potential problem.

In the acute phase, cocaine blocks neuronal reuptake of norepinephrine and dopamine, which causes sympathetic nervous system stimulation. Hypertension, cardiac arrhythmias, and ischemia (possibly due to coronary artery vasospasm) may occur in persons without prior abnormalities.[46] Seizures, cerebrovascular accident, and hyperthermia may also occur. These patients should never undergo elective ambulatory surgery. Chronic cocaine abusers may have these acute problems; as well, there may be cardiomyopathy, nasal septal atrophy, and "crack lung," i.e., pulmonary changes such as decreased compliance and chronic granulomatosis from inhaled impurities.

The opioid abuser may have a history or signs of endocarditis, hepatitis, and chronic pulmonary changes (from suppression of cough reflex and reduced mucociliary clearance).[46,47] In addition, there is a risk of withdrawal symptoms; manifestations include tremor, muscle aches, perspiration, rhinorrhea, hot and cold flashes, fever, and gastrointestinal distress. Pain management can be controversial in the patient with a history of substance abuse. Significantly higher amounts of narcotics may be necessary. Certainly, alternatives to opioids should be used where feasible, but adequate amounts of pain medication should not be withheld merely from fear of contributing to addiction.

Individuals with acute alcohol intoxication (Box 3-16) may have impaired airway reflexes and multiple metabolic abnormalities; these patients are not acceptable for elective surgery. Patients with a history of alcohol abuse should be questioned carefully about other manifestations, such as liver disease, withdrawal symptoms, or history of cardiomyopathy or arrhythmia, and bleeding tendency. Liver disease in the alcoholic patient may range from fatty infiltration to alcoholic hepatitis to cirrhosis; elective surgery should be postponed in the patient with acute abnormalities such as alcoholic hepatitis.

Immunosuppression

The ambulatory surgery setting provides a viable option for the immunocompromised patient requiring a variety of procedures related to their disease. Outpatient surgery offers a short hospital stay, reduced exposure to nosocomial infection and other

---

Box 3-16 *Considerations in Alcohol Abuse*

Acute

Increased aspiration risk
Metabolic abnormalities
Combativeness
Alcoholic hepatitis

Chronic

Cirrhosis
Coagulopathy
Altered drug volume and kinetics
Pulmonary and extra-pulmonary shunting
Acute and chronic gastritis, pancreatitis
Cardiomyopathy, arrhythmia
Delirium tremens, withdrawal seizures, dementia
Bone marrow depression, folate and thiamine deficiency
Unreliable, social problems

---

iatrogenic illnesses, and adequate postoperative care. Patients can return to their own environment with minimal disruption in their activities of daily living. It is not uncommon for immunocompromised patients with leukemia, or with breast, colon, bladder, ovarian, uterine, skin, head, and neck cancers, to be scheduled for ambulatory procedures. Procedures like central venous access ports, diagnostic evaluations under anesthesia to assess response to chemotherapy or radiation therapy, biopsies, and other related surgeries are frequently necessary. Preoperative evaluation may be accelerated because often these procedures are not scheduled on a purely elective basis.

Cancer Patient

In the patient with cancer, the disease state and the extent of involvement of other organ systems, the presence of coexisting medical problems, and the proposed surgical procedure must be considered (Box 3-17). Laboratory tests should be based on the patient's medical status and the effect of oncologic treatment, and may include a complete blood count (including platelets), coagulation studies, liver and kidney function tests, blood glucose and electrolyte levels, chest radiography, ECG, and arterial blood gases. Evaluation of the patient for current and past cancer therapies is important. Radiotherapy, commonly indicated for solid tumors, may cause adhesions, resulting in obstruction and fibrosis. Proper airway evaluation is important, and the possibility of fiberoptic intubation should be considered. Surgical dissection may be more difficult, and potentially may result in more extensive surgery than anticipated (Box 3-18). Immediate or delayed effects of chemotherapy may include tissue necrosis, protracted nausea and vomiting, pancytopenia, tissue edema, aseptic necrosis of the

---

Box 3-17 Considerations for the Outpatient with Cancer

- Myelosuppression
- Cancer-related ectopic hormone production and associated syndromes
- Coexisting medical problems
- Radiotherapy- and chemotherapy-induced organ dysfunction
- Chemotherapy and anesthesia interactions
- Pain management
- Aseptic technique

Box 3-18 Complications of Radiotherapy

Acute

Skin changes, gastrointestinal problems, alopecia, pancytopenia

Intermediate

Bowel obstruction, fistulae

Late

Myocardial fibrosis, radiotherapy-induced coronary artery disease; pericardial effusions; radiation pneumonitis and fibrosis; rib fractures; pleural effusion; hypoxemia; hepatic, renal, central nervous system problems; laryngeal necrosis; and edema

femoral head, stomatitis, cardiac failure, pulmonary toxicity, hepatic dysfunction, nephrotoxicity, and various neuropathies (Table 3-7).

Familiarity with adverse reactions and side effects of oncology drugs allows the anesthesiologist to select an appropriate anesthesia technique for the ambulatory procedure. Patients treated with bleomycin or mitomycin C may be vulnerable to interstitial fibrosis and pulmonary edema, and appropriate intravenous solutions and the minimally effective FiO_2 should be administered. The presence of compromised cardiac function from anthracycline therapy would require avoidance or careful titration of inhaled and intravenous anesthetics that depress the myocardium. The presence of renal or liver disease may affect the choice of anesthetic and muscle relaxant. Peripheral neuropathies should be evaluated before the administration of regional blocks, and signs of central nervous system depression should be identified. Anemia, coagulation disturbances, nutritional deficiencies, and electrolyte abnormalities should be corrected preoperatively.[48]

AIDS Patient

With the increasing prevalence of human immunodeficiency virus (HIV I and II) infection and acquired immunodeficiency syndrome (AIDS), affected patients are now being scheduled for ambulatory procedures. Just as with the patient with cancer, the ambulatory setting decreases the AIDS patient's risk for nosocomial infections, and it provides a minimal disruption in the patient's routine. Associated opportunistic infections, neurologic complications, and other systemic disorders should be sought during the preoperative evaluation (Box 3-19). Patients may have history of pneumonia, gastroenteritis, retinitis, lymphoproliferative disorders, myocarditis, pericardial effusion, cardiomyopathy, or tuberculosis, and should be examined for resolution and treatment of these active symptoms. Multisystem involvement by opportunistic infections (viral, fungal, protozoal, or bacterial), secondary tumor development, encephalopathy, lymphoma, or direct HIV damage can result in altered organ function. Neurologic disorders associated with AIDS may include encephalitis, resulting in memory loss, ataxia, and seizures; peripheral neuropathy, manifested as paresthesias, weakness, and sensory loss; myelopathy, resulting in incontinence; and, less frequently, aseptic meningitis with fever, headache, and cranial nerve palsies.[49] Consequently, the use of spinal or other regional techniques may be questionable. Additionally,

Table 3-7 Chemotherapeutic Agents and Associated Side Effects

Agent	Side effect	Cancer
Alkylating Agents		
Cyclophosphamide (Cytoxan) Nitrogen mustard Chlorambucil	*General:* Rapid destruction of tumor mass resulting in increased production of purine and pyridine metabolites, uric acid nephropathy, bone marrow suppression *Specific:* Cyclophosphamide: Pancytopenia, hemorrhagic cystitis, water retention, pulmonary fibrosis, plasma cholinesterase inhibition Nitrogen mustard: Pancytopenia, tissue necrosis	Lymphoma, breast, ovarian, melanoma, multiple myeloma
Antimetabolites		
Methotrexate 5-fluorouracil (5-FU)	*General:* Bone marrow suppression, severe diarrhea, nausea and vomiting, renal tubal toxicity, acute and chronic hepatotoxicity	Gastrointestinal, pulmonary, sarcoma, leukemia

Cytarabine (cytosine arabenoside and ARA-C)
Mercaptopurine

Specific:
Methotrexate: respiratory depression, hepatic and renal dysfunction, tissue necrosis
5-fluorouracil and cytarabine: diarrhea, pancytopenia, hemorrhage, enteritis
Mercaptopurine: nephrotoxicity

Plant Alkaloids

Vincristine (Oncovin)
Vinblastine (Velban)

Specific:
Neuropathy, hyponatremia
Bone marrow suppression

Hodgkin and non-Hodgkin lymphoma, testicular carcinoma, choriocarcinoma, breast, renal, carcinoma, acute leukemia, lung, Wilm's tumor, neuroblastoma

Antineoplastic Antibiotics

Anthracyclines (Adriamycin and daunorubicin)
Bleomycin, mitomycin C

Specific:
Stomatitis, cardiac failure, acute and chronic cardiac toxicity
Pulmonary fibrosis, skin pigmentation, pulmonary toxicity from high FiO_2, exfoliative dermatitis, Raynaud's phenomenon

Lymphoma, breast, lung, thyroid, ovarian

Continued.

Table 3-7 Chemotherapeutic Agents and Associated Side Effects—cont'd

Agent	Side effect	Cancer
Miscellaneous		
Cisplatinum (Cisplatin)	Myelosuppression, nephrotoxicity, nausea and vomiting	Testicular, ovarian, bladder, head, and neck
Prednisone	Aseptic necrosis of femoral head, diabetes	Acute lymphoblastic leukemia, lymphoma, multiple myeloma, breast, chronic lymphocytic leukemia
Paclitaxel (Taxol)	Cardiotoxicity, neurotoxic, pancytopenia, nausea and vomiting	
Immunogenic		
Interferon	Hypotension, sepsis, hypothermia, sudden decompensation (total body failure, sepsis)	Melanoma, Kaposi's sarcoma, leukemia, lymphoma, Immunodeficiency syndromes
Growth factors	Leaky capillary syndrome, adult respiratory distress syndrome (ARDS), thrombosis	

Box 3-19 Considerations for the Patient with AIDS

- Opportunistic infections
- Cardiomyopathy, pleural effusions, myocarditis
- Diarrhea, esophagitis, dysphagia
- Pancytopenia
- Renal and liver involvement
- Neurologic impairment, neuropathies
- Difficult venous access

---

these patients may be on zidovudine (azidothymidine, AZT) treatment, chemotherapy for associated non-Hodgkin's lymphoma, or other drug therapies that may produce anemia, granulocytopenia, and thrombocytopenia. Associated gastrointestinal manifestations include chronic diarrhea, esophagitis, and dysphagia, and these contribute to electrolyte and volume disturbances. Hyponatremia occurs frequently in hospitalized patients with AIDS, and should be resolved before ambulatory surgery. HIV-associated nephropathy can further complicate the course. Patient history and physical examination should dictate the particular preoperative tests necessary, which frequently include complete blood count (with platelets), coagulation studies, serum electrolytes, renal and liver function tests, chest x-ray, and ECG. The preoperative evaluation and planning of appropriate anesthesia depends on the system-related disorders, drug therapy, and procedure. Many diagnostic procedures and central line placements can be performed under monitored sedation and local anesthesia infiltration. The use of dopaminergic antagonists (e.g., metoclopramide and droperidol) may further exacerbate AIDS dementia complex and should be avoided.[49] Vascular access may be difficult, especially in patients with a history of intravenous drug abuse. Guidelines for health care workers for management of patients with HIV infection follow the Centers for Disease Control (CDC) suggestion to assume that every patient is contagious for a blood-borne pathogen and to adopt universal blood and body fluid precautions for all patients, regardless of whether they are known to be infected or not.[50] Consequently, the ambulatory surgery facility does not need isolation areas, but precautions to avoid occupational acquired infections should be instituted. Needle-free intravenous infusion sets with stopcocks can be used, and needles should not be recapped or bent before discarded.

As with all immunosuppressed patients, adherence to proper aseptic technique is critical to reduce perioperatively acquired infection. Frequent hospitalizations may make these patients particularly anxious or even demanding on the facility, and the ambulatory surgery staff should be particularly sensitive to their needs. Additionally, these patients may have tolerance to routine doses of analgesics, and appropriate postoperative pain treatment should be instituted before discharging the patient.

Summary

As ambulatory surgery continues to grow, so will the variety of patients presenting for elective surgery. To be acceptable candidates for outpatient surgery, patients should have their medical diseases well controlled, accept the responsibilities of postoperative care after discharge, and be accompanied by a responsible adult. Accordingly, proper selection criteria need to be developed by the ambulatory surgery facilities to ensure delivery of high-quality medical services and to maintain patient safety. Management dilemmas of common adult ambulatory patients, including the problems of geriatric patients, patients with cardiovascular and pulmonary disease, diabetes, morbid obesity, renal failure, rheumatoid arthritis, substance abuse, and immunosuppression are highlighted.

References

1. Stiff JF: Evaluation of the geriatric patients. In Rogers MC, editor: Principles and practice of anesthesiology, St Louis, 1993, Mosby, pp. 480-92.
2. Meridy HW: Criteria for selection of ambulatory surgical patients and guidelines for anesthetic management: a retrospective study of 1553 cases. Anesth Analg 1982; 61:921-6.
3. Gold BS, Kitz DS, Lecky JH et al: Unanticipated admission to the hospital following ambulatory surgery. JAMA 1989; 262:3008-10.

4. Freeman LN, Schachat AP, Manolio TA et al: Multivariate analysis of factors associated with unplanned admissions in "outpatient" ophthalmic surgery. Ophthalmic Surg 1988; 19:719-23.

5. Kantelip JP, Sage E, Duchene-Marullaz P: Findings on ambulatory electrocardiographic monitoring in subjects older than 80 years. Am J Cardiol 1986; 57:398-401.

6. Chung FF, Chung A, Meier RH et al: Comparison of perioperative mental function after general anaesthesia and spinal anaesthesia with intravenous sedation. Can J Anaesth 1989; 36:382-7.

7. Chung F, Lavelle PA, McDonald S et al: Cognitive impairment after neuroleptanalgesia in cataract surgery. Anesth Analg 1989; 68:614-8.

8. American Heart Association: 1991 heart and stroke facts, Dallas, 1991, American Heart Association.

9. Polk SL, Roizen MF: Patient factors influencing anesthesia: cardiovascular, neurologic, endocrine, and gastrointestinal. In Liu PL, editor: Principles and procedures in anesthesiology, Philadelphia, 1992, JB Lippincott, pp. 28-35.

10. Goldman L, Caldera DL: Risks of general anesthesia and elective operation in the hypertensive patient. Anesthesiology 1979; 50:285-92.

11. Charlson ME, MacKenzie CR, Gold JP et al: Intraoperative blood pressure. What patterns identify patients at risk for postoperative complications? Ann Surg 1990; 212:567-80.

12. Yurenev AP, Dequattro V, Devereux RB: Hypertensive heart disease: relationship of silent ischemia to coronary artery disease and left ventricular hypertrophy. Am Heart J 1990; 120:928-33.

13. Stone JG, Foex JW, Sear J et al: Risk of myocardial ischemia during anesthesia in treated and untreated hypertensive patients. Br J Anaesth 1988; 61:675-9.

14. Mangano DT, Browner WS, Hollenberg M et al: Perioperative myocardial ischemia during noncardiac surgery. N Engl J Med 1991; 324: 1594-5.

15. Fleisher LA, Barash PG: Preoperative cardiac evaluation for noncardiac surgery: a functional approach. Anesth Analg 1992; 74:586-98.

16. Mangano DT, London MJ, Tubau JF et al: Dipyridamole thallium-201 scintigraphy as a preoperative screening test: a reexamination of its predictive potential. Circulation 1991; 84:493-502.

17. Rosenfeld BA, Rogers MC: Risk stratification in post-myocardial infarction patients: is six months too long to wait? J Clin Anesth 1991; 3:85-7.

18. Shah KB, Kleinman BS, Sami H et al: Re-evaluation of perioperative myocardial infarction in patients with prior myocardial infarction undergoing noncardiac operations. Anesth Analg 1990; 71:231-5.

19. Durand PG, Lehot JJ et al: Calcium-channel blockers and anaesthesia. Can J Anaesth 1991; 38:75-89.

20. Mangano DT: Perioperative cardiac morbidity. Anesthesiology 1990; 72:153-84.

21. Mangano DT, Browner WS, Hollenberg MT et al: Association of perioperative myocardial ischemia with cardiac morbidity and mortality in men undergoing noncardiac surgery. N Engl J Med 1990; 323:1781-8.

22. Mangano DT, Silciano D, Hollenberg M et al: Postoperative myocardial ischemia: therapeutic trials using intensive analgesia following surgery. Anesthesiology 1992; 76:343-53.

23. Shah KB, Kleinman BS, Rao TLK et al: Angina and other risk factors in patients with cardiac diseases undergoing noncardiac operations. Anesth Analg 1990; 70:240-7.

24. Charlson ME, Mackenzie CR, Gold JP et al: The preoperative and intraoperative hemodynamic predictors of postoperative myocardial infarction or ischemia in patients undergoing noncardiac surgery. Ann Surg 1989; 210:637-48.

25. Warner MA, Shields SED, Chute CG: Major morbidity and mortality within one month of ambulatory surgery and anesthesia. JAMA 1993; 270:1437-41.

26. Goldman L, Caldera DL, Nussbaum SR et al: Multifactorial index of cardiac risk in noncardiac surgical procedures. N Engl J Med 1977; 297:845-50.

27. Detsky AS, Abrams HB, Forbath N et al: Cardiac assessment for patients undergoing noncardiac surgery, a multifactorial clinical risk index. Arch Intern Med 1986; 146:2131-4.

28. Carabello BA: Mitral valve disease. Curr Probl Cardiol 1993; 18:423-78.

29. Twersky RS, Kaplan JA: Junctional rhythm in a patient with mitral valve prolapse. Anesth Analg 1986; 65:975-8.

30. Chesler E, Gornick CC: Maladies attributed to myxomatous mitral valve. Circulation 1991; 83:328-32.

31. McFadden ET Jr, Gilbert IA: Asthma. N Engl J Med 1992; 327:1928-37.

32. National Heart, Lung, and Blood Institute, National Asthma Education Program: Expert panel report: guidelines for the diagnosis and management of asthma. J Allergy Clin Immunol 1991; 88(Pt 2): 425-534.

33. Galant SP, Bae J: New treatments for asthma. Hospital Physician 1993:21-31.

34. Konig P: Corticosteroid therapy in mild to moderate asthma. J Resp Dis 1992; 13:S35-S44.

35. Weinberger M: Theophylline: when should it be used? J Pediatr 1993; 122:403-5.

36. Udelsman R, Ramp J, Gallucci WT et al: Adaptation during surgical stress. A reevaluation of the role of glucocorticoid. J Clin Invest 1986; 77:1377-81.

37. Warner MA, Offord KP, Warner ME et al: Role of preoperative cessation of smoking and other factors in postoperative pulmonary complications: a blinded prospective study of coronary artery bypass patients. Mayo Clin Proc 1989; 64:609-16.

38. Zibrak JD, O'Donnell CR, Marton K: Indications for pulmonary function testing. Ann Int Med 1990; 112:763-71.

39. Unger RH, Foster DW: Diabetes mellitus. In Wilson Jd, Foster PW, editors: William's textbook of endocrinology, ed 8, Philadelphia, 1992, WB Saunders, pp. 1255-1333.

40. Milaskiewicz RM, Hall GM: Diabetes and anaesthesia: the past decade. Br J Anaesth 1992; 68:198-206.

41. McMurray JF, Jr: Wound healing with diabetes mellitus. Surg Clin North Am 1984; 61:769-70.

42. Hirsch IB, McGill JB, Cryer PE, White PF: Perioperative management of surgical patients with diabetes mellitus. Anesthesiology 1991; 74:346-59.

43. Christiansen CL, Schurizek BA, Malling G et al: Insulin treatment of the insulin-dependent diabetic patient undergoing minor surgery: continuous intravenous infusion compared with subcutaneous administration. Anaesthesia 1988; 43:533-7.

44. Buckley FP: Anesthetizing the morbidly obese patient. ASA Refresher Courses 1990; 18:53-68.

45. Wilson SE, Connall TP, White R, Connolly JE: Vascular access surgery as an outpatient procedure. Ann Vascular Surg 1993; 7:325-9.

46. Kloner RA, Hale S, Alker K, Rezkella S: The effects of acute and chronic cocaine use on the heart. Circulation 1992; 85:407-19.

47. Frost EAM, Seidel MR: Preanesthetic assessment of the drug abuse patient. Anesthesiol Clin North Am 1990; 8:829-42.

48. Desiderio DP: Cancer chemotherapy: complications and interactions with anesthesia. Hospital Formul 1990; 25(2):176.

49. Berkowitz ID: Evaluation of the patient with acquired immunodeficiency syndrome and other serious infections. In Rogers MC, editor: Principles and practice of anesthesiology, St Louis, 1993, Mosby, pp. 410-27.

50. Centers for Disease Control: Update: universal precautions for prevention of transmission of human immunodeficiency virus, hepatitis B virus and other blood-borne pathogens in health-care settings. JAMA 1988; 260:462-4.

4

Management Dilemmas of Pediatric Patients

Hernando De Soto

Pediatric dilemmas
    The premature infant
    Runny nose
    Postintubation croup
    Sickle cell disease
    Heart disease or heart murmur
    Malignant hyperthermia susceptibility
    Down's syndrome
    Cancer
Summary

Surgery and anesthesia in the pediatric patient are commonly performed in the outpatient setting. Most children are healthy and require very minimal preoperative preparation; however, others have significant medical disease. These patients too can benefit from outpatient surgery, i.e., shorter parental separation and shorter exposure to the hospital and its pathogens. Probably the biggest factor in the successful management of these patients is the optimization of their medical situation. Appropriate consultations and laboratory work-ups should be obtained as needed.

This chapter will discuss some of the most common difficult management situations in the pediatric patient that can confront anesthesia clinicians in the ambulatory surgery center.

Pediatric Dilemmas

The Premature Infant

One of the greatest debates in all of anesthesia centers around the question: At what age can ambulatory surgery be performed safely in the premature infant? With the recent advances in neonatal medicine, many premature infants are surviving neonatal intensive care and presenting for surgery very early in their lives. Procedures like inguinal hernia repair and examinations under anesthesia are very common. Because of the obvious medical and financial benefits, tremendous pressure is being placed on anesthesia clinicians to accept these patients for ambulatory surgery.

Many studies have indicated that former premature infants are at greater risk of significant respiratory complications, especially apnea.[1-7] Apneic episodes are inversely proportional to postconceptual age (PCA),[5] which is the sum of gestational age and postnatal age. From these studies, the recommended age at which ambulatory surgery can be performed safely ranges from 40 weeks PCA[7] to 60 weeks PCA.[5]

Naylor et al.[7] have identified risk factors for apnea and bradycardia that can be used as preoperative indicators. These factors include history of apnea and bradycardia, hemoglobin below 10 gm/dl, chronic respiratory disease, and methylxanthine drug therapy at the time of the operation. For years, methylxanthines have been used in the management of apnea in neonatal wards.

Significant discrepancies in study methodology make definitive conclusions difficult. In the available literature, some studies are retrospective, the definitions of apnea are disparate, and there are no studies of a large series of patients undergoing the same operative procedure with the same anesthetic technique, the same anesthesiologist and surgeon, and the same operating room conditions.[8] Furthermore, the total number of cases in all the studies is quite small.

What should we do? Table 4-1 summarizes our recommendations based on PCA and risk factors. These are relative recommendations based on currently available data. Until more extensive

Table 4-1   Postoperative Admission of the Former
Premature Infant

| | Risk factors* | |
Age	No	Yes
Older than 50 weeks PCA	Discharge	Admit
Younger than 50 weeks PCA	Admit	Admit

*Risk factors include prior history of apnea and bradycardia, hemoglobin lower than 10 gm/dl, chronic respiratory disease, and methylxanthine drug therapy.[7]

prospective studies are carried out, it is reasonable to admit all former premature infants less than 50 weeks PCA and monitor them for perioperative apnea (this is a middle ground between the conservative 60 weeks recommended by Kurth and the 40 weeks recommended by Naylor).[6,8] We recommend a pulse oximeter and an apnea monitor for 12 to 24 hours after surgery. If apnea occurs, the monitoring period should be extended for another 24 apnea-free hours.[9] Furthermore, we strongly recommend erring toward the conservative side and admitting any infant under suspicion of deviating from normal respiratory mechanics, regardless of PCA. There are no special laboratory tests routinely ordered before anesthetizing the former premature infant having outpatient surgery; however, we routinely obtain a hemoglobin and hematocrit determination. Anemia (hematocrit less than 30) in former preterm infants may be associated with an increased incidence of postoperative apnea.[10]

Recently, isolated case reports of apnea in full-term infants have appeared in the literature.[11,12] There currently are no data supporting an appropriate age for term children to undergo outpatient surgery. All reported episodes of postoperative apnea in term infants have occurred within the first 5 hours after the operation. We observe term infants younger than 50 weeks PCA for 8 hours after the operation before allowing discharge. For infants more than 50 weeks PCA, routine guidelines for infant discharge are used.

Recent reports have suggested that caffeine base given intravenously after induction can prevent postoperative apnea.[13,14] More studies will be needed before definitive conclusions can be drawn.

Runny Nose

One of the most common problems handled by and debated by pediatric anesthesia clinicians is a runny nose. Some providers believe that any runny nose or cough is cause for cancelling the operation; while others believe that if the child does not look toxic, surgery and anesthesia can be performed safely.

The main concerns in a child with an upper respiratory infection (URI) are significant perioperative respiratory problems such as laryngospasm, bronchospasm, fever, atelectasis, croup, pneumonia, and postoperative hypoxemia.[15,16] A recent study reported an astounding 11.1% chance of having an adverse respiratory event in intubated patients with URI.[17] However, no increase in complications was noted in children undergoing myringotomies without intubation.[18]

An issue to keep in mind is the tremendous implication of cancelling a case. Significant hardships are imposed on the family, surgeon, anesthesia clinician, and institution. Also it is well known that the average child annually experiences three to six colds, each with a 4- to 10-day acute phase and a 2-week convalescence.[19] This hardly allows any time to perform surgery.

Obviously, the important issue here is whether a true viral or bacterial infectious process is present. If infection is present, postponing elective surgery is the safest option. If the runny nose is caused by a noninfectious process, it is safe to proceed. Box 4-1 describes the common differential diagnosis of a runny nose.

The history obtained from the parents is probably the easiest way to distinguish an infectious from a noninfectious process. Box 4-2 shows some important questions to ask the parents. Obviously, a child who is acting differently, and who has a fever and a purulent nasal discharge will most probably have an infectious process.

Box 4-1 Differential Diagnosis of a Runny Nose

- Allergic rhinitis
- Vasomotor rhinitis (crying)
- Teething
- Chronic rhinorrhea from surgical condition
- Infection

Box 4-2 Questions for Parents

1. Does the child or anyone in the family have allergies like hay fever?
2. Do the child's brothers or sisters have a respiratory infection (cold)?
3. Have there been any changes in the child's appetite, sleeping habits, or playing behavior?
4. Is the child acting differently from how he or she usually acts?
5. What did the nasal discharge look like yesterday? Three days ago? Last week? Is it thicker now? Has the color changed? Has blood appeared in the discharge?

A word of advice: Proceed with caution, use your clinical judgment, and individualize each case. Surgery for children who have evidence of bronchospastic disease, high fever, abnormal adventitious sounds, and signs of toxicity should be postponed and rescheduled for a later date. Recent evidence has demonstrated that for patients with a URI, a delay of 1 to 2 weeks after the resolution of symptoms decreases the risk of perioperative hypoxemia to that of healthy patients.[20] A delay of at least 4 weeks is necessary if the lower respiratory tract is involved.[20]

Postintubation Croup

Croup is one of the many causes of pediatric airway obstruction. Croup can be caused by a viral infection (e.g., viral laryngotracheitis) or by airway manipulation (e.g., postintubation croup). The latter form is more commonly encountered by anesthesia clinicians.

Postintubation croup can be mild or severe. It is a symptom complex composed of stridor; retractions (suprasternal, intercostal, or subcostal); a barking, brassy cough; and hoarseness. These symptoms are due to mucosal swelling in the subglottic region of the larynx. Croup primarily occurs in children between 1 and 4 years of age, although it can occur at any age.[21]

Koka et al.,[21] one of the first groups who reported on postintubation croup, found an incidence of 1% in a long series of patients. They described the following contributing factors: age (1 to 4 years), trauma during intubation (more than one attempt), a tight-fitting endotracheal tube (ET), cough (around the ET), changing the patient's position while intubated, long duration of intubation (more than 1 hour), and surgery in the neck region. Surprisingly, history or presence of a URI did not influence the incidence. As previously discussed, this remains controversial.

A more recent study at another institution found the incidence to be significantly lower, 0.1%.[22] They proposed that the current use of standardized nonreactive endotracheal tubes, and the practice of assuring that an air leak is present around the endotracheal tube, may help decrease the incidence of postintubation croup.

Symptoms of croup usually occur soon after extubation (within 1 hour), with maximum intensity within 4 hours and complete resolution within 24 hours.[23] A chest radiograph, although not necessary in all patients with croup, can be diagnostically useful. In the severe form, the subglottic edema appears as a characteristic "pencil" sign in the chest x-ray.

Table 4-2 shows a scoring system for upper airway obstruction described by Downes and Godinez.[24] This can be used to classify croup as mild, moderate, or severe. A normal score is 0, while a maximum score is 10. A patient with a score of 7 or more and who is not responding to medical treatment is a candidate for artificial ventilation. This scoring system is also used in the recovery room to follow patients once treatment has begun and to assess whether their condition is improving or deteriorating.

Table 4-3 shows our recommended treatment for postintubation croup. Racemic epinephrine (RE) is used for its vasoconstrictive properties. Because of its well-known rebound phenomena, it should be used cautiously. Within 2 hours, the clinical effect of the drug dissipates, and sometimes the obstruction is worse than before.[25,26] This necessitates that the anesthesiologist monitor and observe the patient for at least 2 or 3 hours, even after a single dose.

Discharge criteria in the outpatient setting should be individualized. Consideration should be given to the patient's age, history of prematurity, history of croup, Down's syndrome, history of subglottic stenosis, severity of symptoms, need for drug therapy, response to treatment, parent's comfort level, distance from the hospital, and availability of supportive measures, such as a home humidifier.[23]

Sickle Cell Disease

Sickle cell disease (SCD), one of the most common hemoglobinopathies, is an autosomal recessive genetic disease. A point

Table 4-2 Scoring System for Upper Airway Obstruction

	Score		
	0	1	2
Stridor	None	Inspiratory	Inspiratory and expiratory
Cough	None	Hoarse cry	Bark
Retractions and nasal flaring	None	Flaring and suprasternal retractions	Flaring, and suprasternal, subcostal, and intercostal retractions
Cyanosis	None	In air	In 40% oxygen
Inspiratory breath sounds	Normal	Harsh, with wheezing or rhonchi	Delayed

From Downes JJ, Godínez RI: Acute upper airway obstruction in the child. In American Society of Anesthesiologists: Refresher courses in anesthesiology, vol 8, Philadelphia, 1980, JB Lippincott, pp. 29-48. Used with permission.

Table 4-3 Treatment for Postintubation Croup

Mild	One or more of the following: Tender loving care / Humidification / Oxygen / Hydration
Moderate	As above / Add racemic epinephrine (RE) by nebulization: 0.5 ml of 2.25% RE in 2.5 ml of saline / Dexamethasone: 4-8 mg intravenously
Severe	As above. May repeat RE nebulization up to three times / Consider reintubation

mutation results in the substitution of valine for glutamic acid as the sixth amino acid of the β-chain of hemoglobin, transforming Hb A into Hb S. The gene for SCD is most prevalent among people of African, Caribbean, Mediterranean, and West Indian descent. Approximately 8% of American blacks are heterozygous carriers, and one in 600 is homozygous at conception. The pathological manifestations of SCD are due to the altered physical properties of Hb S. Deoxygenated Hb S β-chains polymerize, which leads to red cell distortion (sickling) and rigidity. Sickled red cells have a shorter lifespan and cannot traverse the microvasculature; thus, the patient is at great risk of developing hemolytic anemia and vasoocclusive crises, the hallmarks of SCD. All patients at risk on the grounds of ethnic origin should be screened for SCD before elective surgery.

If adequate precautions are taken, ambulatory surgery and anesthesia can be performed safely in SCD patients. Box 4-3 describes the guidelines for the perioperative management of these patients. Patients should come to the outpatient center early in the morning so that intravenous fluids can be administered to prevent fasting dehydration. In addition, the surgery should be scheduled early in the morning, and both surgeon and anesthesiologist should be experienced enough to expedite the procedure.[27] The operating room temperature should be kept at 80°F or higher to prevent vasoconstriction, which can predispose to sickling.

The issue of preoperative transfusion in these patients is still somewhat controversial. The results of a large multicenter trial are expected soon, but the preliminary data suggest better outcomes

---

Box 4-3 *Perioperative Management in Sickle Cell Disease*

Preoperative transfusion (so that Hb S < 30%) for major surgery
Adequate oxygenation and ventilation
Optimal hydration
Maintenance of temperature homeostasis
Acidosis prevention
For minor surgery, Hb S level is not as important as long as the rest of the management is followed
Adequate pain relief

for patients who receive transfusions. Obviously, clinical judgment should be used to tailor treatment of each individual based on amount of Hb S, type of procedure (major or minor), tourniquet usage, and presence of preexisting cardiac or respiratory disease. The benefits of transfusion must be weighed against the attendant risks, in particular, red cell alloimmunization (which occurs in up to 20% of SCD patients receiving transfusions)[28] and transmission of hepatitis and other blood-borne infections. Moreover, recent studies have shown a direct relationship between hematocrit and frequency of painful crises.[29] A hematologist should be consulted for any SCD patient who is scheduled for surgery and anesthesia in the outpatient setting.

Discharge criteria should be rigorous. Pain can promote sickling, so it should be well controlled. Vomiting can lead to dehydration; therefore, it should also be well controlled. There should be no respiratory distress, and oxygen saturation should be within normal limits. In integrated ambulatory units, if these criteria are met and a follow-up visit within 24 hours of discharge is scheduled, then it would be appropriate to anesthetize these patients. Free-standing centers should refrain from accepting these patients unless the standard of care at the facility is the same as that in the integrated unit, i.e., the presence of hematology consultations and facilities for inpatient care of potential sickling crises.

Heart Disease or Heart Murmur

The child with congenital heart disease (CHD) can be anesthetized safely in the outpatient setting as long as certain issues are kept in mind.

First of all, the anesthesiologist must completely understand the pathophysiology of the particular disease, and the disease should be well compensated. A thorough history, physical examination, and appropriate laboratory studies should be performed. A call to the pediatrician or cardiologist is mandatory because a team effort is necessary for a successful outcome; the patient may have untreated CHD, the heart may have been reconstructed, or a palliative procedure may have been done. If correction was performed, any complications or residual disease should be known, because there may still be the potential for arrhythmia, ventricular dysfunction, residual shunts, residual valvular stenosis or regurgitation, or residual pulmonary hypertension.[30] Drug therapy should be continued, and polycythemia should be

Table 4-4   Consultation in Pediatric Heart Murmurs

	Clinical diagnosis		
	No heart disease	**Possible heart disease**	**Definite heart disease**
Anesthesiologist	Yes	Yes No	Yes
Pediatrician	Yes	No Yes	Yes
Cardiology consult	No	Yes	Yes

From Hannallah RS, Epstein BS: The pediatric patient. In Wetchler BV, editor: Anesthesia for ambulatory surgery, Philadelphia, 1991, JB Lippincott, p. 140. Used with permission.

controlled (beware of prolonged NPO status). Congestive heart failure (CHF), if present, should be well compensated. Obviously, patients with uncomplicated and compensated lesions may be candidates for outpatient surgery, while those with complicated or complex CHD should be admitted as inpatients. Patients with moderate or severe cyanosis (room air O_2 saturation less than 90%) or with uncompensated CHF should be excluded.

A bigger dilemma is the child in whom a heart murmur is first discovered in the outpatient surgical unit. Sometimes this happens minutes before the operation. It now must be determined whether this is an innocent or pathologic murmur. It is imperative that the cause be diagnosed before induction of anesthesia. Thirty percent of all children between the ages of 3 and 7 years have innocent flow murmurs,[31] usually brief systolic ejection murmurs rarely more severe than grade II, and usually exacerbated by exercise, excitement, fever, and positional changes. The cost of a cardiology consult and of cancelling the surgery should be carefully considered. Table 4-4 shows the grid suggested initially by Hannallah, which is currently used at our institution to determine when a cardiology consult is needed.[32]

To improve the recognition of innocent murmurs, one can practice listening for the common functional murmurs described in Table 4-5.[33] Box 4-4 lists clues favoring an organic or pathologic murmur.[34]

In summary, a careful analysis of vital signs, oxygen saturation, growth and development, exercise tolerance, and other associated medical conditions should help determine whether the

Table 4-5   Common Functional Murmurs

Murmur	Age of onset	Location of best auscultation
Pulmonary artery branch murmur	Birth to 6 weeks old	Base of the heart, in the axillae and in the posterior chest
Venous hum	Late infancy to early childhood	Under one or both clavicles when the patient is sitting erect with the head extended; cannot be heard when the patient is supine (unlike the situation common with patent ductus)
Still's aortic vibratory murmur	Early to middle childhood	Best heard in supine patient at apex or left sternal border, has short moaning quality, is louder after exercise and during held expiration
Pulmonary valve area "flow" murmur	Late childhood to adolescence	Best heard in supine patient at right sternal border, and during deep held expiration, especially after exercise

---

Box 4-4 *Clues Favoring a Pathologic Murmur*

History of CHD in parents or siblings
Maternal issues (during pregnancy)
    Rubella syndrome
    Alcohol use
    Teratogenic drug use
History of inappropriate sweating
History of syncope, chest pain, or squatting
Prematurity
Cyanosis
Recurrent pneumonia
Asymmetric facies

murmur is innocent or not. Boxes 4-5, 4-6, and 4-7 show the American Heart Association protocols for antibiotic prophylaxis in the pediatric patient.[35]

Malignant Hyperthermia Susceptibility

Two criteria must be met before accepting a child susceptible to malignant hyperthermia (MH) for outpatient surgery. First of all, dantrolene *must* be available. Second, the facility must have monitoring capabilities, and its laboratory must be able to perform quantitative acid-base determinations. If these criteria are met and a nontriggering anesthetic is used, then the patient can be accepted for outpatient surgery and anesthesia. Drugs to avoid include succinylcholine and the inhalation anesthetics. Box 4-8 lists drugs that have been proven to be safe for use in the MH–susceptible patient. Ketamine and pancuronium bromide, although considered safe drugs, should be used with caution because they induce tachycardia, an early sign of MH that may confuse the diagnosis. The prophylactic use of dantrolene has not been shown to be of benefit.[36] The minimum safe duration of observation of an MH–susceptible patient is not known. Recently it has been reported that a patient who is asymptomatic after a postoperative observation period of at least 4 hours may safely be discharged.[37] The parent should be given specific instructions to check for fever or dark-colored urine, and to report back to the hospital if either appears.

The main defect leading to MH is a leakage of calcium ions from the sarcoplasmic reticulum. This leads to a hypermetabolic state with increased CO_2 production, lactate production, oxygen consumption, and an ensuing metabolic acidosis. Dantrolene blocks this release of calcium and prevents the hypermetabolic state.

Another dilemma presents if trismus or masseter spasm occurs after induction, which most often occurs with inhalation anesthetics or succinylcholine. Two schools of thought exist. Some clinicians believe that the case should be cancelled, the patient monitored for MH, and a muscle biopsy obtained.[38] Others believe that if there are no other signs of MH, a nontriggering anesthetic may be continued, the patient monitored for any sign of MH during surgery, and MH susceptibility should be evaluated following surgery.[39] Controversy exists over the definition of masseter spasm.[40,41,42] At our institution, it is considered a normal response to succinylcholine if the mouth fully opens and

---

Box 4-5 Oral Prophylactic Antibiotic Regimen for Dental, Oral, or Upper Respiratory Tract Procedures in Pediatric Patients

---

Standard regimen:
    Amoxicillin 50 mg/kg
Amoxicillin/penicillin–allergic patients:
    Erythromycin 20 mg/kg
    or
    Erythromycin ethyl succinate
    or
    Stearate
    or
    Clindamycin 10 mg/kg
    (One-half the initial dose is administered 6 hours later.)

Box 4-6 Alternative Prophylactic Antibiotic Regimen for Dental, Oral, or Upper Respiratory Tract Procedures in Pediatric Patients Unable to Take Oral Medications

---

Alternative regimen:
    Ampicillin 50 mg/kg IV or IM
    (Follow up with half dose* 6 hours later)
Ampicillin/penicillin–allergic patients:
    Clindamycin 10 mg/kg IV
    (Follow up with half dose* 6 hours later)
High-risk patients:
    Ampicillin 50 mg/kg IV or IM
    and
    Gentamicin 2.0 mg/kg IV or IM
    (Follow up with half dose* 8 hours later)
High-risk ampicillin/penicillin–allergic patients:
    Vancomycin 20 mg/kg IV over 1 hour
    (No repeat dose necessary)

*Follow-up doses are for intravenous route. Oral administration differs.

Box 4-7 *Prophylactic Antibiotic Regimen for Gastrointestinal or Genitourinary Procedures in Pediatric Patients*

Standard regimen:
　　Ampicillin 50 mg/kg IV or IM
　　(Follow up with half dose IV 8 hours later)
　　and
　　Gentamicin 2.0 mg/kg IV or IM
Ampicillin/penicillin–allergic patients:
　　Vancomycin 20 mg/kg IV over 1 hour
　　and
　　Gentamicin 2.0 mg/kg IV or IM
　　(Follow up with half-dose IV 8 hours later)
Low-risk patients:
　　Amoxicillin 50 mg/kg PO
　　(Follow up with half dose 6 hours later)

Box 4-8 *Drugs Safe to Use in MH–Susceptible Patients*

- Barbiturates
- Ketamine
- Etomidate
- Propofol

- Nitrous oxide
- Narcotics
- Nondepolarizing skeletal muscle relaxants
- Local anesthetics

---

intubation is easy, and surgery may be continued with careful monitoring. Malignant hyperthermia is suspected if the mouth cannot be fully opened and the intubation is difficult, or if the jaw cannot be opened at all ("jaw of steel"), and the anesthetic is stopped. The patient is placed on a monitored bed, and creatine kinase (CK) levels are determined every 6 hours for the next 24 hours. If CKs rise above 20,000 units, then we assume the patient is MH susceptible. Dantrolene is only given if other signs of a hypermetabolic state become evident or if the patient is unstable. We also follow urine myoglobin and force fluids on the patient.

> **Box 4-9 Conditions Associated with Down's Syndrome**
>
> - Congenital heart disease (endocardial cushion defects, ventricular septal defect (VSD), atrial septal defect (ASD), other heart defects)
> - Low birth weight
> - Pulmonary hypertension
> - Pulmonary infections, sensitive airway
> - Airway problems
> - Atlantoaxial instability
> - Obstructive sleep apnea

Down's Syndrome

Down's syndrome, or trisomy 21 syndrome, is a relatively common genetic disorder affecting about 1 in 800 live births.[43] Associated conditions can be many, with significant implications for the anesthesiologist (Box 4-9). Before accepting the child with Down's syndrome into the outpatient surgical unit, the patient's care providers must determine if he or she is physiologically fit for outpatient surgery.

Congenital heart disease (CHD) exists in a significant number of patients with Down's syndrome. Endocardial cushion defects or AV canal syndrome are the most common types, but virtually any kind of CHD may be present. It is imperative that the CHD be well compensated. Some of these patients may have pulmonary hypertension due to the cardiac lesion or to obstructive sleep apnea.[44]

Perhaps the biggest challenge presented by the child with Down's syndrome is the management of the airway. Because of frequent infections or increased secretions, these children have a very sensitive airway, which can make the induction of anesthesia a nightmare. Also they may have midfacial and mandibular hypoplasia,[45] glossoptosis, abnormally small upper airway, and relative tonsillar and adenoidal encroachment.[46] They can have generalized hypotonia with resultant collapse of the airway during inspiration.[44] A thorough history and physical examination is warranted before accepting the patient for outpatient surgery and anesthesia. In the absence of any systemic diseases, laboratory tests would follow the same pediatric recommendations as for any healthy child.

Finally, 10% to 15% of these patients have a tendency toward atlantoaxial instability.[43] Opinions differ about whether these patients should have a neurological examination or cervical spine films before surgery. The American Academy of Pediatrics and the Special Olympics recommend cervical spine evaluation and restriction of activities in children with radiographic evidence of instability.[47] A recent study has shown that radiographs are unnecessary and that a neurologic evaluation is more important for finding evidence of cord compression.[48] Major physical findings include weakness, positive Babinksi sign, increased deep tendon reflexes, and incontinence. Because the consequences of handling an unstable neck can be disastrous, we obtain both a neurology consult and x-rays of the cervical spine. Usually the pediatrician has already obtained the films.

Can the Down's syndrome patient have surgery and anesthesia in the outpatient center? The answer is yes as long as CHD is not a factor, no pulmonary infection exists at the time, a thorough evaluation of the airway is performed, and no neurologic deficits are found. Extreme caution should be exercised when using heavy preoperative and postoperative sedation, and when using intraoperative and postoperative narcotics, because of the risk of airway obstruction and hypoventilation.

Cancer

The pediatric patient with cancer can present a variety of dilemmas to the anesthesia clinician, depending on the particular procedure being performed. Children with cancer undergo frequent painful outpatient procedures, particularly bone marrow examinations and lumbar punctures. Procedure-related pain is a major source of distress to many children and their families, and it is often viewed as the worst aspect of the entire cancer experience.[49] For years, anesthesiologists have been called upon to provide sedation or general anesthesia to alleviate the discomfort. Several regimens have been used with success. These include hypnosis and relaxation techniques,[50] inhaled general anesthesia, ketamine, nitrous oxide,[51] and other drugs such as narcotics, benzodiazepines, and barbiturates. Recently, propofol has been used with success in these patients.[52] Every effort should be made to make these children as comfortable as possible, recognizing the fact that safety should always be the goal. A good airway should be maintained in the spontaneously breathing patient without an endotracheal tube. Because these are outpatients, prolonged sedation should be avoided. A recent study found both midazolam and fentanyl to be excellent choices for these patients.[53] Preoperative testing should be based on the condition of the patient and the chemotherapeutic agents he or she is taking. For example, patients taking cardiotoxic drugs like doxorubicin or cisplatin should have a cardiac evaluation and ECG. A preoperative coagulation profile might be indicated if agents like plicamycin or asparaginase are used. Abnormal values should be investigated further and corrected when possible. Remember, there is no substitute for a complete history and physical examination.

Another difficult situation in the outpatient center is that of the children who must return daily for weeks to receive radiation therapy. They must lie still for 15 to 45 minutes with the anesthesiologist outside the room. Even though experience tells us that endotracheal intubation every day for several days is not dangerous, the potential for trauma is still there, and techniques that do not involve intubation should be sought. Spontaneous respirations should be maintained, and the patient should be monitored with at least a pulse oximeter, electrocardiogram, and noninvasive blood pressure mechanism. Sedation techniques and guidelines are discussed in detail in Chapter 9. The laryngeal mask airway (LMA) has become very popular for airway control in a variety of circumstances, including the child with cancer needing radiotherapy.[54,55] With the LMA, intubation is not necessary, the airway is maintained with the child breathing spontaneously, and minimal experience is needed for successful mask placement. The LMA may soon become the preferred method of handling the airway in these patients. The anesthesiologist should have visual access to the child, either directly or through a camera. Again, propofol has recently been found to meet all the criteria necessary for these patients, it does not prolong the outpatient stay, and it reduces the incidence of nausea and vomiting.[52] The previously described guidelines are also used for laboratory testing of these patients. Every patient is considered individually, and tests are repeated if necessary.

Last, but not least, we need to provide these patients and their parents with tremendous psychological support during our interactions with them.

Summary

Although most children are healthy and can safely undergo outpatient surgery and anesthesia, occasionally the anesthesiologist is faced with management problems in the pediatric population. While there is no conclusive data on the appropriate age for term children to undergo outpatient procedures, the former premature child should be evaluated for risk of apnea and bradycardia. Infants younger than 50 weeks PCA should be admitted as inpatients and observed postoperatively. Older former premature infants without ongoing cardiopulmonary dysfunction may be managed as outpatients. The child with a respiratory infection is at risk for perioperative respiratory problems. The history and physical examination should help the clinician differentiate an infectious from a noninfectious process. In the presence of URI, a delay of 1 to 2 weeks after resolution of symptoms is recommended, and a delay of at least 4 weeks is recommended if the lower respiratory tract is involved. The child with postintubation croup is evaluated, racemic epinephrine may be necessary, and the patient must be placed under observation for at least 3 hours after treatment. With adequate facility and patient preparation, patients with SCD may undergo ambulatory surgery. Adequate hydration, pain management, and oxygenation should be maintained during the hospitalization. Children with CHD can undergo ambulatory surgery as long as the pathophysiology of the disease is recognized and the present status has been evaluated and is compensated. A cardiology consult may be necessary to differentiate an innocent heart murmur from a pathological murmur. Careful evaluation of vital signs, oxygen saturation, growth and development, exercise tolerance, and other associated medical conditions will determine whether the murmur is innocent or not. Adult and pediatric patients who are susceptible to MH may be considered for outpatient surgery. Prophylactic dantrolene is unnecessary. Patients may be evaluated for discharge following an observation period of at least 6 hours, and the parents given specific instructions about signs and symptoms of MH. Distance from a medical facility needs to be determined before safely discharging these patients home. Although not commonly associated with MH, masseter muscle spasm may be a precursor to its development. Controversy exists whether anesthetics should be continued or whether the patient should be treated for MH. The child with Down's syndrome should be evaluated for associated cardiac, renal, and airway problems. Children with cancer often undergo frequent outpatient procedures; therefore, the anesthetic approach should be aggressive toward pain management, and anesthetics that cause minimal side effects, and no tachyphylaxis upon repeated administration, should be chosen.

References

1. Steward DJ: Pre-term infants are more prone to complications following minor surgery than are term infants. Anesthesiology 1982; 56:304-6.

2. Liu LMP, Coté CJ, Goudsouzian NG et al: Life-threatening apnea in infants recovering from anesthesia. Anesthesiology 1983; 59:506-10.

3. Gregory GA, Steward DJ: Life-threatening peri-operative apnea in the ex-"preemie." Anesthesiology 1983; 59:495-8.

4. Welborn LB, Ramirez N, Oh TH et al: Postanesthetic apnea and periodic breathing in infants. Anesthesiology 1986; 65:656-61.

5. Kurth CD, Spitzer AR, Broennle AM, Downes JJ: Postoperative apnea in preterm infants. Anesthesiology 1987; 66:483-8.

6. Malviya S, Swartz J, Lerman J: Are all preterm infants younger than 60 weeks postconceptual age at risk for postanesthetic apnea? Anesthesiology 1993; 78:1076-81.

7. Naylor B, Radhakrishnan J, McLaughlin D: Postoperative apnea in infants. J Pediatr Surg 1992; 27:955-7.

8. Coté CJ: At what post-gestational age in a previously premature infant would it be safe to anesthetize a child as an outpatient? Soc Pediatr Anesth Newsletter 1989; 2(1):2.

9. Spear RM: Anesthesia for premature and term infants: peri-operative implications. J Pediatrics 1992; 120(2):165-76.

10. Welborn LG, Hannallah RS, Luban NLC et al: Anemia and postoperative apnea in former preterm infants. Anesthesiology 1991; 74:1003-6.

11. Tetzlaff JE, Annand DW, Pudimat MA, Nicodemus HF: Postoperative apnea in a full term infant. Anesthesiology 1988; 69:426-8.

12. Coté CJ, Kelly DH: Postoperative apnea in a full term infant with a demonstrable respiratory pattern abnormality. Anesthesiology 1990; 72:559-61.

13. Welborn LG, De Soto H, Hannallah RS et al: The use of caffeine in the control of postanesthetic apnea in former premature infants. Anesthesiology 1988; 68:796-8.

14. Welborn LG, Hannallah RS, Fink R et al: High dose caffeine suppresses postoperative apnea in former preterm infants. Anesthesiology 1989; 71:347-9.
15. Berry FA: The child with a runny nose. In Berry FA, editor: Anesthetic management of difficult and routine pediatric patients, New York, 1990, Churchill Livingstone, pp. 267-83.
16. De Soto H, Patel RI, Soliman IE, Hannallah RS: Changes in oxygen saturation following general anesthesia in children with upper respiratory infection signs and symptoms undergoing otolaryngological procedures. Anesthesiology 1988; 68:276-9.
17. Cohen MM, Cameron CB: Should you cancel the operation when a child has an upper respiratory tract infection? Anesth Analg 1991; 72:282-8.
18. Tait AR, Knight PR: The effects of general anesthesia on upper respiratory tract infections in children. Anesthesiology 1987; 67:930-5.
19. Betts EK: Pediatric outpatient anesthesia. In Rogers MC, editor: Current practice in anesthesiology, Toronto, 1988, BC Decker, pp. 137-9.
20. De Soto H: The effect of a "cold" on arterial oxygenation in children—How long does it last? Anesthesiology 1992; 77:A1166.
21. Koka BV, Jeon IS, Andre JM et al: Postintubation croup in children. Anesth Analg 1977; 56:501-5.
22. Littman RS, Keon TP: Postintubation croup in children. Anesthesiology 1991; 75:1122-3.
23. Hannallah RS: Postintubation croup. Soc Amb Anesth Newsletter 1990; 5(2):5.
24. Downes JJ, Godínez RI: Acute upper airway obstruction in the child. In ASA: Refresher course in anesthesiology, vol 8, Philadelphia, 1980, JB Lippincott, pp. 29-48.
25. Quan L: Diagnosis and treatment of croup. Am Fam Physician 1992; 46(3):747-55.
26. Kelley PB, Simon JE: Racemic epinephrine use in croup and disposition. Am J Emerg Med 1992; 10(3):181-3.
27. Pasternak LR: Case report No. 4. In Wetchler BV, editor: Anesthesia for ambulatory surgery, Philadelphia, 1991, JB Lippincott, pp. 488-9.
28. Davies SC, McWilliams AC, Hewitt PE et al: Red cell alloimmunization in sickle cell disease. Br J Haematol 1986; 3:29-44.
29. Platt OS, Thorington BD, Brambilla DJ et al: Pain in sickle cell disease: rates and risk factors. N Engl J Med 1991; 325:11-6.
30. Hickey PR: The patient with congenital heart disease for noncardiac surgery: anesthesia for the reconstructed and unreconstructed heart. In International Anesthesia Research Society: Review course lectures, Cleveland, 1992, IARS, pp. 51-4.
31. Gibbons PA: My child has a heart murmur. Soc Amb Anesth Newsletter 1990; 5(2):4.

32. Hannallah RS, Epstein BS: The pediatric patient. In Wetchler BV, editor: Anesthesia for ambulatory surgery, Philadelphia, 1991, JB Lippincott, p. 140.

33. McNamara DG: The pediatrician and the innocent heart murmur. AJDC 1987; 141:1161.

34. Moss AJ: Clues in diagnosing congenital heart disease. West J Med 1992; 156:392-8.

35. American Heart Association (AHA) Committee Report: Prevention of bacterial endocarditis. JAMA 1990; 264:2919-22.

36. Hackl W, Mauritz W, Winkler M et al: Anaesthesia in malignant hyperthermia susceptible patients without dantrolene prophylaxis: a report of 30 cases. Acta Anaesthesiol Scand 1990; 34:534-7.

37. Yentis SM, Levine MF, Hartley ES: Should all children with suspected or confirmed malignant hyperthermia susceptibility be admitted after surgery? A 10-year review. Anesth Analg 1992; 75:345-50.

38. Rosenberg H: Management of patient in whom trismus occurs following succinylcholine. Anesthesiology 1988; 68:654-5.

39. Gronert GA: Management of patient in whom trismus occurs following succinylcholine. Anesthesiology 1988; 68:653-4.

40. Van Der Spek AFL, Fang WB, Ashton Miller JA et al: The effect of succinylcholine on mouth opening. Anesthesiology 1987; 67:459-65.

41. Carroll JB: Increased incidence of masseter spasm in children with strabismus anesthetized with halothane and succinylcholine. Anesthesiology 1987; 67:559-61.

42. Flewellen EH, Nelson TE: Masseter spasm induced by succinylcholine in children: contracture testing for malignant hyperthermia: report of six cases. Can J Anaesth 1982; 29:42-8.

43. Berry FA: Miscellaneous potholes. In Berry FA, editor: Anesthetic management of difficult and routine pediatric patients, New York, 1990, Churchill Livingstone, p. 426.

44. Marcus CL, Keens TG, Bautista DB et al: Obstructive sleep apnea in children with Down's syndrome. Pediatrics 1991; 88:132-9.

45. Fink GB, Madaus WK, Walker GF: A quantitative study of the face in Down's syndrome. Am J Orthor 1975; 67:540-53.

46. Southall DP, Stebbens VA, Mirza R et al: Upper airway obstruction with hypoxemia and sleep disruption in Down's syndrome. Dev Med Child Neurol 1987; 29:734-42.

47. Committee on Sports Medicine: Atlantoaxial instability in Down's syndrome. Pediatrics 1984; 74:152-4.

48. Davidson RG: Atlantoaxial instability in individuals with Down's syndrome: a fresh look at the evidence. Pediatrics 1988; 81:857-65.

49. Jay SM, Ozolins M, Elliott CH, Caldwell S: Assessment of children's distress during painful medical procedures. Health Psychol 1983; 2:133-47.

50. Zeltzer L, Le Baron S: Hypnosis and nonhypnotic techniques for reduction of pain and anxiety during painful procedures in children and adolescents with cancer. J Pediatr 1982; 101:1032-5.

51. Miser AW, Ayesh D, Broda E et al: Use of a patient-controlled devise for nitrous oxide administration to control procedure related pain in children and young adults with cancer. Clin J Pain 1988; 4:5-10.

52. Barst S, McDowall R, Pratila M et al: Anesthesia for pediatric cancer patients: ketamine, etomidate or propofol? Anesthesiology 1990; 73:A1114.

53. Sandler ES, Weyman C, Conner K et al: Midazolam versus fentanyl as premedication for painful procedures in children with cancer. Pediatrics 1992; 89:631-4.

54. Grebenik CR, Ferguson C, White A: The laryngeal mask airway in pediatric radiotherapy. Anesthesiology 1990; 72:474-7.

55. Moylan SL, Luce MA: The reinforced laryngeal mask airway in paediatric radiotherapy. Br J of Anaesth 1993; 71(1):172.

5

Pediatric Considerations

Raafat S. Hannallah and Ramesh I. Patel

Children are excellent candidates for ambulatory surgery. Most children are healthy, and most surgeries performed on children are simple procedures associated with prompt recovery. It is not surprising, therefore, that up to 60% of pediatric surgeries in this country are performed as ambulatory procedures.[1] Avoiding hospitalization is particularly advantageous for preschool children, who benefit from the briefer separation from parents, and for infants, who are spared the exposure to the potentially contaminated hospital environment.

Preparation of Children for Ambulatory Surgery

The successful management of pediatric ambulatory patients requires proper selection, screening, and preparation of children before the day of scheduled surgery. Specific criteria for patient screening and selection have been addressed in an earlier chapter. In general, the child should be in good health (ASA class 1 or 2). Patients who have chronic illness do not need to be excluded from ambulatory surgery; however, their medical condition must be optimally controlled before they are acceptable.

Preoperative Fasting

The need for healthy pediatric ambulatory patients to undergo prolonged fasting before elective surgery has been recently challenged.[2] Studies have shown that children who are allowed to drink clear liquids until 2 to 3 hours before anesthesia induction do not have higher gastric volume or acidity than that of children who fast overnight.[3] Accordingly, most pediatric anesthesiologists have now liberalized NPO orders. Solid food—which includes milk, formula, and milk products—is still not allowed on the day of surgery. Breast-fed infants, however, are allowed to nurse up until 4 hours preoperatively.[4] Children may drink clear liquids (up to 10 ml/kg) until 2 to 3 hours before the posted surgical time. The main advantage of these liberal guidelines is that children are not thirsty and irritable while waiting for surgery. In addition, the patients are less likely to become hypotensive or hypoglycemic during anesthesia.

Preoperative Laboratory Testing

Until recently, most children scheduled for surgery required at minimum a hemoglobin (Hb) or hematocrit (Hct) level determination, as well as a urinalysis. Today, most anesthesiologists will not request the latter unless there is a history of genitourinary disease that warrants it. The requirement for Hb or Hct is still controversial. Studies have shown that the incidence of anemia in healthy children is extremely low and does not usually require therapeutic intervention or anesthesia modification.[5,6] Many anesthesiologists are comfortable requesting preoperative Hb or Hct testing only when the medical history suggests that significant anemia may be present, e.g., for infants, for adolescent females, and in the presence of chronic disease.[6] It is interesting to note, however, that some states mandate such testing.

Psychological Preparation

Most ambulatory surgical facilities today have some form of preoperative information or preparation program for children awaiting surgery. Typically, these programs provide reading material to the family, allow for telephone counselling, and organize visits to the facility before the scheduled day of surgery. The program at Children's National Medical Center (CNMC) is described here as an example; however, there is no single method that will be effective at every facility, or even on every child in the same institution.

The first step in the preoperative preparation of children presenting for ambulatory surgery at CNMC occurs when the admitting office contacts the parents shortly after the procedure has been scheduled. An information package is mailed, which includes a coloring book that depicts some basic information about surgery, anesthesia, and being a patient in a hospital. The parents are invited to visit the hospital on the Sunday before the day of surgery, or sooner if they so choose. Often these preoperative visits are also mentioned and promoted by the surgeons when they first counsel the parents about surgery.

The actual visit is conducted by volunteer staff under the direction of child life specialists. The script is reviewed by many health care professionals, including the anesthesiologist. Then during the visit, the children are told what to expect on the day of surgery. They are shown the areas of the hospital where they will be waiting to be taken into the operating room (the preoperative play room); they are allowed to see and handle special anesthesia equipment (face mask and breathing circle); and they are shown the recovery areas, where they will reunite with their parents. A video is also shown to reinforce the ideas presented during the tour.

Although most people believe that these preparation programs are invaluable in allaying the children's anxiety, there is little objective evidence that they are indeed useful. Rosen et al.[7] attempted to examine the CNMC program's effect on children's behavior during induction objectively. Children who participated in the preoperative preparation program were more likely to be cooperative during induction than those who did not. However, they found that only a small percentage of the parents who were invited to come to the tour did in fact participate. Most of the ones who came were extremely motivated parents who admitted to having prepared their children in many other ways. In addition, parents of very young children and parents of children who were coming for repeat surgery were less likely to come for the tour. In the Rosen study, these were the children who were at the highest risk for being upset during induction.

The value of the preoperative visit with the anesthesiologist in allaying the fears of the child and parents cannot be overemphasized, especially for the ambulatory patient who is completely unfamiliar with the surgical routine. A full explanation of the anesthetic plan must be offered to the parents *and* the child, as appropriate for his or her age. Although a brief discussion of the risks associated with anesthesia and surgery is appropriate and often desired by the parents,[8] risks should not be presented in a way that adds to the inevitable apprehension of awaiting surgery on one's child.

Pharmacological Premedication

The use of premedication in pediatric ambulatory surgery has gone full cycle. When the practice of ambulatory surgery first became popular, one of the major modifications of anesthetic routine was to discontinue premedicating these patients. At the time, the most popular drugs were long-acting (e.g., morphine and pentobarbital), had unpredictable effects, resulted in longer recovery, and increased the incidence of postoperative vomiting. In addition, a painful intramuscular injection was required to administer these drugs. Without premedication, the recovery from anesthesia was fast, and patients could be discharged shortly after the conclusion of surgery. It was an efficient approach that very quickly became the routine in most institutions.

However, many anesthesiologists have become alarmed by the number of unpremedicated children who were uncooperative

Table 5-1   Premedication and Preinduction Agents

Drug	Route	Usual dose (mg/kg)
Midazolam	Oral	0.5
	Nasal	0.2
	Rectal	1
Methohexital (10%)	Rectal	25
Ketamine	Oral	6
	Rectal	3
	Intramuscular	2
OTFC (Oralet)	Transmucosal	0.005-0.015

during induction of anesthesia. Quite often it seemed that the psychological welfare of many children was traded for efficiency. The search started for some form of premedication that could preoperatively sedate but not postoperatively delay recovery and discharge from the facility (Table 5-1). With the "discovery" of oral midazolam, sedation again became popular in pediatric anesthesia, even in ambulatory patients. Midazolam 0.5 mg/kg can be administered orally 30 to 45 minutes before induction to facilitate separation from the parents and improve the patient's cooperation with mask induction.[9] Some researchers have found that children can be separated from their parents as early as 10 minutes after receiving midazolam.[10] Unfortunately, the intravenous form of midazolam that is available in the United States is quite unpalatable. Most children will not drink it unless it is mixed with a strong flavoring, e.g., a little sweetened apple juice, gelatin, or cola syrup. Oral midazolam in this dose does not appear to prolong recovery, even after procedures lasting less than 30 minutes.[9] Oral ketamine in a dose of 6 mg/kg appears to be a satisfactory alternative to midazolam. It has been reported to provide predictable sedation within 20 to 25 minutes, and to allow calm separation from parents, without significant side effects.[11] Oral transmucosal fentanyl citrate (OTFC, Oralet) produces preoperative sedation and facilitates inhalational induction, but it is associated with a significant decrease in respiratory rate and SpO_2 (oxygen saturation), and a high incidence of postoperative nausea and vomiting.[12]

Preinduction Techniques

Preinduction techniques are commonly used for last-minute sedation in children who refuse to separate from their parents, or as an alternative to forced mask induction in young children who cannot cooperate with inhalational induction (Table 5-1). The practical difference between premedication and preinduction is in the speed of onset. Useful preinduction drugs should have a quick onset, generally less than 10 minutes. The following is a brief summary of the drugs that are commonly used for preinduction of anesthesia in ambulatory children.

Rectal administration of sedatives

Rectal methohexital administration is one of the oldest preinduction techniques. Methohexital 10% solution, 20 to 25 mg/kg, usually has a 7- to 10-minute onset in most cases.[13] Administration is simple and can be done outside the operating room in a properly equipped holding area to allow onset of sleep in the parents' presence, and, therefore, to eliminate the usual struggle that occurs with separation. Respiratory depression can occur with methohexital, and it is mandatory that a portable oxygen source and appropriate airway equipment be immediately available whenever this technique is utilized. Other concerns include a high incidence of defecation and failure to induce sleep in some patients. Some authors claim better results when a larger volume of a more dilute solution (e.g., 2%) is utilized. Other drugs that can be administered rectally include midazolam (1.0 mg/kg)[14] and ketamine (3 mg/kg).[15] Midazolam can be administered as a 2 mg/ml solution unless the volume exceeds 10 ml, in which case dilution is not necessary. Preinduction of anesthesia with midazolam is very rapid (usually 10 minutes), but, unlike methohexital, it does not reliably result in loss of consciousness. Children receiving rectal midazolam are usually awake but cooperative, and are calmly willing to separate from their parents.[14] Recovery from general inhalational anesthesia is rapid, and discharge from PACU is not delayed.[14] Recovery may be delayed, however, when rectal midazolam is followed by intravenous thiopental induction.[15]

Intramuscular ketamine

In an intramuscular dose of 2 mg/kg, ketamine induces enough sedation for the child struggling with the mask to accept inhalational induction.[16] Onset time is less than 3 minutes, and recovery is not prolonged, even after brief procedures that do not require tracheal intubation.[16] When low-dose ketamine is followed by an

inhalational anesthetic such as halothane, there is minimal likelihood of delirium or bad dreams during recovery.

Intranasal administration of preinduction drugs

Both midazolam (0.2 mg/kg) and sufentanil (2 mcg/kg) have
been used as preinduction drugs to facilitate separation from the
parents and to improve mask acceptance.[17] Although effective, the
technique is rather unpleasant and can be associated with serious
complications, especially if sufentanil is used. Nasal midazolam is
very irritating and induces prolonged crying in almost all the
children who receive it. Sufentanil can result in chest wall rigidity
and oxygen desaturation.

Parents' Presence during Induction

Since one of the main reasons for routine premedication, or for
resorting to preinduction technique, is to facilitate separation of
the child from the parents, some anesthesiologists have found that
they can reduce or even eliminate the need for such agents by
allowing the parents to stay with the child during induction.[18]
Some institutions have specially built induction rooms where the
parents can accompany their children without having to wear
special operating room attire. Others allow selected parents (with
a cover-all gown or scrubs) to walk with the child into the
operating room. In all these situations, the parents are there only
for the early part of the induction and are escorted back to the
waiting area as soon as the child is asleep.

Although unconventional, this approach is gaining a lot of
support and is being requested by many parents. Studies have
shown that children are less upset when the parents are present.[18]
Parent selection and education are essential for the success of this
approach, since anxious parents can make their children even
more upset.[19]

Pediatric Equipment

Most modern anesthetic machines can be used for patients of all
ages. The safe and efficient management of children, however,
requires familiarity with and availability of certain additional
pieces of equipment, and appropriately smaller sizes of airway and
monitoring devices. For practitioners who do not work with

children on a regular basis, or when the surgical schedule includes adults and young children in the same anesthetizing location, it is extremely convenient and time-saving to have a special pediatric cart that contains all these extras in a single place. Assuming the routine availability of a standard basic adult setup, the following additional equipment should be considered.

Airway Equipment

A complete set of smaller sizes of everything is needed. This includes pediatric face masks (and a selection of food flavorings), endotracheal tubes, laryngeal mask airways (LMA), oro- and nasopharyngeal airways, suction catheters, and bite blocks.

Breathing system

The choice between a pediatric circle system or a Mapleson circuit is largely a matter of preference as long as the anesthesiologist is familiar with the advantages and limitations of each. The circle system is readily available on all anesthesia machines; it is a familiar system that is easy to use with mechanical ventilation; it allows the use of economical fresh gas flow rates (FGF); and it helps conserve heat and moisture. However, the circle absorber system is bulky; its large internal volume delays the wash-in and wash-out of anesthetic agents unless a high FGF is used, and its use may result in an increase in dead space and resistance to breathing. On the other hand, Mapleson-classified systems (e.g., Jackson Rees modification) are lightweight and easy to move away from the anesthetic machine; they also allow for quick changes in the inspired anesthetic gas mixtures by adjustment of the dials. They can be used during spontaneous ventilation, with a FGF equal to approximately two to three times the child's minute volume; or during controlled ventilation, with a much lower FGF that allows for controlled rebreathing without CO_2 accumulation using the following formula:[20]

Patients < 30 kg:
  FGF (in ml/min) $= 1000 + 100/weight$ (in kg)

Patients ≥ 30 kg:
  FGF (in ml/min) $= 2000 + 50/weight$ (in kg)

In practice, a FGF of 3 liters is used for younger children, and 6 liters for older patients.

Airway maintenance

Many pediatric ambulatory procedures are superficial, do not require intense muscle relaxation, and, especially when general anesthesia is supplemented with a regional block, do not require the deep anesthesia that can significantly depress ventilation. Patients undergoing these types of procedures (e.g., hernia repair) can be managed quite successfully with mask anesthesia. When LMAs of appropriate sizes are available (Table 5-2 and Fig. 5-1),

Table 5-2   Size of Laryngeal Mask Airways

LMA size	Patient weight (kgs)	Cuff volume (ml)
1	< 6.5	2-5
2	6.5-25	5-10
2.5	20-30	15
3	25-50	20
4	> 50	20-30

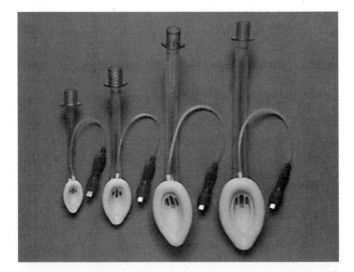

Fig. 5-1 Four sizes of Intavent laryngeal mask airway (LMA). (Courtesy Gensia Pharmaceuticals, Inc.)

***Table* 5-3**   Recommended Tracheal Tube Sizes by Age

Age		Internal diameter (mm)	
Term newborn		3.0	n o n c u f f e d
6 months		3.5	
12 months		4.0	
18-24 months		4.5	
4 years	c	5.0-5.5	
6 years	u	5.5-6.0	
8 years	f	6.0-6.5	
10 years	f	6.5	
12 years	e	7.0	
14 years	d	7.5	
Adult		8.0-9.5	

Children of the same age vary in tracheal size. Occasionally a size 0.5 mm smaller or larger may be required. Cuffs are generally not used with tube sizes smaller than 5.0. General formula for children over 2 years:

$$\text{Tube size mm ID} = \frac{\text{Age (yr)}}{4} + 4.0$$

$$\text{Oral length (cm)} = 12 + \frac{\text{Age}}{2}$$

$$\text{Nasal length (cm)} = 15 + \frac{\text{Age}}{2}$$

they can be used in these patients. Laryngeal mask airways are especially useful for brief procedures in which the airway needs to be maintained without interfering with the surgical field, e.g., lacrimal duct probing or ophthalmic examination.

If an endotracheal tube is to be used in pediatric ambulatory patients, careful attention must be given to selecting a tube appropriately sized for the age of the child (Table 5-3), avoiding traumatic instrumentation, and ensuring the presence of a leak to minimize the possibility of postintubation croup. Children who develop postintubation croup must be treated aggressively with cool mist as soon as the symptoms are apparent, which is usually within the first 30 minutes of extubation. If racemic epinephrine inhalation is used, the child must be closely monitored for 2 to 3 hours afterwards to detect possible rebound edema and symptoms.

Should this happen, repeat treatment is indicated, and overnight admission to a hospital for observation may be required. A general approach to airway maintenance is discussed in Chapter 4.

Monitoring Equipment

A precordial or an esophageal stethoscope should be used to monitor heart rate, heart sounds, and breath sounds; an appropriately sized cuff wide enough to cover about two thirds of the upper arm should be used to monitor blood pressure; and an ECG should be used to detect arrhythmias. Temperature, oxygen saturation, and expired CO_2 should be monitored, and if muscle relaxants are used, neuromuscular function monitoring is strongly recommended. Additional monitoring techniques should be available when indicated, e.g., arterial blood gases if malignant hyperthermia is suspected.

Anesthetic Agents and Techniques

The ideal anesthetic technique for pediatric ambulatory patients would provide rapid, smooth onset; ease of adjustment of anesthetic depth during surgery; prompt emergence; as well as rapid recovery free of pain, vomiting, and unpleasant side effects. Usually a combination of agents and techniques are used to achieve most of these goals.

Inhalational Anesthetics

Inhalational induction is the most popular pediatric anesthesia technique in this country. When the patient is cooperative, and when the anesthesiologist enjoys working with children, the onset is usually smooth and rapid. Recovery is quick after short procedures. Unfortunately, up to 10% to 15% of all children—especially those without adequate preoperative sedation—will not cooperate with attempted mask induction.[1] Some of the reluctance can be overcome with gentle persuasion, distraction, or the use of pleasant food flavorings (e.g., bubble gum) to conceal the plastic smell of the anesthetic mask or the pungent odor of the anesthetic agent. If in spite of all attempts the child continues to struggle and refuse the mask, an alternative induction or preinduction technique should be chosen. This is definitely preferable to forced mask induction, which can be extremely unpleasant and psychologically traumatic for the child.[1]

Halothane

Halothane is the most commonly used inhalational anesthetic for pediatric patients. It is usually combined with nitrous oxide to provide rapid and smooth onset, and, following operations lasting 1 hour or less, quick recovery. Halothane can be used repeatedly in children with minimal concern about hepatic dysfunction. However, it sensitizes the myocardium to the arrhythmogenicity of exogenous catecholamines or elevated arterial CO_2, which can lead to the development of ventricular arrhythmias.

Isoflurane

Although in adult anesthesia practice, isoflurane is considered by many to be the standard inhalational agent, it is not commonly used as an induction agent in pediatric ambulatory patients. Isoflurane has a pungent odor that makes inhalational induction more difficult and that is associated with more airway irritation than halothane.[21] Although its blood solubility is slightly lower than that of halothane, there is no clinically significant difference in the speed of recovery when either agent is used for the usually short (< 1 hour) procedures typically performed in ambulatory patients.[22] Isoflurane does not interact with catecholamines to the degree that halothane does, and is frequently used if epinephrine must be infiltrated by the surgeon to improve hemostasis.

Enflurane

Enflurane has physical characteristics very similar to isoflurane; however, because of its pungency, it is not a very popular agent for pediatric ambulatory patients.

Desflurane

Desflurane has chemical and physical characteristics that are extremely attractive for ambulatory surgical patients. The low solubility (close to that of nitrous oxide) should allow for very fast induction and recovery, as well as ease of control of anesthetic depth. Desflurane is also a very stable, minimally metabolized molecule. However, early experience with desflurane indicates that it is not a suitable induction agent for pediatric patients.[23] The drug has a mildly pungent odor, but compared to halothane, it results in an unacceptably high incidence of airway irritation, moderate-to-severe coughing, and laryngospasm leading to desaturation severe enough to require emergent use of succinylcholine in many patients. Therefore, desflurane is not indicated for initial anesthesia induction in children. Desflurane, however, can be easily introduced following another induction agent, typically halothane. Welborn et al. found that after a brief period of halothane induction, desflurane administration resulted in the same rapid emergence and recovery as when desflurane was used for both induction and maintenance.[24] In addition, desflurane maintenance resulted in significantly faster emergence and recovery than when halothane was used. Desflurane maintenance after halothane induction is particularly useful in patients undergoing otolaryngology procedures (e.g., tonsillectomy, adenoidectomy) when the timing of the end of surgery cannot be accurately predicted, and when rapid awakening and return of airway reflexes is desirable. The ultimate place of desflurane in other types of pediatric ambulatory surgery remains to be established.

Sevoflurane

Sevoflurane has solubility characteristics closer to those of desflurane than to isoflurane. The drug has a very pleasant smell, which makes it the least irritating inhalational induction agent available.[21] Sevoflurane can therefore be used for both induction and maintenance of anesthesia in children. To date, the most extensive clinical experience with sevoflurane has been in Japan.[25] Early investigations in the United States have shown the drug to result in smooth induction with no airway irritation, and significantly faster emergence and recovery, when compared with halothane.[26] Sevoflurane metabolism results in the release of free fluoride ions. The clinical significance appears to be negligible, especially in children undergoing short ambulatory surgical procedures. It is reported that sevoflurane has replaced halothane as the main inhalational agent for children in Japan.[25] Its acceptance in this country remains to be established.

Intravenous Anesthetics (Table 5-4)

Until recently, intravenous anesthesia has not been widely used for pediatric ambulatory surgery. Most available agents led to a longer recovery than that of halothane; and to administer the agent, children had to be subjected to the trauma of venipuncture. The recent introduction of propofol, short-acting opioids, and muscle relaxants into clinical anesthesia has eliminated most concerns about delayed recovery. It is hoped that the

Table 5-4   Pediatric IV Induction Agents

Drug	Dose (mg/kg)
Thiopental	4-6
Methohexital	1.5-2
Propofol*	2.5-3.5

*To minimize pain on injection, use large antecubital veins or mix with 1 mg of lidocaine for every ml or propofol.

availability of EMLA (eutectic mixture of local anesthetics: lidocaine and prilocaine), which can be used to perform painless venipuncture in children,[27] will encourage more anesthesiologists to offer, and more children to accept, intravenous induction. The use of EMLA in Europe and Canada has already increased the acceptance of intravenous induction in children. In ambulatory patients, its use requires careful planning, since at least 1 hour of contact time under an occlusive dressing is required for full effect. In most cases, EMLA should be applied to two potential sites, so that a back-up site is available in case the first venipuncture is not successful. In institutions where preoperative laboratory testing is required, it makes sense to offer the children having blood drawn the option of having their required venipuncture under EMLA, and leaving an intravenous cannula in place to be used later for anesthesia induction. Although EMLA does produce skin anesthesia, it does not eliminate the fear of needles in children who have been previously accustomed to expect pain. Only time and repeated successful use can eliminate that fear.

Sodium thiopental

Until recently, sodium thiopental has been the principal intravenous agent in pediatric patients. To induce sleep, healthy children require a slightly higher dose (4 to 6 mg/kg) than adults. Recovery following short procedures is slightly more prolonged when compared with that seen with halothane anesthesia.[28]

Methohexital

Methohexital (1.5 to 2 mg/kg) results in slightly faster recovery than thiopental. Like other oxybarbiturates, however, methohexital administration is associated with a high incidence of pain on injection, hiccups, and involuntary movement that can be quite difficult to control.

Propofol

Propofol is now the standard intravenous induction agent in adult ambulatory patients. It is soon becoming so in children. Propofol 2.5 to 3.5 mg/kg can be used for induction in children who accept venipuncture.[29] Pain on injection can be minimized or even prevented by using the large antecubital veins. If the hand veins must be used, lidocaine can be mixed with propofol (1 mg lidocaine per ml of propofol) immediately before its injection, with excellent results. When propofol induction is followed by halothane maintenance, recovery is significantly faster than when thiopental induction is followed by halothane.[28] Recovery is fastest if propofol induction is followed by propofol infusion for the maintenance of anesthesia.[28] Because of their higher volume of distribution and increased clearance, children require a higher infusion rate (125 to 300 mcg/kg/min) than adults. This is especially true for younger children, and during the early part of maintenance.

Propofol anesthesia has been consistently shown to be associated with an extremely low incidence of postoperative vomiting, even following surgical procedures that normally result in vomiting, e.g., strabismus surgery.[30-32]

Adjunct Agents (Table 5-5)

Muscle relaxants

Muscle relaxants are not routinely used in ambulatory patients because of the brief, superficial nature of most types of surgery performed on these patients. Muscle relaxants may be used to facilitate tracheal intubation, or as a part of a balanced technique to allow the use of the lightest possible level of anesthesia.

When muscle relaxation is indicated for tracheal intubation only, it is desirable to use the shortest-acting agent available. Succinylcholine has the fastest onset and shortest duration of action of all available agents. In young children, succinylcholine rarely produces fasciculations or muscle pains. It also can be administered intramuscularly when intravenous access is not readily obtainable. However, many anesthesiologists avoid using succinylcholine in children who were induced with halothane to prevent possible confusion about ruling out masseter spasm in the small number of patients in whom incomplete relaxation is

Table 5-5   Adjunct Agents

Agents	Dose (mg/kg)	Route
Muscle Relaxants		
Succinylcholine	2	IV
	5-6	IM
Rocuronium	0.6-0.8	IV
Mivacurium	0.2	IV
Atracurium	0.5	IV
Vecuronium	0.1	IV
Opioids		
Fentanyl	0.5-2 (mcg/kg)	IV
Alfentanil	15-30 (mcg/kg)	IV
Antiemetics		
Metoclopramide	0.15	IV
Droperidol	25-75 (mcg/kg) (max. 2.5 mg)	IV
Ondansetron	0.15 (max. 4 mg)	IV
Promethazine	12.5-25 mg (total)	PR
Prochlorperazine	2.5-5 mg (total)	

observed.[33] Moreover, succinylcholine has been associated with hyperkalemic cardiac arrest in apparently healthy infants and young children who have Duchenne's muscular dystrophy without obvious clinical signs.

Intermediate-acting relaxants are particularly suitable for use in pediatric ambulatory patients (Table 5-5). Of those, mivacurium seems to be particularly attractive, because its very short duration of action and spontaneous degradation often makes pharmacological antagonism unnecessary after a single intubating dose in a surgical procedure that lasts 20 minutes or longer.[34] The avoidance of pharmacological antagonism may decrease the incidence of gastrointestinal disturbances, including nausea and vomiting, in those patients. For longer procedures, atracurium or vecuronium, and more recently rocuronium, have been extensively used, although pharmacological antagonism is almost always indicated with these agents.

Opioids

Short-acting opioids, e.g., fentanyl and alfentanil, can be used as a part of the main anesthetic or for postoperative analgesia in pediatric ambulatory patients. With their use, the dose of potent inhalational or intravenous agents can be decreased; therefore, opioids may actually contribute to more rapid awakening. To prevent recovery delay, the shortest acting agent that is appropriate for the particular surgical procedure should be selected (Table 5-5).

Antiemetics

Routine antiemetic prophylaxis is seldom needed in pediatric patients. For children undergoing procedures known to be associated with a very high incidence of postoperative vomiting, e.g., eye-muscle surgery, the use of propofol has been shown to be very effective in preventing this complication.[30-32] Although some of the traditional antiemetic drugs are at least partially effective, their use is associated with significant side effects, such as prolonged recovery and extrapyramidal symptoms (droperidol 50 to 75 mcg/kg), and gastrointestinal disturbances (metoclopramide 0.15 mg/kg). More recently, ondansetron has been reported to reduce vomiting in children following such vomiting-prone procedures as tonsillectomy, where more conventional antiemetics have little or no effect.[35] The ultimate place of ondansetron in the treatment or prophylaxis of postoperative nausea and vomiting, and the optimal dose required for this purpose, remains to be established.

For patients with persistent postoperative vomiting, our current approach is to stop offering oral fluids[36] and ensure adequate intravenous hydration. Intravenous metoclopramide is administered in a dose of 0.15 mg/kg. Occasionally rectal promethazine 0.5 mg/kg (Phenergan 12.5 to 25 mg) or prochlorperazine 0.1 mg/kg (Compazine 2.5 to 5 mg) is administered in the hospital or given to the parents to use at home.

Fluid Management

Most pediatric ambulatory patients undergo brief surgical procedures that are not associated with significant fluid loss. Fluid management in the perioperative period, therefore, is designed to replace any excessive preoperative deficit and anticipated postoperative needs.

Children undergoing very brief (less than 30 minutes) surgical procedures may not need parenteral fluid, as long as they are not excessively starved preoperatively, and as long as they are expected to be able to ingest and retain oral fluids soon after they are awake.[1] For most other children, intraoperative maintenance fluid

***Table* 5-6**   Maintenance Fluid Therapy

Child's weight (kg)	Basic hourly rate (ml)
< 10	wt × 4
10-20	(wt × 2) + 20
> 20	wt + 40

During the first hour of surgery, up to four times the basic hourly rate may be administered as a hydrating solution.

Modified from Oh TH: Formula for calculating fluid maintenance requirements. Anesthesiology 1980; 53:351.

administration can be calculated based on the child's body weight according to standard formulae (Table 5-6).[37] Although hypotonic solutions (e.g., 0.45% or 0.3% sodium chloride) can be used, many anesthesiologists find it much more appropriate to use a solution suitable for replacement, such as Lactated Ringer's, for intraoperative fluid loss (e.g., during tonsillectomy) or for continuing postoperative loss (e.g., from protracted vomiting).

If continuing postoperative loss through vomiting or inability to tolerate oral intake is anticipated, it is advisable to begin replenishing that anticipated deficit early. This will help ensure that the child is well hydrated when ready to go home, and therefore, that discharge is not delayed while "catch-up" fluid administration is instituted.

Adequate parenteral hydration also obviates the need for forcing children to drink fluids before they are allowed to go home. Recent studies confirm that children who are forced to drink before leaving the facility have higher incidence of vomiting and delayed discharge than children who are allowed to drink only when they are thirsty enough to request a drink.[36]

The need to add glucose to parenteral fluid in pediatric ambulatory patients is rather controversial. The incidence of hypoglycemia in otherwise healthy children who have not been subjected to prolonged fast is extremely low. For those who have fasted for a long period, some dilute glucose–containing solution (e.g., Dextrose 2.5% in Lactated Ringer's) may be used.[38]

Postoperative Analgesia

Adequate postoperative analgesia is a key requirement for successful pediatric ambulatory anesthetic management. Anticipation

Table 5-7   Commonly Used Analgesic Drugs and Dosages

Drug	Route	Dose	Duration of action (hrs)
Acetaminophen	PR/PO	10-15 mg/kg*	4-6
Ketorolac	IM/?IV	1 mg/kg (max 30 mg)	6-8
	PO	1 mg/kg (max 10 mg)	4-6
Ibuprofen	PO	5 mg/kg	6-8
Codeine	PO	0.5-1 mg/kg	4-6
Naproxen	PO	10 mg/kg	6-8
Fentanyl	IV	1-2 mcg/kg	0.5-1
Meperidine	IV/IM	0.5-1 mg/kg	2-4
Morphine	IV/IM	0.05-0.1 mg/kg	2-4

*Acetaminophen suppositories are available in 120 mg, 325 mg, and 650 mg sizes. Usually the calculated dose is rounded up or down to the nearest whole or half size suppository.

of the child's requirements, preemptive analgesic therapy, and early postoperative supplementation ensures patient comfort and may even speed recovery and discharge home.

The selection of the specific analgesic drug or technique is not as vital as the awareness that the individual patient's needs can vary tremendously, and that treatment must be individualized and titrated to effect. For some pediatric ambulatory patients, postoperative analgesia can be ensured by continuing to titrate short-acting intravenous opioids during recovery. For most others, postoperative analgesia can be attained by one or a combination of the following methods (Tables 5-7 and 5-8).

Mild Analgesics

Acetaminophen is the most commonly used mild analgesic for pediatric ambulatory patients. For young children, it is often administered rectally (10 to 15 mg/kg or 60 mg/year of age) before the child awakens from anesthesia. Acetaminophen combined with codeine offers more effective control of moderately severe pain or discomfort.[1] Acetaminophen with codeine elixir contains 120 mg acetaminophen and 12 mg codeine per 5 ml. The usual dose is 5 ml for children 3 to 6 years old, and 10 ml for children 7 to 12 years old.

Nonsteroidal Antiinflammatory Drugs (NSAIDs)

Nonsteroidal antiinflammatory drugs, in particular, ketorolac, have proved effective in relieving postoperative pain following minor

Table 5-8 Regional Techniques for Pediatric Ambulatory Surgery

Surgical procedure	Block	Drug	Dose
Inguinal hernia, hydrocelectomy, orchiopexy	Caudal	Bupivacaine 0.25%-0.125%	0.75-1.0 ml/kg
	Ilioinguinal/iliohypogastric	Bupivacaine 0.25%	0.3-0.5 ml/kg
	Instillation	Bupivacaine 0.25%	0.5 ml/kg
		Bupivacaine 0.25%	0.5 ml/kg
Umbilical hernia	Infiltration	Bupivacaine 0.25%	0.3-0.5 ml/kg
	Caudal	Bupivacaine 0.125%	1.25 ml/kg
Circumcision, hypospadias	Caudal	Bupivacaine 0.25%	0.5 ml/kg
	Dorsal nerve	Bupivacaine 0.25%	4-6 ml
	Ring block	Bupivacaine 0.25%	4-6 ml
	Topical (end of surgery)	Lidocaine jelly or ointment (2%)	
T & A	Infiltration	Bupivacaine 0.25% with epinephrine 1:200,00	0.5 ml/kg
	Topical	Lidocaine 10% spray	
Extremities	Peripheral nerve blocks, e.g., axillary	Bupivacaine	2.5 mg/kg
		Lidocaine	5 mg/kg
Airway endoscopy	Topical	Lidocaine	2 mg/kg

operations in children.[39] Early administration immediately following induction seems to provide optimal postoperative analgesia. More studies are required to determine the optimal dose and best route of administration of ketorolac, as well as its efficacy as an analgesic following more painful ambulatory surgical procedures in children.

Regional Anesthesia

The greatest advantage of regional anesthesia in pediatric ambulatory patients is that local infiltration or regional blocks can be administered intraoperatively after induction to help reduce the requirements of other anesthetic agents, and to promote rapid, pain-free recovery without the need for systemic opioids or other potent analgesics. Many of the surgical procedures performed on these patients are amenable to regional anesthetic supplementation (Table 5-8). The choice of the individual block is determined by the type of operation and anesthesiologist familiarity with the available techniques.

Caudal analgesia

Caudal analgesia can be used in patients undergoing inguinal, penile, perineal, or lower limb procedures (Fig. 5-2). The level of block is determined by several formulae that calculate an appropriate volume of the local anesthetic solution (Table 5-8). A dose of bupivacaine in excess of 2.5 mg/kg is seldom required or justified in pediatric outpatients. Bupivacaine 0.25% and 0.125% solutions have been shown to be equally effective in providing supplemental intraoperative anesthesia, as well as residual postoperative analgesia.[40]

Ilioinguinal/iliohypogastric nerve block

This block is very effective in providing postoperative analgesia following operations performed through an inguinal incision, e.g., hernia repair, hydrocelectomy, or orchiopexy. Since the two nerves enter the inguinal canal through the layers of the anterior abdominal wall muscles, the block can be performed by direct infiltration of these muscles medial to the anterior superior iliac spine using 3 to 5 ml of 0.25% bupivacaine solution.[41] Alternatively, the muscles can be infiltrated through the lateral edge of the inguinal incision,[42] or by instillation of bupivacaine directly in the wound to bathe the exposed nerve trunks during dissection.[43]

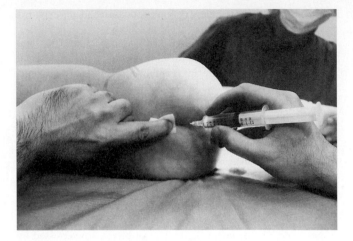

Fig. 5-2 Caudal anesthesia.

Penile blocks

Both dorsal nerve block and ring block around the base of the penis can be used to provide analgesia following circumcision or hypospadias surgery.[44,45] Epinephrine-free solutions must be used. Alternatively, local anesthetic cream or ointment may be applied to the exposed nerve endings of the skin incision after surgical closure has been found effective.[46]

Other blocks

Almost all other regional blocks with which the anesthesiologist is familiar can be adapted for use in children. It is essential, however, that special attention be paid not to exceed the safe dose of the local anesthetic solution (Table 5-8). If the calculated maximum safe dose of a standard concentration results in an inadequate volume, then a more dilute solution or a different block should be chosen. Examples of these group of blocks that are frequently used at CNMC include axillary and femoral nerve blocks.

Local infiltration

For operations that are not amenable to a regional technique, or for minor peripheral procedures, the surgeon must be encouraged to use local infiltration of the wound area before, during, or at the completion of the operation.

Summary

Successful management of pediatric patients undergoing ambulatory surgery is influenced by the proper preparation of children, which should include appropriate screening and limited laboratory testing. Liberalized fasting requirements for children may allow clear liquids up until 3 hours before anesthesia induction. Facilities may differ in their approaches to premedicating children or allowing parents to be present at the time of induction. Preinduction techniques and dosaging are discussed. Monitoring and airway equipment should be appropriate for the child's age and size. Ideal anesthetic technique for pediatric ambulatory patients is one that will provide rapid, smooth onset; ease of adjustment of anesthetic depth during surgery; prompt emergence; and rapid recovery that is free of pain, vomiting, and other side effects. Properties of the inhaled and intravenous agents are discussed. It may be easier to perform painless venipuncture and administer intravenous anesthetics for induction if EMLA cream is used. Techniques and agents are combined to achieve optimum anesthetic conditions.

Most brief pediatric surgical procedures are not associated with significant fluid loss, and fasting periods are shorter; however, for adequate perioperative hydration, the clinician should consider preoperative fluid deficit as well as anticipated postoperative needs. Adequate intraoperative hydration reduces the need for children to ingest fluids before discharge, thereby minimizing dizziness, nausea, and vomiting. For postoperative pain, oral acetaminophen, nonsteroidal antiinflammatory agents, or intravenous opiates may be titrated to effect; this ensures patient comfort and may even speed recovery and discharge. Regional anesthesia in pediatric patients can reduce intraoperative anesthetic requirements and provide postoperative analgesia (i.e., caudal, wound infiltration, upper and lower extremity blocks), and should be strongly encouraged in pediatric ambulatory surgery practices.

References

1. Hannallah RS, Epstein BS: The pediatric patient. In Wetchler BV, editor: Anesthesia for ambulatory surgery, ed 2, Philadelphia, 1991, JB Lippincott, pp. 131-95.
2. Coté C: NPO after midnight for children—a reappraisal. Anesthesiology 1990; 72:589-92.
3. Schreiner MS, Triebwasser A, Keon T: Ingestion of liquids compared with preoperative fasting in pediatric outpatients. Anesthesiology 1990; 72:593-7.
4. Cavell B: Gastric emptying in infants fed human milk or infant formula. Acta Paediatr Scand 1981; 70:639-41.
5. Steward DJ: Screening tests before surgery in children. Can J Anaesth 1991; 38:693.
6. Roy WL, Lerman J, McIntyre BG: Is preoperative haemoglobin testing justified in children undergoing minor elective surgery? Can J Anaesth 1991; 38:700-3.
7. Rosen DA, Rosen KR, Hannallah RS: Anaesthesia induction in children—ability to predict outcome. Paediatric Anaesthesia 1993; 3:365-70.
8. Litman RS, Perkins FM, Dawson SC: Parental knowledge and attitude toward discussing the risk of death from anesthesia. Anesth Analg 1993; 77:256-60.
9. Weldon BC, Watcha MF, White PF: Oral midazolam in children: effect of time and adjunct therapy. Anesth Analg 1992; 75:51-5.
10. Levine MF, Saphr-Schopfer IA, Hartley E et al: Oral midazolam premedication in children: the minimum time interval for separation from parents. Can J Anaesth 1993; 40:726-9.
11. Gutstein HB, Johnson KL, Heard MB, Gregory GA: Oral ketamine preanesthetic medication in children. Anesthesiology 1992; 76:28-33.
12. Friesen RH, Lockhart CH: Oral transmucosal fentanyl citrate for preanesthetic medication or pediatric day surgery patients with and without droperidol as a prophylactic antiemetic. Anesthesiology 1992; 76:46-51.
13. Goresky GV, Steward DJ: Rectal methohexitone for induction of anaesthesia in children. Can Anaesth Soc J 1979; 26:213-5.
14. Spear RM, Yaster M, Berkowitz ID et al: Preinduction of anesthesia in children with rectally administered midazolam. Anesthesiology 1991; 74:670-4.
15. Beebe DS, Belani KG, Chang PN et al: Effectiveness of preoperative sedation with rectal midazolam, ketamine, or their combination in young children. Anesth Analg 1992; 75:880-4.
16. Hannallah RS, Patel RI: Low dose intramuscular ketamine for anesthesia pre-induction in young children undergoing brief outpatient procedures. Anesthesiology 1989; 70:598-600.

17. Karl HW, Keifer AT, Rosenberg JL et al: Comparison of safety and efficacy of intra-nasal midazolam or sufentanil for preinduction of anesthesia in pediatric patients. Anesthesiology 1992; 76:209-15.

18. Hannallah RS, Rosales JK: Experience with parents' presence during anesthesia induction in children. Can Anaesth Soc J 1983; 30:286-9.

19. Bevan JC, Johnston C, Haig MJ et al: Preoperative parental anxiety predicts behavioural and emotional responses to induction of anaesthesia in children. Can J Anaesth 1990; 37:177-82.

20. Rose DK, Froese AB: The regulation of $PaCO_2$ during controlled ventilation of children with a T-piece. Can Anaesth Soc J 1979; 26:104-13.

21. Doi M, Ikeda K: Airway irritation produced by volatile anaesthetics during brief inhalation: comparison of halothane, enflurane, isoflurane and sevoflurane. Can J Anaesth 1993; 40:122-6.

22. Kingston HGG: Halothane and isoflurane anesthesia in pediatric outpatients. Anesth Analg 1986; 65:181-4.

23. Zwass MS, Fisher DM, Welborn LG et al: Induction and maintenance characteristics of anesthesia with desflurane and nitrous oxide in infants and children. Anesthesiology 1992; 76:373-8.

24. Welborn LG, Hannallah RS, McGill WA et al: Induction and recovery characteristics of desflurane and halothane anaesthesia in paediatric outpatients. Paediatric Anaesthesia; in press.

25. Muto R, Miyasaka K, Takata M et al: Initial experience of complete switchover to sevoflurane in 1550 children. Paediatric Anaesthesia 1993; 3:229-33.

26. Greenspun J, Hannallah R, Welborn L, Norden J: Comparison of sevoflurane and halothane in pediatric ENT surgery. Anesth Analg 1994; 78:S140.

27. Soliman IE, Broadman LM, Hannallah RS, McGill WA: Comparison of the analgesic effects of EMLA (eutectic mixture of local anesthetics) to intradermal lidocaine infiltration prior to venous cannulation in unpremedicated children. Anesthesiology 1988; 68:804-6.

28. Hannallah RS, Britton JT, Schafer PG et al: Propofol anaesthesia in paediatric ambulatory patients: a comparison with thiopentone and halothane. Can J Anaesth 1994; 41:12-8.

29. Hannallah RS, Baker SB, Casey W et al: Propofol effective dose and induction characteristics in unpremedicated children. Anesthesiology 1991; 74:217-9.

30. Hannallah R, Britton J, Schafer, P, Norden J: Effect of propofol anesthesia on the incidence of vomiting after strabismus surgery in children. Anesth Analg 1992; 74:S131.

31. Watcha MF, Simeon RM, White PF, Stevens JL: Effect of propofol on the incidence of postoperative vomiting after strabismus surgery in pediatric outpatients. Anesthesiology 1991; 75:204-9.

32. Martin TM, Nicolson SC, Bargas MS: Propofol anesthesia reduces emesis and airway obstruction in pediatric outpatients. Anesth Analg 1993; 76:144-8.

33. Hannallah RS, Kaplan R: Jaw relaxation after a halothane/ succinylcholine sequence in children. Anesthesiology 1994; 81:99-103.

34. Kaplan R, Garcia M, Hannallah R, Norden J: Neuromuscular effects of mivacurium during halothane or sevoflurane anesthesia in children. Anesth Analg 1994; 78:S192.

35. Furst SR, Rodarte A, Demars P: Ondansetron reduces postoperative vomiting in children undergoing tonsillectomy. Anesthesiology 1993; 79:A1197.

36. Schreiner MS, Nicolson SC, Martin T, Whitney L: Should children drink before discharge from day surgery? Anesthesiology 1992; 76:528.

37. Oh TH: Formula for calculating fluid maintenance requirements. Anesthesiology 1980; 53:351.

38. Welborn LG, Hannallah RS, McGill WA et al: Choosing a glucose concentration for routine infusion in pediatric outpatient surgery. Anesthesiology 1987; 67:427-30.

39. Watcha MF, Ramirez-Ruiz M, White PF et al: Perioperative effects of oral ketorolac and acetaminophen in children undergoing bilateral myringotomy. Can J Anaesth 1992; 39:649-54.

40. Wolf AR, Valley RD, Fear DW et al: Bupivacaine for caudal analgesia in infants and children; the optimal effective concentration. Anesthesiology 1988; 69:102-6.

41. Shandling B, Steward DJ: Regional analgesia for postoperative pain in pediatric outpatient surgery. J Pediatr Surg 1980; 15:477-80.

42. Hannallah RS, Broadman LM, Belman AB et al: Comparison of caudal and ilioinguinal/iliohypogastric nerve blocks for control of post-orchiopexy pain in pediatric ambulatory surgery. Anesthesiology 1987; 66:832-4.

43. Casey WF, Rice LJ, Hannallah RS et al: A comparison between bupivacaine instillation versus ilioinguinal/iliohypogastric nerve block for postoperative analgesia following inguinal herniorrhaphy in children. Anesthesiology 1990; 72:637-9.

44. Soliman MG, Tremblay NA: Nerve block of the penis for postoperative pain relief in children. Anesth Analg 1978; 57:495-8.

45. Broadman LM, Hannallah RS, Belman AB et al: Post-circumcision pain—a prospective evaluation of subcutaneous ring block of the penis. Anesthesiology 1987; 67:399-402.

46. Tree-Trakan T, Pirayavaraporn S, Lertakyamanee J: Topical anesthesia for relief of post-circumcision pain. Anesthesiology 1987; 67:395-9.

6

Preoperative Preparation

Carmen R. Green and Sujit K. Pandit

Preoperative Instructions

Once outpatient surgery has been scheduled, it is important to give the patient clear instructions about what to do during the perioperative period. A health professional, usually a registered nurse, certified nurse anesthetist, or another trained person, may give instructions in person or over the telephone. In addition, a written copy of the instructions (or a booklet) is also given to the patient. Many hospitals and facilities have produced short video presentations about what to expect on the day of operation, which they show the patients (and the parents if the patient is a child) during a visit with the surgeon. Box 6-1 contains some instructions that must be given to the patient before an operation.

Fasting Instructions

It is known that aspiration of acidic gastric contents is an important cause of perioperative morbidity and mortality; as a result, overnight fasting has become a standard anesthetic practice. However, a number of recent studies show that the gastric emptying time for clear liquids is very different than that for solid foods. Although after ingestion, solid food takes as long as 6 to 8 hours to leave the stomach, clear liquids leave the stomach within 2 hours. Ingestion of food or drink immediately stimulates stomach activity; solid foods must be broken down to semisolid chyme (2 μm particle size) to pass through the pylorus, while liquids can pass almost immediately. Furthermore, it has been shown that patients who are allowed clear liquids up until 2 to 3 hours before induction are more cheerful, less hungry and thirsty, have lower incidence of perioperative headaches, need less intravenous fluids during and after the operation, and have less residual intragastric volume and acidity.[1] In fact, there is evidence that ingestion of clear liquids 2 to 3 hours before induction increases

---

Box 6-1 Instructions Before Outpatient Operations

- Time of scheduled operation and when to arrive at the facility
- Remember to wear loose and comfortable clothing
- Must have a responsible adult escort to take the patient home
- Must have a responsible adult at home to take care of the patient overnight
- What to bring and what not to bring
- Fasting instructions
- Instructions about current medications

---

gastric peristalsis and helps empty the stomach of residual acid secretions faster.

A recent survey of U.S. anesthesiologists[2] shows that almost 70% of pediatric anesthesiologists and about 40% of adult anesthesiologists have liberalized their fasting requirements for clear fluids. Most anesthesiologists allow patients in ASA class 1 or 2 to ingest an unlimited amount of clear liquids until up to 3 hours before elective surgery. Box 6-2 shows the current NPO (*nulla per os,* nothing by mouth) guidelines[3] at the University of Michigan Medical Center. In patients at increased risk for pulmonary aspiration (e.g., those with morbid obesity, diabetes, pregnancy, hiatal hernia, or other gastroesophageal lesions), use of these guidelines is still controversial. Types of common clear liquids allowed are listed in Box 6-3. It should be noted that cow's milk is *not* a clear liquid and should not be allowed. Although breast milk is not technically a clear liquid, it is functionally a clear liquid because it is rapidly emptied from the stomach. Therefore, most of the surveyed pediatric anesthesiologists allow breastfeeding until 2 to 4 hours before induction; however, this remains controversial.

Use of Current Medications

Most of the patient's current prescribed medications are needed to maintain homeostasis of the patient's physiological condition.

Box 6-2 *Fasting Guidelines Before Elective Operations in* ASA *Class* 1 *or Class* 2 *Patients*

Solid Food

No solid food on the day of operation (8 hours fasting)

Clear Liquid

Adults and children greater than 3 months of age: unlimited amounts of clear liquid up to 3 hours before the operation

Infants (less than 3 months of age): clear liquids up to 2 hours before operation

Oral Medication

For both adult and children, required oral medications may be taken up to 1 hour before the induction, with one-half cup of water

Box 6-3 *Common Clear Liquids Allowed Before Operation*

Children	**Adult**
Water	Water
Apple juice	Apple juice
Carbonated beverage	Black tea or coffee
Jell-O	Carbonated beverage
Broth	
(Breast milk)	

Interruption of these medications may actually be dangerous to the patient's overall health. Primary among these are antihypertensive drugs, coronary artery dilators, bronchodilators, anticonvulsants, and tricyclic antidepressants. These drugs should be continued through the morning of the operation. Certain other drugs like diuretics, anticoagulants, and insulin are usually withheld on the morning of operation and given in the operating room, if necessary, under the direct supervision of the anesthesiologist. Patients on digitalis glycosides and diuretics may be at an increased risk for hypokalemia, which may precipitate digitalis toxicity and dangerous intraoperative arrhythmias. Because of their long half lives (digoxin half life is 36 to 40 hours, digitoxin half life is 5 to 9 days) and narrow therapeutic range, digitalis glycosides should be withheld on the day of surgery. Whether it is necessary to stop some antidepressant medications (e.g., monoamine oxidase [MAO] inhibitors) is controversial. Several recent studies and surveys[4] suggest that MAO inhibitors may be continued as long as the anesthesiologist is fully aware of their possible disastrous interactions with some vasopressors and with some narcotics (e.g., meperidine). There is also controversy regarding continuation of aspirin therapy for patients with coronary artery disease. Chronic use of aspirin products can cause a bleeding tendency and can prolong the bleeding time. A thorough preoperative history and assessment about bleeding tendency will reveal the extent of the problem. Box 6-4 lists recommended preoperative disposition of chronic medications.

Box 6-4 Disposition of Current Medications Before Outpatient Operation

Continue

Antihypertensive
Beta adrenergic blockers
Calcium channel blockers
ACE inhibitors
Vasodilators
Bronchodilators
Antiseizure medications
Tricyclic antidepressants
MAO inhibitors (controversial)
Corticosteriods
Thyroid preparations
Anxiolytics

Discontinue or Withhold

Diuretics
Insulin
Digitalis
Anticoagulants (may change to a short-acting agent like heparin)

> ### Box 6-5 *Purposes of the Nurse's Phone Call the Day Before the Operation*
>
> - Provide reassurance
> - Confirm the time of the scheduled operation and time of arrival at the facility
> - Instruct what to bring (medications, eye glass case, insurance card) and what not to bring (unnecessary money, jewelry, etc.)
> - Restate the fasting instructions
> - Ask about any recent changes in the health status (e.g., upper respiratory tract infection)
> - Instruct about the use of prescribed and current medications
> - Emphasize the need to bring a responsible adult escort (old enough to have a valid driving license) to take the patient back home
> - Emphasize the importance of having a responsible adult at home during the 24 hours following surgery
> - Note the telephone number where the patient can be reached that night in case of any changes in schedule

The Day Before the Operation

Whenever possible, a health care professional, usually a registered nurse or a CRNA should call the patient to give any last-minute instructions, get up-to-date information about the patient's condition, answer any questions, repeat and reinforce previous instructions, and provide reassurance (Box 6-5).

Preanesthetic Evaluation on the Day of the Operation

Regardless of the method of screening or preanesthetic evaluation done earlier, the anesthesiologist must perform a final assessment on the day of the operation. At this time, after reviewing the screening and preoperative records, the anesthesiologist must take a quick history, perform a final focused physical examination, and go over the anesthetic and postanesthetic care plans with the patient (Box 6-6).

Box 6-6 *Purposes of Final Evaluation by the Anesthesiologist*

- Reassure patient
- Establish or re-establish patient-doctor relationship and rapport
- Review health questionnaire
- Review other screening or preanesthetic records and laboratory findings
- Note the current and any recent changes in health status
- Obtain and review previous anesthetic history
- Review family history of anesthetic complications
- Note history of drug allergy
- Ask about last meal, drink, and medications taken
- Take history of current and prescribed medications
- Note history of any other chemical use
- Perform a short physical examination including examination of the heart, lung, blood pressure, and airway
- Note the relevant available laboratory findings
- Perform necessary laboratory tests (e.g., blood sugar for diabetics, serum potassium for patients receiving diuretics)
- Explain the anesthetic and postanesthetic care plans
- Answer any questions and obtain informed consent
- Provide pharmacologic premedication, if necessary

The holding room nurse also should take a pertinent history that includes the patient's allergies; the last time the patient ate or drank anything; the patient's current health status; whether the patient wears dentures, eyeglasses, or contact lenses; the name of the patient's escort; and telephone numbers where the patient can be reached. The clinician should also note the patient's heart rate, blood pressure, respiratory rate, temperature, and, if available, room air oxygen saturation (SaO_2).

Preoperative Medication

Preoperative medications are given for many reasons (Box 6-7). This discussion focuses on adults, while specific pediatric

---

Box 6-7 Purposes of Preoperative Medication

Primary Purposes

Allay anxiety
Reduce gastric acidity and residual volume
Decrease histamine activity
Reduce oral and airway secretions
Minimize nausea and vomiting
Control infection

Secondary Purposes

Produce amnesia
Produce sedation
Provide analgesia
Reduce anesthetic requirement
Reduce vagal activity
Reduce anesthetic requirement
Provide hemodynamic stability

---

premedicants are addressed in Chapter 5. Several things must be considered before ordering preoperative medications (Box 6-8).

Antianxiety Premedicants

Explanation of the procedure and reassurance by the anesthesiologist during the preoperative period goes a long way in relieving patient anxiety.[5] Nevertheless, most patients remain anxious before an operation.[6,7] Controversy has long existed about whether a preoperative antianxiety agent should be administered to anxious patients undergoing outpatient surgery.[8] The older anxiolytic agents were associated with delayed discharge and recovery. However, when midazolam, a rapid-onset short-acting, water-soluble benzodiazepine, was introduced, these problems were solved. An ideal outpatient premedicant should have rapid onset of action and a short elimination half life. Midazolam, with an elimination half life of 2.5 hours, is the most common premedicant used in the United States.[8] Instead of using a fixed dosing regimen, it is best to titrate the drug to effect, by increments of 0.5 mg to 1 mg. Since the onset of action is rapid (1 to 2 minutes),

Box 6-8 *Questions to Ask Before Any Preoperative Medication Is Ordered*

- Does this patient need a pharmacological premedicant in addition to the psychological preparation and suggestions?
- Is this patient at a high risk for acid aspiration?
- Is this patient at a high risk for postoperative nausea and vomiting?
- Does this patient need a drying agent?
- Does this patient need any histamine receptor blockers (H_1 and H_2) to prevent allergic reactions?
- Does this patient need antibiotic prophylaxis?

titration is easy. Rarely does an average adult need more than 2 mg; elderly patients need even less, often only 0.5 mg. Midazolam can also be administered intramuscularly (0.07 to 0.1 mg/kg), orally (0.5 to 0.75 mg/kg), or intranasally (0.2 mg/kg) in pediatric and adult patients. Oral midazolam has a very bitter taste that can be masked by mixing it with a sweetened clear liquid, like cola, or grape or apple juice. When the midazolam dose is in the upper limits of the dose range, the discharge time may be delayed because of long anterograde amnesia and diminished psychomotor function, which may be undesirable in the adult ambulatory patient.[9,10]

Oral diazepam (5 to 10 mg) may be given 1 hour preoperatively; patients may take this dose at home before leaving for the facility, as long as they are not driving. Although diazepam has a long elimination half life (about 20 hours), this dose is well tolerated by healthy, young adults. Long-acting agents (e.g., lorazepam) are not recommended, mainly because of their extremely long sedative and amnesic effects. Triazolam and the formulation of temazepam currently available in the United States are not recommended for outpatient premedication because of unpredictable duration. Short-acting narcotics (e.g., fentanyl 0.5 to 1.0 µg/kg, sufentanil 0.15 to 0.2 µg/kg) are occasionally used as antianxiety premedicants when benzodiazepines are

---

Box 6-9 *Ideal Anxiolytic Premedicant for Outpatient Surgery*

- Rapid onset of action
- Nonirritating to tissue when given intravenously or intramuscularly
- Short elimination half life
- Nonactive metabolites
- Brief, if any, amnesic effect
- Effective orally (in children)
- Devoid of side effects (e.g., nausea, vomiting, dizziness, and sedation)

---

inappropriate.[11] Innovative ideas like transdermal or transmucosal administration systems (e.g., fentanyl) for outpatients are now available; however, these are not desirable because of the high incidence of nausea and vomiting, pruritus, long latency, and high cost.

Box 6-9 lists the characteristics of an ideal antianxiety premedicant. Box 6-10 lists the common antianxiety premedicants for outpatient surgery in adults.

Sedative, Amnesic, and Analgesic Premedicants

Except in a very small number of extremely anxious patients, neither sedation nor amnesia is a desirable feature of a premedicant. In fact, prolonged sedation and anterograde amnesia in the immediate postoperative period is certainly unwarranted because the patient must remember the postoperative instructions given to them. However, the pediatric patient differs from the adult patient: Amnesia may actually be desirable in children, since it is the parents who are responsible for understanding the postoperative instruction.[10] Midazolam in small doses causes anterograde amnesia, but fortunately, the duration of this amnesia is fairly short, about 30 minutes. Analgesic premedicants (e.g., fentanyl 1 to 2 µg/kg, sufentanil 0.15 to 0.2 µg/kg) are indicated when a painful procedure is contemplated before the induction of anesthesia (e.g., regional anesthetic blocks).[11]

Box 6-10 *Preoperative Medicants for Anxiolysis in Adult Outpatient Surgery*

Most Common Premedicant

Midazolam intravenously (titrate to effect in increments of 0.5 to 1 mg; total dose is usually no more than 2 to 3 mg)

Other Premedicants

Midazolam: intramuscularly (0.08 to 0.1 mg/kg)
              intranasal (0.2 mg/kg)
Fentanyl intravenously (0.5 to 1.0 µg/kg)
Sufentanil intravenously (0.15 to 0.2 µg/kg)
Ketamine intramuscularly (2 to 4 mg/kg) in belligerent patients
Diazepam orally (5 to 10 mg) 1 hour before operation

Alpha$_2$ adrenergic agonists (e.g., clonidine, dexmedetomidine) have been utilized preoperatively as premedicants and as adjuncts during the intraoperative period.[12] These drugs reduce anesthetic requirements by virtue of their analgesic effects. Oral clonidine (200 to 300 µg, approximately 3 µg/kg) has been used to provide sedation and anxiolysis while maintaining hemodynamic stability. Clonidine in larger doses and as transdermal patch may be associated with prolonged postoperative sedation. The optimal dose of dexmedetomidine for premedication of the ambulatory patients is 0.3 to 0.6 µg/kg intravenously or 1.0 mg/kg intramuscularly. The incidence of side effects (e.g., sedation, dry mouth, and hypotension) increase when higher doses of clonidine and dexmedetomidine are used.

Medications to Prevent Acid Aspiration

The incidence of serious pulmonary aspiration is rare in healthy adults undergoing elective outpatient surgery: less than 1:25,000.[13] Over the last decade, studies and anesthesiologists' experience have disproved earlier reports that outpatient surgery patients were at higher risk for acid aspiration than were inpatient surgery patients. These reports stemmed from an erroneous assumption that a residual gastric volume of 25 ml or greater, along

Box 6-11 Patients at Higher Risk for Pulmonary
          Acid Aspiration

- Morbidly obese patients
- Insulin dependent and non-insulin-dependent diabetic patients
- Pregnant patients
- Patients with a history of hiatal hernia or other gastro-esophageal dysfunction
- Patients at the extremes of age
- Patients who smoke[14]
- Patients with high anxiety
- Patients with an anticipated difficult airway

with a pH of 2.5 or less, automatically places a patient at a higher risk for acid aspiration. According to this false assumption, the majority of the patients scheduled for any surgery (inpatient or outpatient) are at high risk for pulmonary aspiration. Actually, the incidence of pulmonary aspiration in ASA class 1 or 2 patients undergoing elective surgery is extremely rare. Thus, routine aspiration prophylaxis for all outpatient surgical candidates is neither cost-effective nor appropriate. However, some patients are perceived to be at a higher risk for pulmonary acid aspiration (Box 6-11). These patients and other high-risk patients should be pretreated (Box 6-12). A dose of an oral H_2 antagonist the night before surgery and another dose the morning of surgery gives the best result. A prescription for this drug should be given to patients during the preoperative visit so that they can take it at home. An intravenous H_2 antagonist may be administered within 1 hour before surgery. However, rapid intravenous infusion of cimetidine may result in cardiac arrhythmias (e.g., bradycardia). The H_2 blocker may be combined with metoclopramide, which has anti-emetic properties, increases the lower esophageal sphincter pressure, and may prevent gastric regurgitation.[15] A clear antacid is best given just before the operation in patients who are at risk (see Box 6-12) but were not prepared appropriately with a H_2 blocker and/or metoclopramide.

Box 6-12 Drugs for Acid Aspiration Prophylaxis

H_2 Antagonists

Ranitidine
   150 mg orally about 2 hours before operation
   50 mg intravenously about 1 hour before operation
Cimetidine
   300 to 400 mg orally about 2 hours before operation
   300 mg intravenously about 1 hour before operation
      (Dosage may need to be reduced for patients
      with renal insufficiency.)
Famotidine
   20 to 40 mg orally 2 hours before operation
   20 mg intravenously about 1 hour before operation

Gastrokinetic Agents

Metoclopramide
   10 mg intravenously about 30 minutes before
      operation
   10 mg orally about 1 hour before operation

Clear Antacids

Sodium citrate (or Bicitra)
   15 to 30 ml orally about 15 minutes before operation
   (Allow thorough intragastric mixing by rolling the patient from side to side.)

Antiemetic Premedicants and Prophylaxis

Nausea and vomiting is still a significant problem following outpatient surgery. Box 6-13 lists the conditions that predispose to postoperative nausea and vomiting (PONV).

Strategy to control postoperative nausea and vomiting

Nausea and vomiting is the most disliked postoperative sequelae by both patients and PACU nurses. Specific postoperative treatment modalities are discussed in Chapter 11. It has been shown by many authors that PONV, even when treated, significantly prolongs recovery room stay and discharge time. This delay in discharge from PACU impacts the smooth operation of the facility, thus increasing the cost of health care. As a result, prevention of

Box 6-13 *Factors That Predispose to* PONV

- Female gender
- Infants and small children
- Certain operations:
      Eye surgery, especially strabismus surgery
      Laparoscopy
      Middle ear surgery
      Tonsillectomy/adenoidectomy
      Abortion
- Inappropriate mask and bag ventilation
- Intraoperative narcotic use
- Nitrous oxide and narcotic combination
- Operation during the days of menstruation and ovulation
- History of motion sickness
- History of previous PONV or chemotherapy
- Obesity
- Oral intake attempted too early in the postoperative period
- Postoperative ambulation attempted too early, especially after narcotic use
- Postoperative hypotension

PONV is certainly a better strategy than treating after it occurs. However, routine PONV prophylaxis for all outpatients is neither cost-effective nor desirable, as most currently used antiemetics are not always effective, and they do have undesirable side effects. Box 6-14 lists strategies to prevent PONV.

A prophylactic antiemetic should be considered for any patient who appears to be at high risk for PONV when other strategies may not be adequate. The incidence of nausea and vomiting for similar situations vary tremendously among various facilities and even among anesthesiologists practicing in the same facility. Thus, each anesthesiologist's plan must be based on his or her own experience and track record. Box 6-15 gives a list of common antiemetics that are used for prophylaxis.

Box 6-14 **Strategies to Prevent PONV**

- Provide smooth, elegant anesthesia (by an experienced and caring anesthesiologist)
- Use propofol anesthesia
- Prevent gastric distention
- Ensure adequate preoperative and intraoperative intravenous hydration
- Limit usage of intraoperative narcotic; instead use regional blocks
- Provide prompt treatment of pain during recovery
- Avoid sudden movements in the PACU
- Avoid attempting oral intake and ambulation too early
- Avoid orthostatic hypotension in PACU
- Provide prophylactic antiemetic for high-risk patients

Box 6-15 **Prophylactic Antiemetic Drugs**

Droperidol
    10 to 20 µg/kg intravenously at the time of induction
Metoclopramide
    10 mg intravenously at the end of operation
Ondansetron
    4 to 8 mg intravenously during the operation
Hydroxyzine
    1.0 to 1.5 mg/kg intramuscularly in preoperative period
Ephedrine
    25 to 50 mg intramuscularly during the operation or in
        the postoperative period

Droperidol, a butyrophenone, a dopaminergic antagonist, is by far the most common and probably the most effective prophylactic antiemetic used in the United States. While a dosage of 10 to 20 µg/kg is usually effective,[16] in certain situations such as strabismus surgery, a dose of 50 to 75 µg/kg has been recommended. Droperidol has a long latency and a long duration of action. Thus, it should be given toward the beginning of the operation rather than near the end. Nevertheless, it is unwise to give droperidol during the preoperative period, since it can cause extreme anxiety and restlessness in the patient waiting for surgery. Droperidol is also associated with extrapyramidal side effects, agitation, and dysphoria.

Metoclopramide, also a dopaminergic antagonist, is a proven antiemetic when used in large doses in patients receiving cancer chemotherapy. However, the effectiveness of smaller doses in the outpatient surgery setting is rather controversial. It appears to be most effective when given at the end of surgery, or on arrival to the PACU in an intravenous dose of 10 mg. Rapid administration of metoclopramide, like that of droperidol, may also result in extrapyramidal side effects, flushing, intestinal cramps, and agitation. There is some indication that metoclopramide hastens recovery from anesthesia.[16]

Ondansetron, a serotonin 5-HT$_3$ receptor antagonist, has been recently approved as an antiemetic for PONV. Like metoclopramide, it has been used successfully for antiemetic prophylaxis before cancer chemotherapy. Available results indicate that it is an effective intravenous antiemetic in a dose of 4 to 8 mg, but that it is probably no more effective than droperidol.[17] However, ondansetron has no cardiovascular and psychological side effects. At this time, ondansetron is very expensive (a 4.0 mg dose costs about $17.00), making it a poor choice for routine antiemetic prophylaxis. Many anesthesiologists reserve its use as a last-resort rescue medication to treat PONV when other methods have failed.

Hydroxyzine is an effective antiemetic that also provides sedation, especially when combined with a small amount of narcotic. However, prolonged sedation may be a disadvantage in the outpatient setting. In addition, intramuscular injection of hydroxyzine is painful and may cause tissue irritation. Intramuscular ephedrine has also been a useful antiemetic agent during the intraoperative and postoperative period, especially when symptoms of low blood pressure accompany nausea and emesis.

Many other medications, especially antihistaminics, phenothiazines, anticholinergics, and transdermal scopolamine, are also used for antiemetic prophylaxis before outpatient surgery. Their effectiveness is variable, and all seem to have undesirable side effects. Nonpharmacological methods such as acupuncture and acupressure have been advocated for PONV, but their effectiveness has not been established in any large study.

Box 6-16 Anticholinergic Premedicants

Atropine
    0.4 to 0.6 intramuscularly or intravenously; causes tachycardia, crosses blood-brain barrier, possible central cholinergic syndrome
Scopolamine
    0.4 to 0.6 mg intramuscularly or intravenously; has prolonged sedative and amnesic effect; postoperative agitation is common in older adults because of its central effect; should not be used for outpatient surgery
Glycopyrrolate
    0.2 to 0.3 mg intravenously or intramuscularly; does not cross the blood-brain barrier; causes less tachycardia than atropine

---

Anticholinergic Premedicants

Anticholinergics (e.g., atropine, scopolamine, and glycopyrrolate) are sometimes used to dry oral and airway secretions, especially when difficult airway intubation is anticipated (Box 6-16). Scopolamine should be avoided in outpatient surgery because of its long onset of action and prolonged sedative and anterograde amnesic effect. When drying of oral secretions is desired, glycopyrrolate, a quaternary amine compound, is a better choice because it does not cross the blood-brain barrier, and because it has no central nervous system effect. It also causes less tachycardia than does atropine. Drying agents must be given about 30 minutes before the intended time of effect, usually in the holding room. In the pediatric population, atropine may be used as prophylaxis against bradycardia, which is particularly common after administration of succinylcholine. When atropine (10 to 20 µg/kg) is utilized preoperatively for this purpose, it has been shown to be efficacious only when given intravenously immediately before induction. Intravenous atropine has a duration of action of approximately 30 minutes.

Miscellaneous Premedicants

Reduction of anesthetic requirements and provision for intraoperative hemodynamic stability

The secondary goals of premedication are to reduce anesthetic requirements and provide for intraoperative hemodynamic stability. The medications most commonly employed for these purposes are alpha$_2$ adrenergic agonists (e.g., clonidine 5 to 15 µg/kg orally, intramuscularly, or intravenously; dexmedetomidine 0.3 to 0.6 mg/kg).

Histamine receptor blocking agents

A patient with a history of multiple allergies may benefit from pretreatment with a combination of H$_1$ blockers (e.g., diphenhydramine 25 to 50 mg orally, intramuscularly, or intravenously; hydroxyzine 1.0 to 1.5 mg/kg intramuscularly) and H$_2$ blocking agents (ranitidine or famotidine, dosage described previously).

Corticosteriods

The use of small doses of steroids for a short period of time (e.g., dose pack) can suppress the hypothalamic pituitary axis for up to 12 months. It is clear that a patient who requires exogenous corticosteroids for health maintenance may not be able to respond to major stressors (e.g., surgery) and thus replacement steroid therapy may be necessary to prevent intravascular collapse due to adrenal insufficiency. However, it is controversial whether patients undergoing minor surgery need steroid replacement, and what the dosage should be if they do. We believe that patients who have received corticosteroids during the immediate perioperative period and patients on steroid therapy for longer than 1 month within the last 6 months should be considered for preoperative corticosteroid replacement administration. Chapter 3 discusses the relative potencies of the exogenously administered corticosteroids (see Table 3-4). In general, a 70 kg patient should receive an intravenous 100 mg dose of hydrocortisone phosphate before minor procedures. Patients on long-term cortisone or hydrocortisone replacement therapy should either double the dose or increase it by 20 mg the night before surgery, and resume the normal dose on the first postoperative day.[18] For minor operations, this regimen should obviate the need for perioperative intravenous hydrocortisone, although it is highly recommended that hydrocortisone 100 mg be available in the operating room and in the PACU in case of acute adrenal insufficiency.

Selective beta$_2$ agonists

Beta$_2$ agonist nebulizers (e.g., albuterol) are commonly utilized for the management of asthma, chronic bronchitis, exercise-induced bronchospasm, and other medical problems associated with hyperreactive airways. Patients who have respiratory diseases will often report that stressful situations (e.g., surgery), environmental allergens, and temperature changes may exacerbate their symptoms. Even patients who report that they are well controlled with minimal use of nebulizers may become symptomatic during stressful perioperative episodes that predispose them to bronchospasm and laryngospasm. In light of this, these patients should be instructed to continue using their inhalers through the morning of operation and to bring their inhalers to surgery since they may need to self-administer their medication (2 puffs) before induction.

Prophylactic Antibiotics

Preoperative antibiotics are used to prevent infection in the surgical wound and to prevent bacterial endocarditis in patients with certain preexisting cardiac lesions. Antibiotics used to prevent surgical wound infection are usually ordered by the surgical team; however, it is often the anesthesiologist who administers them. Many antibiotics have anesthetic implications, primarily allergic reactions (especially after penicillin), histaminic reactions (e.g., vancomycin), drug interactions (e.g., aminoglycosides with nondepolarizing muscle relaxants).

Prophylaxis against bacterial endocarditis is often the responsibility of the anesthesiologist. Any patient who has an organic cardiac lesion, such as mitral valve prolapse, valvular disease, or rheumatic heart disease, should be considered for antibiotic prophylaxis. According to the recommendations of the American Heart Association, the only patients with mitral valve prolapse who should receive antibiotic prophylaxis are those with valvular regurgitation (Box 6-17).[19] Recommended medications, dosage, and timing are briefly described in Boxes 6-18 to 6-20. With the discharge instructions, a prescription should be given for the remaining antibiotic regimen, and the importance of completing the antibiotic course for preventing endocarditis should be stressed. This is usually done by the surgeon, but the anesthesiologist should make certain that it is done.

Preparation for Anesthesia

General Preparation

The preparation for anesthesia really begins when the anesthesiologist-patient rapport is established. The patient wants

Box 6-17 Endocarditis Prophylaxis Recommendations[19]

Cardiac Conditions That Require Endocarditis Prophylaxis

- Prosthetic cardiac valves
- Previous bacterial endocarditis
- Most congenital cardiac malformations
- Rheumatic and other acquired valvular dysfunction, even after surgery
- Hypertrophic cardiomyopathy
- Mitral valve prolapse with valvular regurgitation

Surgical Procedures That Require Endocarditis Prophylaxis

- Tonsillectomy and/or adenoidectomy
- Surgical operations that involve intestinal or respiratory mucosa
- Rigid bronchoscopy
- Sclerotherapy for esophageal varices
- Esophageal dilation
- Cystoscopy
- Urethral dilation
- Urethral catheterization, if urinary tract infection is present
- Urinary tract surgery, if urinary tract infection is present
- Prostatic surgery
- Incision and drainage of infected tissue
- Dental procedures likely to cause gingival or mucosal bleeding

Procedures That May Not Require Endocarditis Prophylaxis

- Injection of local intraoral anesthetic
- Tympanostomy tube insertion
- Endotracheal intubation
- Flexible bronchoscopy
- Endoscopy
- Dental procedures not likely to induce gingival bleeding

Box 6-18 *Standard Prophylactic Regimen Recommendations for Dental, Oral, or Upper Airway Procedures in Adult Patients at Risk*[19]

Standard Regimen

| Amoxicillin | 3.0 g orally, 1 hour before procedure; 1.5 g 6 hours after initial dose |

In Amoxicillin/Penicillin-Allergic Patients

| Erythromycin | Erythromycin ethyl succinate 800 mg, or erythromycin stearate 1.0 g orally 2 hours before procedure; then half the dose 6 hours after the initial dose |

or

| Clindamycin | 300 mg orally 1 hour before procedure; then 150 mg 6 hours after the initial dose |

Box 6-19 *Alternate Prophylaxis Regimen for Adult Patients Unable to Take Oral Medications*[19]

Standard Regimen

Ampicillin: 2.0 g intravenously or intramuscularly 30 minutes before procedure, then amoxicillin 1.0 g orally, 6 hours after initial dose

Ampicillin/Amoxicillin/Penicillin-Allergic Patients

Clindamycin: 300 mg intravenously 30 minutes before the procedure; then 150 mg orally, 6 hours after the initial dose

Patients Who Are Considered High Risk

Ampicillin, gentamicin, and amoxicillin: Ampicillin 2.0 g intravenously and gentamicin 1.5 mg/kg (not to exceed 80 mg) 30 minutes prior to procedure; then amoxicillin 1.5 g orally 6 hours after the initial dose (Alternatively, the parenteral dose may be repeated 8 hours later.)

Ampicillin/Amoxicillin/Penicillin-Allergic Patients

Vancomycin 1 g infused intravenously over 1 hour starting 1 hour before procedure; no repeated dose necessary

---

Box 6-20 *Prophylaxis Regimen for Genitourinary and Gastrointestinal Procedures in Adults*[19]

Standard Regimen

Ampicillin, gentamicin, and amoxicillin
    Ampicillin 3 g intravenously plus gentamicin 1.5 mg/kg (not to exceed 80 mg), then amoxicillin 1.5 g orally 6 hours after initial dose (Alternatively, the parenteral regimen can be repeated 8 hours after the initial dose.)

Ampicillin/Amoxicillin/Penicillin-Allergic Patients

Vancomycin and gentamicin
    Vancomycin 1.0 g infused intravenously over 1 hour, plus gentamicin 1.5 mg/kg (not to exceed 80 mg), 1 hour before procedure; may be repeated 8 hours after initial dose

Alternate Low-Risk Patient Regimen

Amoxicillin
    3 g orally 1 hour before procedure; then 1.5 g 6 hours after initial dose

---

to feel that he or she is being well cared for and is safe from harm, while the anesthesiologist has the responsibility of providing this care and protecting to the best of his or her abilities. This requires that the anesthesiologist be thorough and vigilant about setting up the work environment (e.g., medication preparation) by confirming the proper functioning of the anesthetic equipment. This attention to detail is critical whether a local, regional, or general anesthetic technique is planned.

Intravenous Access and EMLA Cream

Intravenous access should be obtained in all but the rare patient undergoing ambulatory surgery, regardless of the anesthetic technique that is selected. A catheter connected to intravenous fluids should be used to provide hydration to compensate for the preoperative fast. Most adult patients will require at least 6 ml/kg of intravenous fluids during the preinduction period. Acceptable intravenous fluids include Lactated Ringer's, normal saline, and Normosol. Diabetics may need dextrose-containing salt solutions. Patients receiving a central regional blockade (i.e., spinal or epidural) will require up to 1 liter of intravenous crystalloid fluid before proceeding with the introduction of the local anesthetic. The size of the intravenous catheter in an adult patient should be at minimum a 20-gauge angiocatheter, but optimally, an 18-gauge catheter. In very brief procedures (e.g., breast biopsy) even a butterfly needle may be appropriate for intravenous access. Ideally the catheter should be placed in the nondominant upper extremity away from the elbow joint. Discomfort that commonly accompanies insertion of the catheter can be minimized by prior intradermal infiltration of lidocaine using a tuberculin syringe with a 30-gauge needle.

One of the major advances in the intravenous induction of anesthesia in the pediatric population has been the introduction of EMLA (eutectic mixture of local anesthetic). EMLA has made venous cannulation virtually painless. It has been particularly useful in pediatrics,[20] but it is also being used in the adult population. EMLA cream is applied to the skin surface overlying the anticipated venipuncture site. For EMLA to be effective, it must be applied to the skin under an occlusive dressing for at least 60 minutes.

The Anesthetic Plan

The next step is the initiation of the anesthetic plan as discussed previously with the patient. The choice of appropriate technique is determined by anesthesiologist recommendation and patient preference. For instance, some patients may absolutely refuse a regional or MAC (monitored anesthesia care) for a procedure (e.g., breast biopsy) that is easily managed by these techniques, and their wishes for general anesthesia should be respected and accepted if general anesthesia is safe. Likewise some patients will request regional anesthetic techniques for surgical sites that are not usually done under regional blockade (e.g., diagnostic laparoscopy with laser), or the patient may not be a candidate for regional block or MAC because of a coexisting disease process.

The major difference between general anesthesia and regional anesthetic techniques or MAC is the level of consciousness. For regional techniques, peripheral (e.g., ankle block) or conduction blockade (e.g., subarachnoid or epidural block) of the surgical site is provided. Like regional anesthesia techniques, MAC procedures use minimal sedation to keep the patient comfortable while maintaining the level of consciousness. However, MAC procedures depend upon the surgeon infiltrating the surgical site with local anesthetic. General anesthesia renders the patient unconscious for the intraoperative events. Common anesthetic techniques for outpatient procedures are discussed in Chapter 2. Despite the differences between general, regional, and MAC anesthetic techniques, they all require the anesthesiologist to ensure an adequate airway, so that general anesthesia may be induced if necessary. Therefore, the routine preparation for all anesthetic techniques is the same, i.e., preparation for a possible general anesthetic.

Equipment and Monitoring

The current recommendations for anesthetic machine, equipment, and medication check-out are briefly described in Box 6-21. Box 6-22 is a modification of the American Society of Anesthesiologist standards for basic intraoperative monitoring.[21] It describes the basic intraoperative monitoring checklist that should be completed before the induction of anesthesia. Pediatric equipment is described in Chapter 5.

Airway Management

Face Mask

General anesthesia without tracheal intubation can be provided for many outpatient surgeries, including dilatation and curettage, cone biopsy, perineal operations, orthopedic or general surgery on extremities and trunk, inguinal hernia repair, and hydrocele operations. During these operations, the airway can usually be managed via an appropriate size face mask and possibly with an oropharyngeal (Guedel) or a nasopharyngeal airway.

Tracheal Intubation

The indications of tracheal intubation during outpatient surgery are listed in Box 6-23.

Airway management under special circumstances

The endotracheal tube is most commonly inserted orally. However, there are many other endotracheal tube options as well as methods of insertion. For many surgical procedures (e.g., oral surgery), nasal endotracheal intubation may be necessary so that adequate surgical access can be provided. For laser ENT procedures additional preparation is necessary because the anesthesiologist

Box 6-21 Standard Anesthesia Machine, Equipment, and Medications

Standard Anesthetic Machine Check

- Attach an anesthetic breathing system with a properly sized face mask, and confirm the ability to provide positive pressure ventilation of the lungs with oxygen.
- Check anesthetic breathing system valves.
- Calibrate oxygen analyzer with air and oxygen, and set alarm.
- Check soda lime for color changes and liquid level of vaporizers.
- Confirm function of mechanical ventilator and audible disconnect alarm.
- Confirm availability of end-tidal CO_2 monitor.
- Confirm availability and function of wall suction.
- Check position of flowmeters, vaporizer, and monitor (alarm) settings.

Standard Drugs Available for Any Anesthetic Technique

- Lidocaine
- Propofol or barbiturate
- Atropine
- Catecholamine to treat an allergic reaction (epinephrine) and a sympathomimetic
- Depolarizing (succinylcholine) and nondepolarizing muscle relaxant
- Antagonist for muscle relaxants (anticholinesterase) and narcotics (e.g., naloxone)

Standard Equipment

- Angiocatheter for vascular cannulation and intravenous fluid with connecting tubing
- Suction catheter
- Oral (No. 3 to 5) and/or nasal airway (No. 28 to 34) with lidocaine lubricant to ease insertion
- Face masks of assorted sizes
- Laryngeal mask airways of assorted sizes
- Laryngoscope (MAC 3 is the most commonly used, but other sizes and makes may be necessary depending upon the circumstances.)
- Endotracheal tube (6.5 to 8.0 mm for women, and 8.0 to 9.0 mm for men) with lubricated stylet available
- Latex gloves

Box 6-22 Checklist Before the Induction of All Anesthetics

- Intravenous access
- Oxygen analyzer present and inspired oxygen measured
- Pulse oximeter placed for continuous monitoring
- ECG placed for continuous evaluation
- Blood pressure cuff placed and cycled at least every 5 minutes
- Peripheral nerve stimulator placed (only for general anesthesia with muscle relaxants)
- Capability to auscultate breath and cardiac sounds
- Temperature monitoring capabilities available
- Baseline ECG, blood pressure, pulse rate, and pulse oximetry data recorded

---

Box 6-23 Indications for Tracheal Intubation During Outpatient Surgery

---

- Allow easier surgical access (e.g., operations in the head and neck area)
- Secure the airway where an existing anatomic problem or the operative procedure may compromise the airway when the patient is anesthetized (e.g., operation in the airway, anatomic abnormality of head and neck)
- Protect the airway where pulmonary aspiration is probable (e.g., patients considered to have a full stomach, diabetics, pregnant patients, operation in the oropharynx, increased intraabdominal pressure as in laparoscopic procedures)
- Provide surgical relaxation by using a neuromuscular blocking agent (e.g., laparoscopic procedure, laparotomy, or thoracoscopy)
- Where controlled ventilation is necessary (e.g., intrathoracic or intracranial procedure)

and the surgeon must share the same airway, and because there is a potential for airway fire. Under these special circumstances, a metal, a wrapped metal, or an impregnated endotracheal tube should be considered. Although red rubber endotracheal tubes are less flammable than the polyvinyl chloride endotracheal tubes, they are more flammable than the other materials and should not be used unless wrapped with metal. Additional measures to diminish the risk of fire include injecting saline or lidocaine into the endotracheal cuff.

Laryngeal Mask Airway (LMA)

With the recent introduction of the laryngeal mask airway (LMA), we now have an alternative method to manage the airway during outpatient anesthesia. Laryngeal mask airway (LMA), developed by Dr. A. I. J. Brain of Britain, is a boat-shaped miniature face mask that is attached to a short endotracheal tube (Fig. 6-1).[22] The mask, when properly placed and inflated with air, sits directly on the laryngeal inlet. The distal end of the tube is connected to the anesthetic circuit. The LMA is made entirely of surgical silicone, which can be resterilized many times by autoclaving. The LMA is usually placed blindly into the mouth of either a deeply anesthetized patient or a topically anesthetized awake patient.

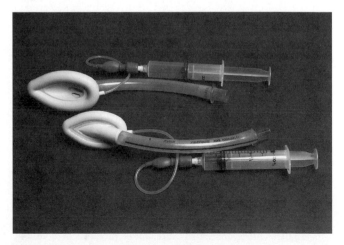

Fig. 6-1 Laryngeal mask airway (LMA).

In general, there are three indications for LMA: (1) in the spontaneously breathing anesthetized patient, in place of a face mask; (2) in place of an endotracheal tube, as long as the inflation pressure is not more than 20 cm of water when ventilation is controlled; and (3) in the patient who has an expected or unexpected difficult airway or tracheal intubation that requires management. The major concern with LMA is that it does not protect against gastric regurgitation and pulmonary aspiration. Thus, LMA should not be used (1) where gastric regurgitation and pulmonary aspiration is probable, and (2) where controlled ventilation is likely to require a high-inflation pressure, more than 20 cm H_2O, e.g., bronchospastic disease or morbid obesity (Box 6-24).

LMA is supplied in five sizes, 1, 2, 2.5, 3, and 4. The smaller three sizes (Nos. 1, 2, and 2.5) are for pediatric use; No. 3 is suitable for small adults and No. 4 for average and large adults. Because propofol tends to relax the jaw and pharyngeal muscles better than thiopental, deep propofol anesthesia is ideal for the insertion of a LMA. After testing the LMA for leaks and fully deflating the cuff, the posterior aspect of the appropriate size LMA is lubricated with a water-soluble lubricant. The LMA can be inserted either after an adequate general anesthesia (more common), or after a good topical anesthesia of the mouth and the upper airway. The patient may be completely anesthetized with propofol or volatile anesthetic and placed in the classical supine "sniffing" position. The LMA is then inserted into the mouth blindly in the midline, with concavity forward, by pressing on the anterior shaft with the tip of the index finger toward the hard palate and guiding it toward the pharynx. When the upper esophageal sphincter is reached, a characteristic resistance is felt. Depending on the size of LMA, the cuff is inflated with 10 to 30 ml of air, and then the tube is attached to the anesthetic circuit. A No. 3 LMA requires 20 ml, and a No. 4 LMA requires 30 ml of air for cuff inflation. Alternatively, especially in children, the LMA may be inserted back-to-front (i.e., like insertion of a Guedel airway), with the cuff either partially inflated or deflated, and then turned counterclockwise 180 degrees while advancing it in the hypopharynx. End tidal CO_2 should be observed in the monitor, either as the patient breathes spontaneously or on gentle intermittent positive pressure ventilation. Anesthesia can then be maintained either with a continuous infusion of propofol or a volatile anesthetic agent. At the end of the operation, the LMA may be left in place until the patient is awake; this prevents aspiration of

---

Box 6-24 Outpatient Surgery LMA Indications and Contraindications

---

Indications

- In spontaneously breathing patients, in place of face mask or endotracheal tube
- In place of endotracheal tube, during controlled ventilation, as long as the inflation pressure does not exceed 20 cm H_2O
- To manage an expected or unexpected airway management problem, e.g., difficult intubation

Contraindications

- When gastric regurgitation and pulmonary aspiration is probable
- When controlled ventilation is likely to require high inflation pressure (more than 20 cm H_2O), e.g., bronchospastic disease, morbid obesity

---

accumulated pharyngeal secretions. However, it should be remembered that regurgitation of stomach contents and pulmonary aspiration are possible while the LMA is in place, especially when the patient is waking up and coughs and bucks.

Innumerable case reports and anecdotes have been published where LMA has been a lifesaver in cases of expected or unexpected airway failure. In such a situation, the LMA may be used either in place of an endotracheal tube, or a 6.0 mm endotracheal tube may be inserted (blindly or with the help of a fiberoptic bronchoscope) in the trachea through the lumen of the LMA after the LMA has already been placed. Accordingly, an entire set of LMAs should be available during general anesthesia for outpatient surgery.

This alternative form of airway management offers many potential benefits for outpatients having surgery. In patients who do not need an endotracheal intubation, the LMA provides more reliable airway control than does the face mask, and it frees up the anesthesiologist's hands. In cases where it is used as an alternative to an endotracheal tube, there are less hemodynamic alterations. Whether the LMA causes less airway trauma or sore throat is still debatable. Nevertheless, the use of LMA in outpatient anesthetic practice is likely to increase.

Summary

Adequate preoperative preparation of the adult patient starts when the patient is scheduled for surgery, and continues until the actual performance of the procedure. Fasting requirements have been modified for children and appropriately selected adults, and changes are being adopted regularly. Identifying the use of chronic medications (e.g., cardiac, diabetic, pulmonary) is important so that the homeostasis of the patient's physiological condition can be maintained during the perioperative period. Patients are generally contacted the day before surgery to give final instructions, to update their medical status, to answer unanswered questions, and to provide reassurance. Regardless of the method of preoperative evaluation, the anesthesiologist will need to perform a final assessment of the patient on the day of the procedure. Preoperative medication can be used in the ambulatory period. Agents with rapid onset, short duration, and minimal side effects should be selected. Midazolam, both in adults and pediatric patients, is the benzodiazepine of choice for preoperative medication. Analgesic premedicants with opiates or with nonsteroidal antiinflammatory agents may be useful in reducing perioperative analgesic requirements. Because the risk of acid aspiration is low, only selected patients at risk should receive prophylactic treatments with H_2 antagonists, gastrokinetics, or nonparticulate antacids. Additionally, routine prophylaxis against PONV is neither cost-effective or desirable. Strategies to prevent PONV are discussed. Occasionally some patients may need preoperative preparation with histamine-blocking agents, corticosteroids, or prophylactic antibiotics for protection of the surgical wound and bacterial endocarditis. Recommendations are discussed. Preoperative preparation must also include anesthetic machine, equipment, and medication check-outs following the ASA Recommendations for intraoperative monitoring. The availability of the LMA has expanded options for airway management in outpatient surgery; however, it does not protect against gastric regurgitation and pulmonary aspiration. The LMA may offer many potential benefits for outpatients in reducing sore throat, and in preventing complications of laryngoscopy and muscle relaxants.

References

1. Agarwal A, Chari P, Singh H: Fluid deprivation before operation: the effects of a small drink. Anaesthesia 1989; 44:632-4.
2. Green CR, Pandit SK, Schork MA, Wayne VW: Current NPO trends in the United States: results of a national survey. Anesthesiology 1993; 79:A1088.
3. Goresky GV, Maltby JR: Fasting guidelines for elective surgical patients. Can J Anaesth 1990; 37:493-5.
4. Stack CG, Rogers P, Linter SPK: Monoamine oxidase inhibitors and anesthesia. Br J Anaesth 1988; 60:222-7.
5. Egbert LD, Battit GE, Turndorf H, Beecher HK: The value of the preoperative visit by an anesthetist: a study of doctor-patient rapport. JAMA 1963; 185:553-5.
6. Twersky RS, Lebovits AH, Lewis M, Frank D: Early anesthesia evaluation of the ambulatory surgical patient: does it really help? J Clin Anesth 1992; 4:204-7.
7. McCleane GJ, Cooper R: The nature of pre-operative anxiety. Anesthesia 1990; 45:153-5.
8. Shafer A, White PF, Urquhart ML, Doze VA: Outpatient premedication: use of midazolam and opioid analgesics. Anesthesiology 1989; 71:495-501.
9. Philip BK: Hazards of amnesia after midazolam in ambulatory surgical patients. Anesth Analg 1987; 66:97-8.
10. Twersky RS, Hartung J, Berger BJ et al: Midazolam enhances anterograde but not retrograde amnesia in pediatric patients. Anesthesiology 1993; 78:51-5.
11. Pandit SK, Kothary SP: Intravenous narcotics for premedication in outpatient anesthesia. Acta Anaesthesiol Scand 1989; 33:353-8.
12. Aanta R, Kanto J, Scheinin M et al: Dexmedetomidine, an alpha$_2$ agonist, reduces anesthetic requirements for patients undergoing minor gynecologic surgery. Anesthesiology, 1990; 73:230-5.
13. Federated Ambulatory Surgery Association: FASA special study I, Alexandria, Va, 1986, FASA.
14. Wright DJ, Pandya A: Smoking and gastric juice volume in outpatients. Can Anaesth Soc J 1979; 26:328-30.
15. Pandit SK, Kothary SP, Pandit UA, Mirakhur RK: Premedication with cimetidine and metoclopramide: effect on the risk factors of acid aspiration. Anesthesia 1986; 41:486-92.

16. Pandit SK, Kothary SP, Pandit UA et al: Dose-response study of droperidol and metoclopramide as antiemetics for outpatient anesthesia. Anesth Analg 1989; 68:798-802.
17. Berghuis PA, Gortiski WJ, Mandell DK et al: Comparison of ondasetron, ephedrine and droperidol for treatment of postoperative nausea and vomiting. Anesthesiology 1993; 79:A7.
18. Byyny RL: Preventing adrenal insufficiency during surgery. Postgrad Med 1980; 67:219-25.
19. Dajani AS, Bisno AL, Chun KJ et al: Prevention of bacterial endocarditis: recommendations by the American Heart Association. JAMA 1990; 264:2919-22.
20. Soliman IE, Broadman LM, Hannallah RS, McGill WA: Comparison of the analgesic effects of EMLA (eutectic mixture of local anesthetics) to intradermal lidocaine infiltration prior to venous cannulation in unpremeditated children. Anesthesiology 1988; 68:804-6.
21. ASA: Standards for basic anesthetic monitoring. Approved by House of Delegates in October 1986. Amended on October 13, 1993.
22. Brain AJ: Development of laryngeal mask—a brief history of the invention, early clinical studies and experimental work from which the laryngeal mask evolved. Euro J Anaesthesiol 1991; Suppl 4:5-17.

General Anesthesia 7

Beverly K. Philip

General anesthesia techniques are commonly used to provide anesthesia for ambulatory surgery. While it may appear easy to provide an acceptable outcome for ambulatory patients, it is considerably more difficult to provide an excellent outcome. To provide this higher level of care, one must first define the specific needs of the ambulatory patient and then tailor a general

203

anesthetic plan to meet those needs. These needs begin with efficient anesthesia practice: a rapid induction and a prompt awakening
timed to match the end of surgery. The maintenance phase of
anesthesia must be adequate to control physiologic responses and
to interfere with patient memory, but excess depth must be avoided
so as not to prolong awakening or recovery. The recovery period
should be as brief as possible, and be associated with minimal
postanesthetic sequelae, such as sore throat, nausea, dizziness, and
headache.[1] The anesthesia should also enable the patient to return
rapidly to normal activities, with minimal reliance on postanesthesia staff or support at home.

General anesthesia should be specifically tailored for ambulatory
surgery by choosing the appropriate anesthetic agents and using
them correctly. When deciding whether to incorporate any particular agent in the armamentarium for ambulatory anesthesia, certain
criteria should be met. These desiderata have not changed appreciably in the last decade.[2] Anesthetic agents should provide rapid,
smooth, pleasant induction; minimal or no excitement; readily
controllable depth; no increase in secretions; rapid, smooth, pleasant
emergence; minimal nausea or vomiting; rapid return to rational
behavior; and early return to appropriate status of ambulation.

Induction of Anesthesia

(Preoperative preparation and premedication have been discussed
in Chapter 6.)

Induction of general anesthesia in ambulatory patients should
aim for the same patient goals given above. These goals can be
reached either through the use of an inhalation induction or, more
often, an intravenous induction, and both are successful if used
appropriately. With either technique, it is important that the
patients be told about the events they will experience during the
induction sequence, because it is this portion of anesthesia they
are likely to remember.[3A] Several intravenous induction agents are
available for clinical ambulatory use (Table 7-1).

Thiopental

Sodium thiopental is a thiobarbiturate available in a 2.5% solution, with a pH between 10 and 11. This alkaline pH is
responsible for the pain experienced during intravenous injection.
Extravasation of thiopental may cause tissue necrosis; intraarterial

Table 7-1   Pharmacokinetics of Intravenous Induction Agents[3B-5]

	Distribution half life (minutes)	Elimination half life (hours)	Clearance (ml/kg/min)	Volume of distribution (l/kg)
Thiopental	2-8	5-12	3.4-3.6	1.5-2.5
Methohexital	5-6	2-4	10.9-12.1	1.1-2.2
Midazolam	7-10	2-4	4.0-8.0	1.1-1.8
Etomidate	2-4	2-5	11.5-25.0	2.3-4.5
Ketamine	11-17	2-3	17.5-19.1	2.5-5.0
Propofol	2-8 (fast) 34-64 (slow)	3-11	24.0-33.0	2.5-5.0

injection may result in thiopental crystal formation and local norepinephrine release—which may culminate in thrombosis and severe ischemia of the extremity. Therapy for intraarterial injection involves intravascular dilution and perivascular infiltration with local anesthetic, sympathetic block of the extremity to reduce vasoconstrictor tone, and anticoagulation with heparin.[2] The high pH of this drug solution also causes it to precipitate easily when mixed with other, more acidic anesthetic agents.

Thiopental is used to induce anesthesia in doses of 3 to 6 mg/kg, with the higher doses for the young, healthy, unpremedicated patient. A single bolus of 2.6 mg/kg produced sleep lasting for 120 seconds in volunteers; 5 minutes later they were able to walk and answer questions.[6] However, larger doses lead to a prolonged recovery time. A 4 mg/kg loading dose, with a 428 mg infusion for a 21-minute procedure, resulted in recovery times of 10 minutes until awakening, 20 minutes until orientation, and 1.9 hours until fit for discharge. Initial awakening after thiopental is due to redistribution from the brain,[7] rather than to metabolism and excretion. In obese patients, the dose (per kg) should be approximately 15% less than that in thin or muscular individuals, because of the smaller proportion of lean body weight in these individuals.[8]

Induction and recovery from anesthesia with thiopental are smooth, and the drug is associated with minimal side effects. Thiopental lowers myocardial stroke volume and cardiac output, with dilation of capacitance vessels. Thiopental, like other barbiturates, does not sensitize the myocardium to catecholamines. Thiopental is a respiratory depressant that causes decreased tidal volume, and brief periods of apnea may occur after larger, induction doses. Intraocular pressure is reduced after thiopental.[9]

Methohexital

Methohexital is an oxybarbiturate available in a 1% solution with an alkaline pH of 10.6. Methohexital is approximately 2.5 times as potent as thiopental. Induction is rapid, but it is associated with side effects, including cough and hiccup in 28% of patients, and tremors and involuntary muscle movements in 38% of patients.[10] This can be reduced by the prior administration of a small amount of opioid.

Methohexital has been compared with thiopental for induction and recovery. Comparing kinetic parameters, the distribution half lives are similar after a single intravenous bolus of either agent.[11] However, the drugs differ in their clearance and elimination half lives, with methohexital's much shorter half life due to its greater hepatic clearance. Recovery after methohexital 0.88 mg/kg or thiopental 2.5 mg/kg has been compared using clinical indices and a driving stimulator.[6] Seventy-eight percent of the methohexital subjects had completely recovered by 35 minutes after injection, whereas only 34% of the thiopental subjects had recovered. Recovery of fine motor coordination after methohexital 2 mg/kg required 45 to 90 minutes, compared with 105 to 210 minutes after thiopental 5 mg/kg.[12] Despite its minor side effects, methohexital appears preferable to thiopental whenever more rapid recovery from anesthesia is desired, and particularly when large doses are used.

Midazolam

Midazolam is a unique benzodiazepine, for it is available in an aqueous formulation; its water solubility is a property due to the opening of its diazepine ring at pH less than 4.0.[13] Midazolam is most commonly used for premedication and intraoperative sedation, but it may also be used as an induction agent for general anesthesia in ambulatory surgery. Doses of 0.2 to 0.35 mg/kg will produce sleep within 2 minutes. This induction time can be shortened by the preadministration of an opioid, but it remains significantly longer than that of the barbiturate induction agents. Loss of consciousness with midazolam should be confirmed both by the inability to open eyes on command, as well as by the loss of the lash reflex. There is a wide variability in induction dose requirements. Both dose requirement and dose variability are decreased in the elderly.

The use of midazolam as an induction agent in the ambulatory setting is limited by its relatively long effects. After doses of 0.2 mg/kg for ambulatory laparoscopy, awakening can be achieved within 20 minutes.[14] However, recovery is prolonged compared with that of thiopental. Times to awakening, orientation, ambulation, and return of cognitive functioning are significantly longer with midazolam than with thiopental.[15] A period of postoperative amnesia may also occur; caution must be observed not to give discharge instructions during this time. The use of midazolam as an induction agent for ambulatory surgery patients should be reserved for longer cases where its residual effects will have time to dissipate.

Flumazenil, a specific benzodiazepine receptor antagonist, can reverse the central nervous system effects of therapeutic benzodiazepines in a dose-related fashion.[15] Flumazenil is effective in reversing residual sedation after benzodiazepine-induced general anesthesia, as well as after excess benzodiazepine sedation. Intraoperative amnesia generated by a benzodiazepine is retained when postoperative amnesia is terminated by the use of flumazenil. Flumazenil can also reverse or prevent the benzodiazepine component of apnea induced by midazolam-opioid combinations. However, doses adequate to reverse sedation (the usual clinical endpoint) may be inadequate to completely reverse respiratory depressant effects or amnesia.[16] The half life of flumazenil is approximately 1 hour, compared with 2.5 hours for midazolam. The potential for resedation exists, and resedation has occurred after larger doses of benzodiazepine. If significant resedation occurs, it is usually seen by 1 hour after administration of the antagonist.[17] Flumazenil may be given in 0.2 mg increments until the desired level of awakening is reached, to a maximum total dose of 1 mg. Flumazenil can be used to awaken patients after midazolam-induced general anesthesia,[14] and although they can then be cared for in less intensive recovery settings, patients should not be discharged prematurely before the effect of flumazenil has worn off.

Etomidate

Etomidate is an imidazole compound solubilized with propylene glycol. It is used in doses of 0.2 to 0.4 mg/kg. Etomidate causes no significant cardiovascular effects, respiratory depression, or histamine release. Times to induction and to awakening are similar to those of thiopental.[18] Recovery using psychomotor tests is comparable to that after thiopental; however, both are longer than that after methohexital. Disadvantages of etomidate administration include involuntary muscle movement (70%), severe pain on injection (50%), and high incidence of postoperative nausea and vomiting (PONV) (55%, compared with 15% after thiopental). Coadministration of lidocaine or preadministration of an opioid may decrease the injection pain. Etomidate is also associated with a transient suppression of adrenal steroidogenesis for 4 to 8 hours.[19] Although etomidate may be useful with those ambulatory patients for whom cardiovascular stability is imperative, its general use for ambulatory anesthesia is uncertain.

Ketamine

Ketamine is a phencyclidine derivative that can be used for induction at a dose of 1 to 2 mg/kg. Ketamine is also effective when given intramuscularly at a dose of 2 to 4 mg/kg. Anesthesia with ketamine is associated with adequate airway tone, adequate ventilation, somatic analgesia, and a dissociated mental state. Ketamine causes sympathetic nervous system stimulation, with a rise in blood pressure, intracranial pressure, and heart rate. However, the use of ketamine for ambulatory surgery patients is limited by its psychomimetic and other side effects that may persist after discharge. Compared with thiopental, ketamine is associated with more dreams and more unpleasant dreams, as well as a higher incidence of nausea, vomiting, headache, and dizziness.[20] The use of ancillary sedatives, especially benzodiazepines, can ameliorate the psychomimetic effects, but recovery may be prolonged, and sedatives do not eliminate the other undesired side effects that persist after discharge. Ketamine is a useful adjunct for the care of uncooperative mentally handicapped patients, but it should only be used with specific indications in the routine adult ambulatory surgery patient.

Propofol

Propofol is an alkyl phenol compound that is insoluble in water and formulated as a lipid emulsion of soybean oil, glycerol, and egg phosphatide. Studies with the earlier formulation in Cremophor-EL demonstrated a high incidence of anaphylactoid reactions; the current product rarely causes allergic reactions and may be given to patients with egg (protein) allergy. Doses of 2.0 to 2.5 mg/kg are used to induce anesthesia in healthy adults. A larger induction dose of 2.5 to 3.5 mg/kg is required in children.[21-25] The adult dose should be reduced by 25% to 50% in elderly or debilitated patients to avoid the most prominent side effect: hypotension. Propofol causes cardiovascular depression by a combination of direct myocardial effects and vasodilation. Heart rates are low because of depression of the baroreceptor reflex and decreased sympathetic outflow.[26] The concurrent administration of propofol with the "fentanils" (fentanyl, sufentanil, alfentanil, remifentanil, and newer synthetic compounds) or with succinylcholine has resulted in severe bradycardia.[27] The cardiovascular effects of propofol are more pronounced in older patients. Propofol also causes greater suppression of airway reflexes than does thiopental, which permits better toleration of endotracheal and laryngeal mask intubation.[28] The incidence of prolonged (longer than 60 seconds) apnea after induction of sleep is greater with propofol than with the barbiturates,[29] which must be kept in mind when preservation of spontaneous ventilation is an anesthetic goal. Another common side effect is pain on injection, which can be reduced by coadministration of lidocaine or injection into a large vein.[30]

Propofol has achieved widespread popularity as an induction agent for ambulatory anesthesia for three prominent reasons: one is that its effect dissipates rapidly. The pharmacokinetics of propofol follow a three-compartment model with rapid-phase and slower-phase distribution half lives; it is the former that is associated with initial patient awakening. Propofol also has a clearance rate that is greater than hepatic blood flow, implying nonhepatic clearance sites, such as the lung. Because propofol has high lipid solubility, the potential for accumulation in fatty tissue exists and may contribute to delayed recovery after prolonged administration. The elimination half life of this drug is very long and increases after extended administration, but it represents less than 1% of a drug dose. The pharmacokinetic promise of propofol has been borne out in clinical recovery data. Compared with thiopental, time to eye opening and time to date-of-birth response were significantly faster with propofol, 4.8 ± 0.45 minutes vs. 9.6 ± 0.74 minutes, and 5.8 ± 0.34 vs. 10.6 ± 0.74 minutes, respectively.[31]

Postoperative side effects such as headache and drowsiness were also less with propofol. With propofol, in a total dose of 3.0 mg/kg, instead of thiopental 7.0 mg/kg, the time to respond was reduced from 18.0 ± 6.2 minutes to 13.9 ± 2.6 minutes, and the time to stand steadily was reduced from 62.0 ± 29.0 to 33.0 ± 6.9 minutes. Psychomotor test performance remained below control for 5 hours for propofol, as compared with 1 hour for thiopental.[32] However, the time to initial awakening is similar after single doses of propofol or methohexital.[33] In pediatric patients, induction (3.0 mg/kg) and maintenance of anesthesia (50 to 150 µg/kg/min) with propofol, as compared with those with thiopental/halothane, resulted in faster recovery and discharge.[34,35]

The second reason for widespread use of propofol is its lower incidence of postoperative nausea. Propofol/nitrous oxide anesthesia, as compared with thiopental/isoflurane, resulted in more patients having no emesis and a decrease in the time to tolerate oral fluids.[36] It may be particularly useful in procedures prone to produce postoperative vomiting.[37,38] Propofol appears to have direct antiemetic effect, even at subhypnotic doses.[39,40] The third reason for its widespread use is the high degree of patient satisfaction, due to the rapid return to a clear-headed state, minimal side effects, and elation produced by the drug.[41]

Maintenance

Nitrous Oxide

Nitrous oxide is a commonly used component of general anesthesia. Although it is an incomplete anesthetic if used alone, it reduces the needed concentrations of other potent inhaled agents in a direct MAC-additive fashion. It also reduces the need for other concomitantly administered intravenous anesthetics, and thus its administration results in fewer side effects from those drugs. Nitrous oxide has a low blood gas solubility; therefore, both induction and emergence with this agent are rapid (Table 7-2). Uptake of nitrous oxide is aided by the concentration effect. When nitrous oxide is given in high concentrations, its uptake from the alveoli results in an augmented inspired volume. In a similar fashion, nitrous oxide increases the uptake of other more potent inhaled agents (second gas effect). However, since the MAC of nitrous oxide is high (greater than 100%), overpressure cannot be used to supplement its lack of potency. Induction with nitrous

***Table* 7-2**   Pharmacokinetic Properties of Inhaled Anesthetic Agents[4,5,42]

	MAC (% in oxygen)	Vapor pressure at 20°C (mm Hg)	Partition coefficients at 37°C	
			Blood-gas	Brain-blood
Nitrous oxide	105-110	(Gas)	0.47	1.1
Halothane	0.75	243	2.3	2.6
Enflurane	1.68	175	1.9	1.5
Isoflurane	1.15	250	1.4	2.6
Desflurane	6.0	664	0.42	1.3
Sevoflurane	2.0	160	0.67	1.7

oxide is also limited by the need to simultaneously give adequate inspired concentrations of oxygen.

In addition to low solubility, nitrous oxide has several other advantages: It is nonflammable; easy to deliver (it is a gas); and inexpensive, especially when purchased in bulk. There are several potential disadvantages to the drug. Because nitrous oxide is insoluble and is delivered in high concentrations, it can diffuse readily into gas-containing spaces in the body. This occasionally leads to dilation of distensible gas-filled structures, such as the bowel. However, the relative importance of this effect among other factors that dilate the bowel is unclear. In a blind study of laparoscopic cholecystectomy, there was no difference in the reported bowel distension or operating conditions, and the surgeon was unable to identify whether nitrous oxide or air was being given.[43] Similarly, the use of nitrous oxide is restricted with tympanoplasty procedures. Diffusion of nitrous oxide into the nondistensible, closed middle ear space can increase pressure there and cause the tympanoplasty graft to detach; therefore, nitrous oxide should be discontinued before the graft is placed. Nitrous oxide has little depressant effect on the respiratory or circulatory system. However, it causes direct sympathetic nervous system stimulation,[44] and may ameliorate the cardiodepressant effects of other anesthetic agents.

Controversy exists regarding the contribution of nitrous oxide to PONV. One group of outpatients undergoing minor gynecological

***Table* 7-3**   Pharmacokinetic Properties of Opioids[5,49,50]

	Distribution half life (minute)	Elimination half life (hour)	Clearance (ml/kg/min)	Volume of distribution (l/kg)
Fentanyl	13.4	3.6	11.6	4.2
Sufentanil	17.7	2.7	13.0	1.7
Alfentanil	11.6	1.6	6.4	0.86
Remifentanil	0.94	0.16	41.2	0.39

procedures received fentanyl followed by isoflurane in oxygen and had a 3.2% incidence of nausea and vomiting, whereas the group with a comparable anesthetic and 60% nitrous oxide had a 25% incidence of nausea and vomiting.[45] However, other studies have not found an association between the use of nitrous oxide and the development of PONV.[46,47] Potentially, nitrous oxide could contribute to perioperative nausea and vomiting via gastrointestinal distention or increased middle ear pressure,[48] as well as possible interaction with the endogenous opioid receptor system. However, the effect of nitrous oxide may be outweighed by the many other factors which increase or decrease perioperative nausea and vomiting. Because of its overall utility, beneficial effects, and minimal side effects, nitrous oxide remains widely used.

Opioids

Techniques involving opioids are a mainstay of ambulatory general anesthesia. Timing of administration is important. In general, the opioids should be given early in the procedure to coincide with the timing of maximal surgical and anesthetic stimulation during surgery and anesthesia, and to decrease the amount of time after the operation for the undesired opioid side effects to remit. In general, long-acting opioids should not be used, to avoid prolonged side effects. Comparative pharmacokinetic parameters of opioids appropriate for ambulatory anesthesia are found in Table 7-3; a comparison of effect site concentration simulations will provide additional insight.[51]

In the ambulatory surgery setting, fentanyl is the most commonly used opioid and, because it is available in generic form, the least expensive as well. Fentanyl doses of 1 to 2 µg/kg are recommended for the ambulatory patient. The use of fentanyl compared with halothane as an adjunct to nitrous oxide resulted in less abdominal pain in the facility and, after returning home, without an increase in the frequency of nausea or vomiting.[52] Onset of analgesia after intravenous administration is rapid (within 2 minutes), and duration of analgesia is adequately short, approximately 45 minutes. Unfortunately, the duration of respiratory depression is longer. Respiratory depression requiring ventilatory support with recurrence of somnolence have occurred after 30 minutes to 4 hours in recovery. Doses of 1.3 µg/kg caused depression of the slope of the CO_2 response curve comparable in magnitude and in duration to that caused by 0.12 mg/kg of morphine, with both responses remaining below 80% of control 4 hours after administration.[53] Furthermore, respiratory depression may recur; a fall in CO_2 response slope to less than 50% of control value has been reported 90 minutes to 2 hours after anesthesia with fentanyl.[54] This may be due to reappearance of fentanyl either from gastric juice reabsorbed in the small intestine, or from peripheral sites, such as muscle.

Bradycardia is another side effect of fentanyl. Opioid-induced bradycardia is mediated through stimulation of the central vagal nucleus, and can be seen with all opioids except meperidine. Rigidity is a supraspinal phenomenon that has been reported with many opioids, but it appears to be more common with the fentanils.[55] Rigidity occurs in the chest, extremities, and larynx, and it may interfere with ventilation by bag and mask. Partial glottic rigidity to complete glottic closure have been reported. Moderately high doses of fentanyl (3.9 µg/kg) have caused rigidity in 4% of a series of patients undergoing minor gynecologic surgery.[56] Fentanyl has minimal hemodynamic effect.

Sufentanil is a structurally related opioid with approximately 10 times the potency of fentanyl, and a therapeutic index 100 times that of the older drug. Sufentanil has similar onset and duration of effect as fentanyl, with the typical opioid side effects, when using the small doses (0.25 µg/kg to 0.75 µg/kg) appropriate for an ambulatory surgery patient. Recovery after outpatient arthroscopy using sufentanil 1 µg/kg has been compared with using isoflurane 0.9% as supplements to methohexital/nitrous oxide anesthesia.[57] Time to eye opening was significantly shorter in the sufentanil group, and p-deletion test scores were normalized faster (60 versus 120 minutes). Fewer sufentanil group patients required an analgesic in the PACU (0 versus 3/20), but they experienced more symptoms requiring antiemetic therapy

(9/20 versus 3/20). In a comparison of sufentanil infusion (total dose 13.02 ± 2.35 µg) with fentanyl infusion (93.28 ± 4.88 µg) to supplement thiopental/nitrous oxide for dilatation and curettage, the sufentanil group showed less postoperative nausea and less analgesic need, with similar awakening and discharge time.[58]

Alfentanil is a short-acting analog of fentanyl. Its redistribution half life is slightly shorter than that of fentanyl, but the elimination half life of alfentanil is significantly more rapid, because it has a much smaller volume of distribution. Two factors that contribute to the smaller volume distribution of alfentanil are its lower lipid solubility and its higher protein binding. With alfentanil, the termination of clinical effect is primarily due to drug elimination, and thus the duration of alfentanil effect is less dependent on the size and timing of the dose than with fentanyl.[49]

Intraoperative side effects and clinical recovery times of alfentanil have been compared with those of fentanyl.[59] Patients receiving fentanyl for brief outpatient gynecologic procedures showed a higher incidence of chest wall rigidity and ventilatory depression; those receiving alfentanil showed a higher incidence of mild bradycardia and moderate hypotension, but there was no significant difference in the incidence of PONV, dizziness, or excessive drowsiness. Immediate recovery times (awakening and orientation) were shorter with alfentanil 15 to 40 µg/kg than fentanyl 1.5 to 6 µg/kg.[59,60] In later recovery parameters after larger doses of both drugs (alfentanil 15 µg/kg, or fentanyl 5 µg/kg), the group receiving alfentanil showed faster improvement in times to ambulation and in function at home.[61]

Because of the rapid dissipation of effect, bolus dosing with alfentanil for maintenance of anesthesia causes unstable effects. Ausems and colleagues[62] showed that bolus doses of alfentanil for maintenance of anesthesia produced repeated motor and hemodynamic responses. A preferable technique is to provide alfentanil by continuous variable infusion. For outpatient gynecological procedures, the administration of alfentanil by infusion rather than by intermittent bolus resulted in lower average opioid doses utilized, less intraoperative respiratory depression and muscular rigidity, and significantly shorter times for awakening and orientation.[59]

Alfentanil has typical opioid side effects. Respiratory depression occurs but is briefer than after fentanyl. The mean plasma alfentanil concentration at which spontaneous respiration resumes after anesthesia has been determined to be 226 ± 10 ng/ml.[62]

However, delayed respiratory depression and respiratory arrest have been reported approximately 60 minutes after the cessation of prolonged intraoperative alfentanil infusions. At the time of one respiratory arrest, the plasma alfentanil concentration was 95 ng/ml.[63] The alfentanil concentration at the time of the respiratory arrest suggests that the respiratory depression that may be seen during recovery is not due to the reappearance of alfentanil from peripheral storage sites, but rather may be a function of decreased stimulation in the PACU and the effects of sleep per se. Alfentanil also exhibits the typical opioid side effect of rigidity, which may involve the larynx and pharyngeal structures as well as chest and extremities, and may interfere with the ability to ventilate. This is more common with higher doses, but may be seen at doses appropriate for ambulatory general anesthesia. Other typical opioid side effects associated with alfentanil include nausea and vomiting, which occur at rates comparable with fentanyl,[59] and vagally mediated bradycardia.

Remifentanil is another piperidine derivative currently in development. In addition to its opioid structure, remifentanil has an ester linkage that can be metabolized by blood and tissue esterases, resulting in an ultra-short terminal half life of only 10 minutes.[64] Remifentanil clearance is three to four times greater than hepatic blood flow, which is consistent with extensive extrahepatic metabolism, and clearance is constant, and independent of dose or weight.[50] The volume of distribution is small and also dose-independent, which suggests widespread extravascular distribution. The time required for a 50% decrease in effect site concentration has been calculated to be 3.65 minutes for remifentanil, 33.9 minutes for sufentanil, and 58.5 minutes for alfentanil.[65] The potency ratio of bolus doses of remifentanil to alfentanil is approximately 20:1, and the potency ratio of infusions of remifentanil to alfentanil is approximately 10:1. The duration of analgesia and respiratory depression after single equipotent boluses of remifentanil and alfentanil are similar.[65,66] Cardiovascular depression and histamine release are minimal. Remifentanil is a typical μ-receptor agonist opioid that has the typical opioid side effects, including respiratory depression, rigidity, and nausea and vomiting; the relative frequency of nausea and vomiting compared with that of the other opioids has yet to be determined. The issue of providing adequate postoperative analgesia, possibly using a continued infusion, is also undergoing evaluation. The very rapid onset and offset of effect, which is independent of duration of administration, suggests that remifentanil may prove useful as an opioid infusion for ambulatory procedures, with little risk of prolonged recovery.

Butorphanol is an opioid with mixed κ-receptor agonist as well as μ-receptor antagonist activity. It has analgesic and sedative properties, and does not cause profound respiratory depression. Butorphanol has been compared with fentanyl as the narcotic component of general anesthesia for ambulatory gynecologic laparoscopy.[67] Patients received equianalgesic doses of butorphanol (20 μg/kg) or of fentanyl (1 μg/kg), together with nitrous oxide and isoflurane. Postoperatively there were no differences in analgesic need. Patients who received butorphanol reported more postoperative sedation during the first 45 minutes of recovery, but discharge times were not different. On the first postoperative day, more subjects who received butorphanol were satisfied with their anesthesia experience. Other studies involving higher doses of butorphanol have shown prolonged sedative effects and delayed discharge. Comparable increased doses of fentanyl as the opioid have also been shown to prolong recovery.

Nalbuphine, another mixed agonist/antagonist opioid, has also been compared with fentanyl as the opioid component of ambulatory gynecologic anesthesia.[68] Patients were given equianalgesic doses of fentanyl (1.5 μg/kg) or nalbuphine (300 μg/kg). Postoperative analgesic need and patient assessment of postoperative analgesia were similar in both groups. However, use of nalbuphine was associated with increased nausea, increased length of stay, increased dreaming, and increased incidence of unpleasant dreams. In that study, another patient group was given a higher nalbuphine dose (500 μg/kg) to provide increased analgesia; this resulted in further increases in dreaming, unpleasant dreaming, and nausea, without a difference in postoperative analgesic requirement. Nalbuphine can also be used to reverse postoperative opioid-induced respiratory depression with better postoperative analgesia, compared with naloxone.[69] The duration of both of these mixed agonist/antagonist opioids is long (3 to 4 hours), and their benefits should be carefully weighed against their side effects.

Propofol

Propofol may be used for maintenance of anesthesia and given as repeated boluses of 0.5 to 1.0 mg/kg. However, when given by intermittent bolus technique, the rapid changes in blood concentrations result in frequent changes in anesthetic depth; therefore, propofol may be more effectively given by continuous variable infusion. The infusion regimen usually begins with a postinduction rate of 200 μg/kg/min, followed by a decrease to 100 μg/kg/min, which is then titrated to effect. When propofol is given for maintenance of anesthesia with nitrous oxide, mean infusion rates have been 112.2 to 149.4 μg/kg/minute.[70] Early recovery times after ambulatory procedures are faster when propofol infusion is used for maintenance of anesthesia, rather than isoflurane[71] or enflurane,[72] even when all groups receive propofol for induction. Infusions of propofol cause less hemodynamic disturbance than do bolus doses. Maintenance of anesthesia with propofol 108 μg/kg/min and nitrous oxide 67% resulted in a decrease in systolic arterial pressure to 55% of awake value, and a drop in cardiac output to 74% of awake value in healthy, premedicated adults. Mild respiratory depression was also noted, with elevations of arterial pCO_2 to 52 mm Hg.[73] Even when propofol induction and maintenance was supplemented with appropriate doses of isoflurane, prompt recovery was achieved.[74]

Potent Inhaled Agents

Commonly, ambulatory general anesthesia includes the simultaneous administration of nitrous oxide, an opioid, and one of the potent inhaled anesthetic agents (Table 7-2). Rapidity of induction with the potent inhaled agents can be enhanced by the use of overpressure—the administration of MAC multiples to quickly achieve surgical anesthetic concentration of the agents in the brain. In fact, the use of appropriate comparable overpressure is the most effective technique to produce rapid induction. The inspired concentrations needed to reach 1 MAC in the alveoli within several breaths can be calculated.[42] This inspired concentration is 4.1 MAC (3.3%) for halothane, 3.4 MAC (5.7%) for enflurane, 2.6 MAC (2.9%) for isoflurane, 1.5 MAC (9.2%) for desflurane, and 1.8 MAC (3.7%) for sevoflurane. Solubility becomes the limiting factor when equal MAC multiples of the various agents are administered. The concentration effect is not an important factor with potent agents, because high concentrations cannot be given.

Among the currently available anesthetics, halothane has a pleasant odor and is not irritating to the airway. It can therefore be given easily by mask inhalation. However, blood gas solubility and blood tissue solubility are high, which results in significant uptake into fat and relatively slow emergence. Halothane does depress the myocardium, but it causes limited change in heart rate and decrease in systemic resistance.[75] It sensitizes the heart to both exogenous and endogenous catecholamines, and arrhythmias may occur. Halothane produces increased respiratory rate, decreased tidal volume, and bronchodilation at depth. Intraocular pressure is reduced. Halothane can trigger malignant hyperthermia. Most importantly, halothane undergoes significant metabolic degradation (10% to 20%), generating compounds that may cause halothane-associated hepatic toxicity. With the other presently available agents that have less potential for toxicity, halothane use is limited in adult outpatients.

Enflurane's lower blood gas and blood tissue solubilities should result in faster emergence from anesthesia. Although times to recovery (response to name) were faster with enflurane than halothane,[76] there was no difference in postoperative complaints or psychomotor function. Airway pungency is more than with halothane. Approximately 2% to 3% of an inhaled enflurane dose is metabolized;[77] enflurane-associated hepatitis is rare. Enflurane metabolism generates inorganic fluoride. Myocardial depression is similar to that which occurs with halothane, but a more marked decrease in systemic vascular resistance also occurs. Enflurane does not sensitize the heart to catecholamines. Intracranial, intraocular, and respiratory effects are similar to those of halothane, but with less tachypnea. Bronchodilation is also produced at deeper levels of anesthesia. Uniquely, enflurane is associated with seizure activity at higher concentrations (greater than 4%) in the presence of hypocarbia.

Isoflurane has a lower blood-gas partition coefficient and is eliminated faster than halothane. However, it does have a more pungent odor, which limits its use for induction and slows the speed at which surgical anesthesia can be established unless preceded by an intravenous induction agent. Isoflurane is associated with myocardial depression and decreased systemic vascular resistance. Myocardial steal has been reported with isoflurane in patients with coronary artery disease; this redistribution of blood flow from already compromised areas may cause ischemia.[78] Isoflurane does not sensitize the heart to catecholamines, but tachycardia is seen in some patients. Intracranial and intraocular pressures as well as effects on respiratory rate and tidal volume are similar to those seen with halothane. Though recovery is rapid, the use of isoflurane for ambulatory procedures has been associated with higher postanesthetic side effects.[79] Compared with patients who received enflurane or halothane, patients who received isoflurane required more analgesics in the PACU, and on the first postoperative day, they reported more dizziness, nausea, coughing, and headache. However, isoflurane does undergo less metabolism, less than 1% of the administered dose.[80] Because of this, immediate or delayed toxic effects with this agent are unlikely, and it enjoys widespread use.

Desflurane, which became available in 1992, differs from isoflurane with notably lower blood-gas and tissue-blood partition coefficients. Induction with desflurane is expectedly very rapid. Peripheral vascular resistance is decreased more than with isoflurane,[75] and desflurane may have more neuromuscular depressant effects.[81] Myocardial effects of this drug are similar to those of isoflurane. Desflurane does not sensitize the heart to catecholamines. However, evidence suggests that rapid changes in inspired desflurane concentration, whether at induction or during the anesthetic, results in sympathetic nervous system discharge.[82] The result can be significant tachycardia and hypertension (compared with isoflurane); desflurane should be used with caution in patients who would be at risk to such changes. Desflurane is also associated with considerable airway pungency, which prohibits its use for induction in pediatric patients and severely restricts its use for inhalation induction in adults. Coughing is an issue at emergence. Wake-up times after desflurane have been determined for different inhaled concentrations, for procedures lasting 90 minutes to 4 hours.[83,84] Emergence times are linearly related to the desflurane concentration used for anesthesia, and are significantly faster than with isoflurane from 0.5 to 1.25 MAC. Recovery studies after discontinuation of the inhaled agent show significantly shorter times to eye opening and ability to follow commands, compared with those shown after isoflurane.[83] Studies have compared induction and maintenance with desflurane/oxygen to induction and maintenance with propofol/nitrous oxide. Patients who received only desflurane and oxygen showed significantly faster initial wakening; times to intermediate recovery (sitting in chair, standing, and fitness for discharge) were no longer different, by 90 minutes after anesthetic end.[85,86] Postoperative nausea and vomiting, and pain, are similar in patients who received desflurane or isoflurane; patients who received propofol for induction or maintenance experienced less nausea. Another advantage of desflurane is its very low rate of in vivo degradation, which suggests a lack of renal or hepatic toxicity. Desflurane's high vapor pressure necessitated the development of a new heated, pressurized vaporizer for its administration.

Sevoflurane has a low blood-gas partition coefficient, which should translate into rapid induction and emergence with this agent. It was released for general use in Japan in 1990, and it is currently undergoing clinical trials in North America. Sevoflurane has dose-dependent cardiovascular and respiratory depressant effects similar to those of enflurane and isoflurane, and neuromuscular effects similar to those of isoflurane. Drug-induced hypotension and tachycardia are less than with isoflurane, and sevoflurane does not sensitize the heart to catecholamines. A unique feature of sevoflurane is a lack of airway pungency, and it can be inhaled without coughing or breathholding by children and adults. It appears to be a suitable alternative for inhalational induction and maintenance in neonates, infants, and children.[87] Recovery comparisons of sevoflurane with isoflurane for the maintenance of propofol-induced general anesthesia revealed significant faster early wake-up parameters (times to eye opening, command, and orientation) for sevoflurane without an earlier need for first analgesic, and with less postoperative somnolence and nausea.[88] Time to sit up without dizziness or nausea was also significantly faster with sevoflurane, although discharge time was not different. Like all inhalants, sevoflurane can trigger malignant hyperthermia.[89] Drawbacks associated with sevoflurane are related to its degradation and metabolism. At alkaline conditions and elevated temperatures, sevoflurane undergoes degradation to several olefin compounds; the potential toxicity of these compounds is under evaluation.[90] In vivo, sevoflurane is metabolized to products including inorganic fluoride. However, evaluation of sensitive renal concentrating ability has been performed after sevoflurane anesthetic administration to volunteers, and no renal dysfunction has been demonstrated.[91] This may be related to the rapid elimination of sevoflurane and, therefore, rapid decline in inorganic fluoride concentrations, which results in a limited kidney dose exposure. Both desflurane and sevoflurane have the potential for changing ambulatory practice.[92,93]

Endotracheal Intubation

(Airway management and preparation for endotracheal intubation and its alternatives are discussed in Chapter 6.)

The indications for endotracheal intubation are generally the same for all patients: to help maintain the airway, to provide positive pressure ventilation, and to decrease the risk of aspiration. However, there are morbidities associated with endotracheal intubation that are more pertinent to the ambulatory patient, and these should be kept in mind. Postoperative sore throat is a major problem. In the outpatient, the incidence of sore throat after any tracheal intubation has been reported at 40% to 65%. In comparison, the incidence of sore throat after general anesthesia *without* an endotracheal tube is 15% to 20%,[94] and this has been attributed to breathing dry gases, use of oral and nasal airways, and use of anticholinergic agents. The incidence of sore throat after intubation can be reduced by choosing an appropriate endotracheal tube. The use of a low-volume, high-pressure cuff (rather than a high-volume, low-pressure cuff, as may be used for long-term intubations) has reduced the incidence of sore throat from 46% to 25%; it appears that the area of cuff abrading the trachea is the contributory factor.[95] The incidence of sore throat after intubation can also be reduced by using a smaller diameter tube.[96] In women, substitution of a 6.5 OD (outside diameter) for a 8.5 OD tube reduced the incidence of sore throat from 48% down to 22%, as well as the incidence of hoarseness from 33% down to 18%. The potential increase in airway resistance generated by these smaller tubes is not an issue for brief intraoperative intubations in ambulatory surgery patients. Succinylcholine also causes sore throat without endotracheal intubation.[94] After pretreatment with curare, an incidence of sore throat of 45%, and of hoarseness of 10%, have been reported in nonintubated patients who received succinylcholine. This was ascribed to residual discomfort in the striated muscles of the larynx.

Neuromuscular Blocking Agents

Depolarizing Agents

Succinylcholine is a benchmark for neuromuscular blocking agents used in ambulatory anesthesia. Succinylcholine is a membrane-depolarizing agent that acts at the postjunctional nicotinic cholinergic receptor. Block occurs because the depolarized membrane cannot respond to subsequent acetylcholine stimulation. Succinylcholine may be given to adults as a 1 to 1.5 mg/kg bolus to facilitate endotracheal intubation, or by continuous infusion to provide continued relaxation for short procedures. Onset after intubating doses occurs within 1 to 2 minutes, and the duration is short as 5 minutes after a bolus dose. Continuous infusion is titrated to maintain at least 1 out of 4 twitches. Succinylcholine action is terminated by hydrolysis by plasma pseudocholinesterase. Therefore, patient conditions that decrease the type and amount of pseudocholinesterase enzyme will prolong the clinical action of the drug. This is seen in ambulatory patients taking anticholinesterase medications for glaucoma or myasthenia gravis, or patients taking chemotherapeutic drugs such as nitrogen mustard and cyclophosphamide, as well as in patients with a genetically atypical enzyme.

The use of succinylcholine has associated drawbacks. The potential side effect of particular concern for ambulatory surgery patients is the production of postanesthetic muscle pains. Churchill-Davidson first reported the increased incidence of myalgias in patients who ambulated shortly after their procedure (67%), compared with patients who remained at bed rest for 48 hours (13.9%).[97] The intensity of pain was also greater in ambulatory patients, with 66% of outpatients describing the pain as severe, compared with 20% of inpatients. Many approaches have been evaluated to lessen postsuccinylcholine myalgia. Diazepam, calcium gluconate, and self-taming with succinylcholine have limited efficacy. Pretreatment with small doses of pancuronium caused a reduction in visible fasciculations that was not associated with a reduction in postanesthetic myalgia.[98] Small doses of gallamine, metocurine, or atracurium are effective, but the prior administration of D-tubocurarine 3 mg causes the most consistent reduction in symptoms. Interestingly, the substitution of succinylcholine by vecuronium did not lower the incidence of myalgia seen after outpatient diagnostic laparoscopy, and the distribution and duration of pains were similar in both groups.[99] The presence of myalgias after laparoscopy independent of the neuromuscular blocking agent used suggests a significant contribution from factors related to the surgical procedure itself, such as abdominal distension and manipulation, residual intraperitoneal gas, and positioning of the patient.

Other potential side effects of succinylcholine are increased intraocular pressure, increased intragastric pressure, malignant hyperthermia, and hyperkalemia. Patients who are particularly susceptible to hyperkalemia following administration of succinylcholine are now being seen in the ambulatory setting. These include patients with burns; neuromuscular disorders, such as Guillain-Barré disease and amyotrophic lateral sclerosis; and nerve injuries or spinal cord trauma. Succinylcholine has caused rhabdomyolysis, hyperthalmia, and cardiac arrest in children and adolescents with undiagnosed myopathies. Succinylcholine can also be associated with severe bradycardia. Especially when given in combination with other vagotonic agents (e.g., alfentanil, sufentanil, propofol), sinus arrest has been reported.[100] This occurs particularly when the surgical procedure itself also generates vagal stimulation (e.g., gynecologic outpatient surgery). Despite its many side effects, succinylcholine remains a widely used neuromuscular blocking agent because of its rapid effect and low cost.

Nondepolarizing Agents

(See Table 7-4 for dosing recommendations and Table 7-5 for pharmacokinetic properties.)The side effects associated with succinylcholine have encouraged the development of short-acting, nondepolarizing neuromuscular blocking agents. Nondepolarizing agents act by combining with the nicotinic cholinergic receptors in the postjunctional membrane, but do not activate the receptor or directly block the channel. The nondepolarizing neuromuscular blocking agents fall into two general structural groups, and the drugs with short-to-moderate durations of both groups are

Table 7-4   Dosing Recommendations for Nondepolarizing Neuromuscular Blocking Agents

	Intubating dose (mg/kg)	Maintenance bolus (mg/kg)	Maintenance infusion (µg/kg/min)
Atracurium	0.4	0.1	5-9
Mivacurium	0.2	0.1	6-7
Vecuronium	0.1	0.010-0.015	1
Rocuronium	0.6	0.1-0.2	4-16

Table 7-5   Pharmacokinetics of Neuromuscular Blocking Agents[4,5]

	Distribution half life (minutes)	Elimination half life (minutes)	Clearance (ml/kg/min)	Volume of distribution (l/kg)
Atracurium	2	17-22	5.0-6.0	0.15-0.18
Mivacurium		2-3	53-99	0.15-0.27
		22 (*cis-cis*)	4.2	
Vecuronium	4	65-75	3.6-4.5	0.3-0.4
Rocuronium	1-2	84	4.2	0.25

appropriate for use in ambulatory surgery patients. Atracurium and mivacurium represent the benzylisoquinoline group, and vecuronium and rocuronium represent the steroidal group. For all agents, the dose should be reduced when given with potent inhalational anesthetics. To enhance recovery, reversal of their effects is usually needed with anticholinesterases (e.g., neostigmine, edrophonium), anticholinergics (e.g., glycopyrrolate atropine), and appropriate monitoring.

Atracurium has a time to onset of 2 to 3 minutes, and a time to 25% recovery of 35 to 45 minutes, when given in routine intubating doses of 0.4 mg/kg ($ED_{95} \times 2$). This drug undergoes spontaneous degradation at body pH and temperature, in addition to undergoing ester hydrolysis. Atracurium is therefore useful for ambulatory patients with significant hepatic or renal disease. At higher doses, atracurium causes histamine release from mast cells. At doses of 0.3 to 0.4 mg/kg, no patients responded with histamine release, while at a dose of 0.5 mg/kg, 30% responded, and at 0.6 mg/kg, 50% responded.[101] Slowing the rate of injection reduces the incidence of histamine-associated cardiovascular effects. A disadvantage of atracurium is the relatively long onset, compared with that of succinylcholine. Several techniques have been developed to reduce this time. One technique is to increase the initial intubating dose, but this is of limited utility with atracurium because of the histamine-related side effects generated. Another approach is the use of a priming dose. For atracurium, a dose of 0.05 mg/kg may be given 3 to 5 minutes before induction and the intubating dose of 0.3 mg/kg. For maintenance of neuromuscular blockade, atracurium may be given by intermittent boluses of approximately 0.1 mg/kg, or by continuous infusion at a rate of 5 to 9 μg/kg/min.

Mivacurium is the shortest available nondepolarizing agent of the benzylisoquinoline group. It consists of a mixture of three stereoisomers. The *trans-trans* and *cis-trans* isomers represent 95% of the mixture and are equipotent; the *cis-cis* isomer has one-tenth potency of the other isomers. An intubating dose of 0.2 mg/kg ($ED_{95} \times 2$) provides intubating conditions in approximately 2 minutes. However, this dose is associated with some histamine release and transient drops in blood pressure. Mivacurium is hydrolyzed by plasma cholinesterase, at a rate approximately 70% to 88% that of succinylcholine.[102] Prolonged recovery has been reported in patients homozygous for atypical pseudocholinesterase enzyme.[103] In patients with normal enzyme, recovery is apparent within 15 minutes; time to 25% control is 20 minutes, and spontaneous full recovery occurs at approximately 30 minutes. A priming approach to reduce further induction time has been done using 0.15 mg/kg, followed in 30 seconds by 0.10 mg/kg.[104] It has been observed that the time at which relaxation occurs at the adductor policis is significantly delayed, compared with relaxation at the diaphragm and larynx;[105] intubation with mivacurium may be best performed when the jaw (masseter) becomes slack. Increasing the initial bolus dose does not appreciably prolong the duration of action of this drug. The short duration of action of mivacurium corresponds well to the length of many ambulatory surgical procedures, and routine use of neuromuscular reversal agents may not be necessary. This may reduce the potential for neostigmine-associated postoperative nausea.[106] However, neuromuscular function should be monitored consistently. Mivacurium may be given by incremental boluses of 0.10 mg/kg, or by continuous infusion for maintenance of neuromuscular blockade at a rate of 6 to 7 μg/kg/min, with recovery at 17 minutes.

Vecuronium is a steroidal neuromuscular-blocking analog of pancuronium. The intubating dose of this drug (0.1 mg/kg [$ED_{95} \times$ 2]) produces intubating conditions in approximately 2.5 to 3 minutes. The duration of action at this dose is approximately 30 minutes, with recovery to 25% of control at 25 to 40 minutes; larger doses prolong the duration of action. Vecuronium is the only neuromuscular blocking agent essentially devoid of cardiovascular side effects. Its use is recommended in ambulatory patients who might be particularly sensitive to changes in blood pressure; however, bradycardic arrest may occur if it is used with other vagotonic agents.[107] Vecuronium is metabolized in the liver and excreted in urine, and its effect may be prolonged in ambulatory patients with significant hepatic or renal disease. If a priming approach is desired to hasten the onset, doses of 0.01 mg/kg followed by doses of 0.05 mg/kg may be used. For maintenance of anesthesia, vecuronium should be given as increments of 0.010 to 0.015 mg/kg. Maintenance neuromuscular block can also be provided by infusion using 1 μg/kg/min, with recovery at approximately 30 minutes.

Rocuronium is another steroidal neuromuscular blocking agent. Intubating doses of 0.6 mg/kg provides satisfactory conditions at 60 to 90 seconds, more rapidly than with vecuronium.[108] For rocuronium, the time to recovery to 25% control is approximately 30 minutes (which is comparable with that of vecuronium), but some drug accumulation may occur with additional dosing. The cardiovascular effects of rocuronium are minimal, possibly with mild increase in heart rate.[109] Rocuronium is excreted by the liver, and duration of action is prolonged in patients with hepatic disease. Maintenance doses are boluses of 0.1 to 0.2 mg/kg every 12 to 24 minutes, or infusion of 4 to 16 μg/kg/min.

Total Intravenous Anesthesia

Total intravenous anesthesia (TIVA) is becoming increasingly popular. Advantages of this technique include avoidance of the side effects of potent inhaled agents and of nitrous oxide, and avoidance of operating room pollution by these agents. The technique may be particularly useful when airway surgery precludes continuous administration of an inhaled anesthetic, and when the administration of 100% oxygen is desired. Disadvantages of TIVA include the need to use separate hypnotic and analgesic drugs, and the purchase, maintenance, and utilization of the additional infusion technology. Available technology ranges from simple drip-counting devices to computer-controlled, population kinetics–determined infusion devices,[110] with widely varying costs. Most commonly, syringe pumps with either simple preprogrammed or programmable infusion rates are employed. Anesthetic drugs described for TIVA use in ambulatory surgery patients include combinations of alfentanil, propofol, midazolam, and/or ketamine, with a neuromuscular blocking agent. Recommended doses for intravenous administration of commonly used drugs in ambulatory surgery are provided in Table 7-6.

Early TIVA techniques involved bolus administration of intravenous drugs. Holmes et al. described a technique involving fentanyl 100 μg followed by midazolam 0.15 mg/kg for ambulatory cystoscopy. The awakening time was 16.7 minutes after this large dose of midazolam.[111] More recently, the combination of midazolam and alfentanil with flumazenil has been suggested for total intravenous anesthesia,[112] using alfentanil 0.03 mg/kg followed by midazolam 0.3 mg/kg for ambulatory dilatation and curettage lasting 11.6 ± 0.5 minutes. The addition of flumazenil 0.5 mg after this regimen reduced the time to eye opening from 21.2 ± 4.5 minutes to 0.5 ± 0.1 minutes, and the time to give correct birthdate from 28.0 ± 4.3 minutes to 0.80 ± 0.1 minutes. Psychomotor effects were not completely reversed; however, current flumazenil dosage recommendations go up to 1.0 mg.

Midazolam or propofol infusions have been compared when given with alfentanil for TIVA for longer 90-minute procedures.[113] The propofol infusion consisted of a loading dose of 2 mg/kg and an infusion of 150 μg/kg/min for 30 minutes, then 75 μg/kg/min thereafter; the midazolam infusion consisted of a loading dose of 0.42 mg/kg followed by an infusion of 0.125 mg/kg/hour. Both groups received alfentanil, starting with a bolus of 25 μg/kg followed by an infusion of 50 μg/kg/hour (0.83 μg/kg/min), which was varied by patient response. Times to awakening after these techniques were 8.5 ± 4.6 minutes in the propofol group, compared with 16.9 ± 5.2 minutes in the midazolam group. However, the midazolam doses used here may be excessive, because they were determined in a study using only midazolam infusion without an opioid; the synergistic effects of the combination of midazolam and alfentanil may result in a 67% reduction in the dose of midazolam necessary to produce sleep.[114] Nonetheless, propofol remains the hypnotic of choice for TIVA in the ambulatory setting.

A recommended ambulatory surgery regimen of drugs for TIVA consists of propofol with alfentanil, plus a neuromuscular blocking agent. The technique begins with a bolus of alfentanil 10 μg/kg, with a simultaneous infusion begun at 1.0 μg/kg/min. Sleep induction is accomplished with propofol 2.0 mg/kg, which is followed by an infusion of 200 μg/kg/min for 5 to 10 minutes,

Table 7-6 Intravenous Anesthesia Infusions

Intravenous anesthesia component	Loading dose (µg/kg)	Maintenance infusion (µg/kg/min)	Stop infusion prior end of case (min)	Plasma drug concentration (minor surgery)
Analgesic				
Alfentanil	10-30	0.5-2.0	15-30	100-300 ng/ml
Fentanyl	2-4	0.02-0.08*	45-60	2-5 ng/ml
Sufentanil	0.25-0.75	0.005-0.01	15-30	0.3-1.5 ng/ml
Sedative/hypnotic†				
Propofol	1000-2000	120-200	5-10	3-5 µg/ml
Midazolam	100-250	0.25-1.0	15-30	50-250 ng/ml
Methohexital	1000-2000	50-150	10-15	5-10 mg/ml

Recommended infusion schemes are when combined with 65% to 70% N_2O.

*Recommended for long cases *only*.

†Titrated to loss of consciousness.

Adapted from Glass PSA, Shafer SL, Jacobs JR, Reves JF: Intravenous drug delivery systems. In Miller RD, editor: Anesthesia, ed 4, New York, 1994, Churchill Livingstone, pp. 389-416.

depending on blood pressure, then decreased to 100 µg/kg/min. An additional bolus of alfentanil 10 µg/kg can be given before intubation if the initial opioid-induced sedation and bradycardia are not pronounced. A moderate degree of neuromuscular relaxation should also be provided. Anesthesia depth can be controlled by titrating with either agent, but it may be easier to vary the opioid. If hemodynamic signs of light anesthesia develop, the alfentanil should be increased with a bolus of 5 µg/kg followed by an increase in the infusion rate of 0.25 µg/kg/min. Signs of approaching consciousness should be treated with additional propofol. The alfentanil infusion should be terminated 5 to 15 minutes before the end of surgery, and normocapnea maintained. Total anesthesia with propofol and alfentanil also produces less immediate PONV and less likelihood for overnight admission, compared with enflurane and nitrous oxide.[115]

Summary

General anesthesia still remains the most commonly used technique in ambulatory surgery. The development of different sedative-hypnotics, opioids, muscle relaxants, and inhaled agents with pharmacological properties more tailored for the ambulatory patient have encouraged its popularity. Ideally, anesthesia should provide a rapid smooth pleasant induction; minimal or no side effects; a readily controlled depth with a rapid smooth emergence; minimal nausea and vomiting; and a rapid, early return to activities of daily living. These goals can be reached either through the use of inhalational or intravenous agents. Induction of anesthesia with commonly used barbiturates is discussed. The use of midazolam and its antagonist flumazenil is reviewed. The use of ketamine for outpatient surgery is limited by the psychomimetic effects and delayed discharge. Propofol has achieved wide popularity both as an induction and maintenance agent in adult and pediatric patients, and recommendations for its administration are provided. Opioids remain a mainstay of ambulatory anesthesia by providing analgesia and cardiovascular stability, and their administration should be timed to coincide with the maximal surgical and anesthetic stimulation. The side effects of nausea, vomiting, bradycardia, chest wall rigidity, and respiratory depression are common to all synthetic opioids. The use of agonist-antagonists in ambulatory surgery have not gained wide acceptance. Among the potent inhaled agents, desflurane and sevoflurane have significantly lower blood-gas partition coefficients, which promote a faster recovery. Reduction of side-effects related to endotracheal intubation are discussed. Neuromuscular blocking agents should be selected on the time of onset and duration of relaxation that is needed. The use of succinylcholine in both adult and pediatric patients has its associated drawbacks; the most important of these are myalgias and hyperkalemia. The short-acting nondepolarizing neuromuscular blocking agents mivacurium and rocuronium may be good alternatives to succinylcholine in outpatient practice. A review of the intermediate-acting neuromuscular blocking agents is provided. Techniques for TIVA require a knowledge of the pharmacological properties of anesthetics, and the availability of programmable computer-controlled technology. Recommended infusions for common intravenous agents are provided.

References

1. Philip BK: Patients' assessment of ambulatory anesthesia and surgery. J Clin Anesth 1992; 4:355-8.
2. Lichtiger M, Wetchler BV, Philip BK: Management of the adult and geriatric patient. In Wetchler BV, editor: Anesthesia for ambulatory surgery, Philadelphia, 1985, JB Lippincott, pp. 175-224.
3A. Philip BK: Ambulatory anesthesia. Sem Surg Oncol 1990; 6:177-83.
3B. White PF, Shafer AS: Clinical pharmacology and uses of injectable anesthetic and analgesic agents. In Wetchler BV, editor: Outpatient anesthesia, vol 2, Philadelphia, 1988, JB Lippincott, pp. 37-54.
4. Rogers M, Tinker J, Covino B, Longnecker D: Principles and practice of anesthesiology, St Louis, 1993, Mosby, pp. 1053-86, 1151-4, 1518-40.
5. Wood M, Wood A: Drugs and anesthesia, Baltimore, 1990, Williams & Wilkins, pp. 129-78, 179-224, 225-70, 271-318.
6. Elliott CJR, Green R, Howells TH et al: Recovery after intravenous barbiturate anesthesia. Lancet 1962; 1:68-70.

7. Price HL, Kovnat BS, Safer JN et al: The uptake of thiopental by body tissues and its relation to the duration of narcosis. Clin Pharmacol Ther 1960; 1:16-20.

8. Dundee JW, Hassard TH, McGowan WAW, Henshaw J: The 'induction' dose of thiopental. Anaesthesia 1982; 37:1176-84.

9. Mirakhur RK, Sheppard WFI, Darrah WC: Propofol or thiopentone: effects on intraocular pressure associated with induction of anaesthesia and tracheal intubation (facilitated with suxamethonium). Br J Anaesth 1987; 59:431-6.

10. Dundee JW: Clinical studies of induction agents. VII. A comparison of eight intravenous anaesthetics as main agents for a standard operation. Br J Anaesth 1963; 35:784-92.

11. Hudson RJ, Stanski DR, Burch PG: Pharmacokinetics of methohexital and thiopental in surgical patients. Anesthesiology 1983; 59:215-9.

12. Vickers MD: The measurement of recovery from anesthesia. Br J Anaesth 1965; 37:296-302.

13. Philip BK: Pharmacology of intravenous sedative agents. In Rogers MC, Tinker JH, Covino BG, Longnecker DE, editors: Principles and practice of anesthesiology, St Louis, 1993, Mosby, pp. 1087-1104.

14. Philip BK, Simpson TH, Hauch MA, Mallampati SR: Flumazenil reverses sedation after midazolam-induced general anesthesia in ambulatory surgery patients. Anesth Analg 1990; 71:371-6.

15. Philip BK: Flumazenil: the benzodiazepine antagonist. Anesthesiology Clinics North Am 1993; 11:799-814.

16. Pearson RC, McCloy RF, Morris P, Bardhan KD: Midazolam and flumazenil in gastroenterology. Acta Anaesthesiol Scand 1990; 34(Suppl 92):21-4.

17. Philip BK: Drug reversal: benzodiazepine receptors and antagonists. J Clin Anesth 1993; 5:46S-51S.

18. Fragen RJ, Caldwell N: Comparison of a new formulation of etomidate with thiopental side effects and awakening times. Anesthesiology 1979; 50:242-4.

19. Wagner RL, White PF: Etomidate inhibits adrenocortical function in surgical patients. Anesthesiology 1984; 61:647-51.

20. Thompson GE, Remington JM, Millman BS et al: Experiences with outpatient anesthesia. Anesth Analg 1973; 52:881-7.

21. Manschot HJ, Meursing AEE, Axt P et al: Propofol requirements for induction of anesthesia in children of different age groups. Anesth Analg 1992; 75:876-9.

22. Morton NS, Wee M, Christie G et al: Propofol for induction of anaesthesia in children. Anaesthesia 1988; 43:350-5.

23. Hannallah R, Baker S, Casey W et al: Propofol: effective dose and induction characteristics in unpremedicated children. Anesthesiology 1991; 74:217-9.

24. Fisher DM: Propofol in pediatrics: lessons in pharmacokinetic modeling. Anesthesiology 1994; 80:2-5.

25. Kataria BK, Ved SA, Nicodemus HF et al: The pharmacokinetics of propofol in children using three different data analysis approaches. Anesthesiology 1994; 80:104-22.

26. Ebert TJ, Muzi M, Berens R et al: Sympathetic responses to induction of anesthesia in humans with propofol or etomidate. Anesthesiology 1992; 76:725-33.

27. Baraka A: Severe bradycardia following propofol-suxamethonium sequence. Br J Anaesth 1988; 61:482-3.

28. Brown GW, Patel N, Ellis FR: Comparison of propofol and thiopentone for laryngeal mask insertion. Anaesthesia 1991; 46:771-2.

29. Gold MI, Abraham EC, Herrington C: A controlled investigation of propofol, thiopentone and methohexitone. Can J Anaesth 1987; 34:478-83.

30. McLeskey CH, Walawander CA, Nahrwold ML et al: Adverse events in a multicenter phase IV study of propofol: evaluation by anesthesiologists and postanesthesia care unit nurses. Anesth Analg 1993; 77:S3-9.

31. MacKenzie N, Grant IS: Comparison of the new emulsion formulation of propofol with methohexitone and thiopentone for induction of anaesthesia in day cases. Br J Anaesth 1985; 57:725-31.

32. Korttila K, Nuotto EJ, Lichtor JL et al: Clinical recovery and psychomotor function after brief anesthesia with propofol or thiopental. Anesthesiology 1992; 76:676-81.

33. Logan MR, Duggan JE, Levack ID, Spence AA: Single-shot IV anaesthesia for outpatient dental surgery. Br J Anaesth 1987; 59:179-83.

34. Hannallah RS, Britton JT, Schafer PG et al: Propofol anaesthesia in paediatric ambulatory patients: a comparison with thiopentone and halothane. Can J Anaesth 1994; 41:12-8.

35. Borgeat A, Popovic V, Meier D, Schwander D: Comparison of propofol and thiopental/halothane for short-duration ENT surgical procedure in children. Anesth Analg 1990; 71:511-5.

36. Korttila K, Ostman P, Faure E et al: Randomized comparison of recovery after propofol-nitrous oxide versus thiopentone-isoflurane-nitrous oxide anaesthesia in patients undergoing ambulatory surgery. Acta Anaesthesiol Scand 1990; 34:400-3.

37. Martin TM, Nicolson SC, Bargas MS: Propofol anesthesia reduces emesis and airway obstruction in pediatric outpatients. Anesth Analg 1993; 76:144-8.

38. Weir PM, Munro HM, Reynolds PI et al: Propofol infusion and the incidence of emesis in pediatric outpatient strabismus surgery. Anesth Analg 1993; 76:760-4.

39. Borgeat A, Wilder-Smith OHG, Saiah M, Rifat K: Subhypnotic doses of propofol possess direct antiemetic properties. Anesth Analg 1992; 74:539-41.

40. Borgeat A, Wilder-Smith OH, Suter PM: The nonhypnotic therapeutic applications of propofol. Anesthesiology 1994; 80:642-56.

41. Gepts E, Claeys MA, Camu F, Smekens L: Infusion of propofol as sedative technique for colonoscopies. Postgrad Med J 1985; 61(Suppl 3):120-6.

42. Philip JH: GAS MAN—Understanding anesthesia uptake and distribution, Chestnut Hill, 1990, Med Man Simulation.

43. Taylor E, Feinstein R, White PF, Soper N: Anesthesia for laparoscopic cholecystectomy. Is nitrous oxide contraindicated? Anesthesiology 1992; 76:541-3.

44. Ebert TJ, Kampine JP: Nitrous oxide augments sympathetic outflow: direct evidence from human peroneal nerve recordings. Anesth Analg 1989; 69:444-9.

45. Melnick BM, Johnson LS: Effects of eliminating nitrous oxide in outpatient anesthesia. Anesthesiology 1987; 67:982-4.

46. Muir JJ, Warner MA, Offord KP et al: Role of nitrous oxide and other factors in postoperative nausea and vomiting. Anesthesiology 1987; 66:513-8.

47. Korttila K, Hovorka J, Erkola O: Nitrous oxide does not increase the incidence of nausea and vomiting after isoflurane anesthesia. Anesth Analg 1987; 66:761-5.

48. Mann MS, Woodsford PV, Jones RM: Anaesthetic carrier gases. Their effect on middle ear pressure peri-operatively. Anaesthesia 1985; 40:8-11.

49. Philip BK: Opioids in outpatient anesthesia. Anesthesiol Rev 1991; 18(S1):4-8.

50. Glass PSA, Hardman D, Kamiyarna Y et al: Preliminary pharmacokinetics and pharmacodynamics of an ultra-short-acting opioid: remifentanil (GI78084B). Anesth Analg 1993; 77:1031-40.

51. Shafer SL, Varvel JR: Pharmacokinetics, pharmacodynamics, and rational opioid selection. Anesthesiology 1991; 74:53-63.

52. Hunt TM, Plantevin OM, Gilbert JR: Morbidity in gynaecological day-case surgery. Br J Anaesth 1979; 51:785-7.

53. Rigg JRA, Goldsmith CH: Recovery of ventilatory response to carbon dioxide after thiopentone, morphine and fentanyl in man. Can Anaesth Soc J 1976; 23:370-82.

54. Becker LD, Paulson BA, Miller RD et al: Biphasic respiratory depression after fentanyl-droperidol or fentanyl alone used to supplement nitrous oxide anesthesia. Anesthesiology 1976; 44:291-6.

55. Benthuysen JL, Smith NT, Sanford TJ et al: Physiology of alfentanil-induced rigidity. Anesthesiology 1986; 64:440-6.

56. White PF: Use of continuous infusion versus intermittent bolus administration of fentanyl or ketamine during outpatient anesthesia. Anesthesiology 1983; 59:294-300.

57. Zuurmond WWA, van Leeuwen L: Recovery from sufentanil anaesthesia for outpatient arthroscopy: a comparison with isoflurane. Acta Anaesthesiol Scand 1987; 31:154-6.

58. Phitayakoran P, Melnick BM, Vicinie AF: Comparison of continuous sufentanil and fentanyl infusions for outpatient anaesthesia. Can J Anaesth 1987; 34:242-5.

59. White PF, Coe V, Shafer A, Sung ML: Comparison of alfentanil with fentanyl for outpatient anesthesia. Anesthesiology 1986; 64:99-106.

60. Haley S, Edelist G, Urbach G: Comparison of alfentanil, fentanyl and enflurane as supplements to general anaesthesia for outpatient gynaecologic surgery. Can J Anaesth 1988; 35:570-5.

61. Raeder JC, Hole A: Out-patient laparoscopy in general anaesthesia with alfentanil and atracurium: a comparison with fentanyl and pancuronium. Acta Anaesthesiol Scand 1986; 30:30-4.

62. Ausems ME, Vuyk J, Hug CC, Stanski DR: Comparison of a computer-assisted infusion versus intermittent bolus administration of alfentanil as a supplement to nitrous oxide for lower abdominal surgery. Anesthesiology 1988; 68:851-61.

63. Sebel PS, Lalor JM, Flynn PJ, Simpson BA: Respiratory depression after alfentanil infusion. Br Med J 1984; 289:1581-2.

64. Lineberger CK, Ginsberg B, Franiak RJ, Glass PSA: Narcotic agonists and antagonists. Anesthesiology Clinics North Am 1994; 12:65-89.

65. Westmoreland CL, Hoke JF, Sebel PS et al: Pharmacokinetics of remifentanil (GI 87084B) and its major metabolite (GI 90291) in patients undergoing elective inpatient surgery. Anesthesiology 1993; 79:893-903.

66. Egan TD, Lemmens HJM, Fiset P et al: The pharmacokinetics of the new short-acting opioid remifentanil (GI 87084B) in healthy adult male volunteers. Anesthesiology 1993; 79:881-92.

67. Philip BK, Scott DA, Freiberger D et al: Butorphanol compared with fentanyl in general anaesthesia for ambulatory laparoscopy. Can J Anaesth 1991; 38:183-6.

68. Garfield JM, Garfield FB, Philip BK et al: Comparison of clinical and psychologic effects of fentanyl and nalbuphine in ambulatory gynecological patients. Anesth Analg 1987; 66:1303-7.

69. Bailey PL, Clark NJ, Pace NL et al: Antagonism of postoperative opioid-induced respiratory depression: nalbuphine versus naloxone. Anesth Analg 1987; 66:1109-14.

70. Sear JW, Shaw I, Wolf A, Kay NH: Infusions of propofol to supplement nitrous oxide-oxygen for the maintenance of anaesthesia. Anaesthesia 1988; 43S:18-22.

71. Philip BK, Mushlin PS, Manzi D et al: Isoflurane versus propofol for maintenance of anesthesia for ambulatory surgery: a comparison of costs and recovery profiles. Anesthesiology 1992; 77:A44.

72. Ding Y, Fredman B, White PF: Recovery following outpatient anesthesia: use of enflurane versus propofol. J Clin Anesth 1993; 5:447-50.

73. Coates DP, Monk CR, Prys-Roberts C, Turtle M: Hemodynamics effects of infusions of the emulsion formulation of propofol during nitrous oxide anesthesia in humans. Anesth Analg 1987; 66:64-70.

74. White PF, Stanley TH, Apfelbaum JL et al: Effects on recovery when isoflurane is used to supplement propofol-nitrous oxide anesthesia. Anesth Analg 1993; 77:S15-20.

75. Weiskopf RB, Cahalan MK, Eger EI et al: Cardiovascular actions of desflurane in normocarbic volunteers. Anesth Analg 1991; 73:143-56.

76. Stanford BJ, Plantevin OM, Gilbert JR: Morbidity after day-case gynaecological surgery. Br J Anaesth 1979; 51:1143-5.

77. Lewis JH, Zimmerman HJ, Ishak KG et al: Enflurane hepatotoxicity. Ann Intern Med 1983; 98:984-92.

78. Khambatta HJ, Sonntag H, Larsen R et al: Global and regional myocardial blood flow and metabolism during equipotent halothane and isoflurane anesthesia in patients with coronary artery disease. Anesth Analg 1988; 67:936-42.

79. Tracey JA, Holland AJC, Unger L: Morbidity in minor gynaecological surgery: a comparison of halothane, enflurane and isoflurane. Br J Anaesth 1982; 54:1213-5.

80. Davidkova T, Kikuchi H, Fujii K et al: Biotransformation of isoflurane: urinary and serum fluoride ion and organic fluorine. Anesthesiology 1988; 69:218-22.

81. Kelly RE, Lien CA, Savarese JJ et al: Depression of neuromuscular function in a patient during desflurane anesthesia. Anesth Analg 1993; 76:868-71.

82. Ebert TJ, Muzi M: Sympathetic hyperactivity during desflurane anesthesia in healthy volunteers: a comparison with isoflurane. Anesthesiology 1993; 79:444-53.

83. Ghouri AF, Bodner M, White PF: Recovery profile after desflurane-nitrous oxide versus isoflurane-nitrous oxide in outpatients. Anesthesiology 1991; 74:419-24.

84. Smiley RM, Ornstein E, Matteo RS et al: Desflurane and isoflurane in surgical patients: Comparison of emergence times. Anesthesiology 1991; 74:425-8.

85. Van Hemelrijck J, Smith I, White PF: Use of desflurane for outpatient anesthesia. Anesthesiology 1991; 75:197-203.

86. Wrigley SR, Fairfield JE, Jones RM, Black AE: Induction and recovery characteristics of desflurane in day case patients: a comparison with propofol. Anesthesiology 1991; 46:615-22.

87. Lerman J, Sikich N, Kleinman S, Yentis S: The pharmacology of sevoflurane in infants and children. Anesthesiology 1994; 80:814-24.

88. Philip BK, Kallar SK, Bogetz MS et al: Multicenter comparison of sevoflurane with isoflurane in nitrous oxide for ambulatory surgery. Anesthesiology 1993; 79:A40.

89. Ochiai R, Toyoda Y, Nishio I et al: Possible association of malignant hyperthermia with sevoflurane anesthesia. Anesth Analg 1992; 74:616-8.

90. Bito H, Ikeda K: Closed-circuit anesthesia with sevoflurane in humans: effects on renal and hepatic function and concentrations of breakdown products with soda lime in the circuit. Anesthesiology 1994; 80:71-6.

91. Frink EJ, Malan TP, Isner RJ et al: Renal concentrating function with prolonged sevoflurane or enflurane anesthesia in volunteers. Anesthesiology 1994; 80:1019-25.

92. Eger EI: New inhaled anesthetics. Anesthesiology 1994; 80:906-22.

93. Weiskopf R, Eger E: Comparing the costs of inhaled anesthetics. Anesthesiology 1993; 79:1413-8.

94. Capan LM, Bruce DL, Patel KP et al: Succinylcholine-induced postoperative sore throat. Anesthesiology 1983; 59:202-6.

95. Loeser EA, Stanley TH, Jordan W et al: Postoperative sore throat: influence of tracheal tube lubrication versus cuff design. Can Anaesth Soc J 1980; 27:156-8.

96. Stout DM, Bishop MJ, Dwersteg JF, Cullen BF: Correlation of endotracheal tube size with sore throat and hoarseness following general anesthesia. Anesthesiology 1987; 67:419-21.

97. Churchill-Davidson HC: Suxamethonium (succinylcholine) chloride and muscle pains. Br Med J 1954; 74(1):74-5.

98. Brodsky JB, Brock-Utne JG, Samuels SI: Pancuronium pretreatment and postsuccinylcholine myalgias. Anesthesiology 1979; 51:259-61.

99. Zahl K, Apfelbaum JL: Muscle pain occurs after outpatient laparoscopy despite the substitution of vecuronium for succinylcholine. Anesthesiology 1989; 70:408-11.

100. Rivard JC, Lebowitz PW: Bradycardia after alfentanil-succinylcholine. Anesth Analg 1988; 67:900-7.

101. Basta SJ, Savarese JJ, Ali HH et al: Histamine releasing potencies of atracurium, dimethyltubocurarine and tubocurarine. Br J Anaesth 1983; 55:105S.

102. Savarese JJ, Ali HH, Basta SJ et al: The clinical neuromuscular pharmacology of mivacurium chloride (BW B1090U). Anesthesiology 1988; 68:723-32.

103. Ostergaard D, Jensen E, Jensen FS, Viby Mogensen J: The duration of action of mivacurium-induced neuromuscular blockade in patients homozygous for the atypical plasma cholinesterase gene. Anesthesiology 1991; 75:A774.

104. Ali HH, Brull SJ, Witkowski T et al: Efficacy and safety of divided dose mivacurium for rapid tracheal intubation. Anesthesiology 1993; 79:A934.

105. Donati F, Meistelman C, Plaud B: Vecuronium neuromuscular blockade at the adductor muscles of the larynx and adductor pollicis. Anesthesiology 1991; 74:833-7.

106. King MJ, Milazkiewicz R, Carli F, Deacock AR: Influence of neostigmine on postoperative vomiting. Br J Anaesth 1988; 61:403-6.

107. Starr NJ, Sethna DH, Estafanous FG: Bradycardia and asystole following the rapid administration of sufentanil with vecuronium. Anesthesiology 1986; 64:521-3.

108. Wierda JM, de Wit AP, Kuizenga K, Agaston S: Clinical observations on the neuromuscular blocking action of ORG 9426, a new steroidal non-depolarizing agent. Br J Anaesth 1990; 64:521-3.

109. Booth MG, Marsh B, Bryden FM et al: A comparison of the pharmacodynamics of rocuronium and vecuronium during halothane anaesthesia. Anaesthesia 1992; 47:832-4.

110. Jacobs JR, Glass PSA, Reves JG: Technology for continuous infusion in anesthesia. Int Anesthesiol Clin 1991; 29(4):39-52.

111. Holmes CM, Galletly DG: Midazolam/fentanyl—a total intravenous technique for short procedures. Anaesthesia 1982; 37:761-5.

112. Raeder JC, Hole A, Arnulf V, Grynne BH: Total intravenous anesthesia with midazolam and flumazenil in outpatient clinics. Acta Anaesthesiol Scand 1987; 31:634-41.

113. Vuyk J, Hennis PJ, Burm AGL et al: Comparison of midazolam and propofol in combination with alfentanil for total intravenous anesthesia. Anesth Analg 1990; 71:645-50.

114. Vinik HR, Bradley EL, Kissin I: Midazolam-alfentanil synergism for anesthetic induction in patients. Anesth Analg 1989; 69:213-7.

115. Raftery S, Sherry E: Total intravenous anesthesia with propofol and alfentanil protects against postoperative nausea and vomiting. Can J Anaesth 1992; 39:37-40.

Regional Anesthesia

8

D. Janet Pavlin

Regional versus General Anesthesia

Regional anesthesia is an excellent alternative to general anesthesia for outpatient surgery. It enables the anesthesiologist to provide the patient with total comfort at the operative site without obtunding mental function or airway reflexes. From the patients' point of view, regional anesthesia allows them the ability to maintain control of their mental faculties, which may be perceived as less "threatening" than the unconscious state of general anesthesia. In some instances, with regional anesthesia, patients may even watch the surgery on a video screen.

The use of regional anesthesia also bypasses many of the potential sources of minor or major morbidity associated with general anesthesia, i.e., trauma to lips, teeth, pharynx, vocal cords; bronchospasm; aspiration; prolonged somnolence; prolonged paralysis due to aberrant responses to neuromuscular blockers; and potential adverse responses to other anesthetic agents (e.g., malignant hyperthermia). In addition, protracted nausea and vomiting are less common, and postoperative pain is minimized or delayed by regional anesthesia.[1-3] After peripheral nerve blocks, phase I recovery may be unnecessary, and patients can begin mobilizing almost immediately after surgery. This represents a significant saving in terms of patient time and recovery room resources.

Clearly, there are significant benefits to be attained through the use of regional anesthesia. What are the potential negative aspects of regional anesthesia, either real or imagined?

Time. Regional anesthesia takes more time to initiate than does general anesthesia. However, time "lost" in initiating a regional anesthetic may be regained at the end of surgery, because patients can often transfer themselves to a stretcher and proceed immediately to the recovery unit.[1-3]

Equipment. Although the necessity of maintaining supplies and equipment for regional anesthesia is a potential disadvantage, equipment and recovery room costs for it may actually be less than that for general anesthesia.[1]

Personnel. An additional person is frequently required during initiation of a block to provide reassurance, to administer a sedative to the patient, to observe the airway, to maintain the patient in an optimal position, and to aid in controlling a nerve stimulator. These requirements, however, can typically be met without hiring additional personnel; a nurse in a preoperative holding area, or a circulating nurse in the operating room, may serve in this capacity.

Regional Anesthesia Skills

Perhaps the greatest potential disadvantage of regional anesthesia is the need to develop adequate regional anesthesia skills. This relates both to the actual technique, as well as to the skillful management of awake or lightly sedated patients. However, this can be a very positive experience that significantly contributes to the patient's favorable impression of the operative experience, an important "marketing" feature for an institution and the profession of anesthesiology.

Ideally, staffing would be sufficient so that an anesthesiologist can be relieved from a preceding case to establish a regional block in advance of the anticipated surgery. Alternatively, equipment and patients may be prepared by an assistant, while the anesthesiologist completes the previous case. The anesthesiologist can then commence performing a block immediately on completion of a preceding case, thus minimizing turnover time. A routine system of communication between anesthesiologist and surgeon is desirable with regard to what types of block will suffice for each patient—particularly for orthopedic surgeries, in which possible bone graft sites, tourniquet requirements, or procedures of extremely short duration may dictate the most acceptable method of anesthesia. Clearly, regional anesthesia requires a significant commitment to obtain optimal efficiency.

Patient Selection and Consent

The selection of appropriate candidates for regional anesthesia should be based on anesthesiologist skill, patient wishes, surgical requirements, and the underlying condition of the patient. Certain anatomical considerations (morbid obesity, kyphoscoliosis) or behavioral characteristics (drug addiction, extreme anxiety) may make regional anesthesia challenging, if not impossible. Decisions should be individualized and regional anesthesia employed when it will provide the most satisfactory anesthetic for a given patient.

Patients should be provided with a clear explanation of what is entailed with a particular block, of the potential side effects and complications, together with a discussion of the alternative: general anesthetic. It is wise to avoid presenting too many alternatives, as patients may be overwhelmed by a long list of options. Patients should also be informed that sedation will be available and provided as needed. It is wise to ask the patient in advance how sedated he or she wishes to be, because some patients take exception to having been sedated when they clearly wished to remain awake, while others express an extreme dislike at having been awake and able to hear the sounds of the operating room.

General Preparation and Management

The requirements for performing safe regional anesthesia include all that we accept as being necessary for a routine general anesthetic.

Monitoring

Monitoring should include regular automated measurement and display of blood pressure, ECG, and oxyhemoglobin saturation. Oxygen should be administered, and its effectiveness monitored by pulse oximetry. A trained observer should be constantly assessing the adequacy of the patient's airway and ventilation if sedation is given.

Resuscitative Equipment

Resuscitative equipment must be immediately available in case of respiratory and cardiovascular emergencies (Table 8-1). A cardiac arrest cart should be identifiable and ready for use. Venous access is mandatory before instituting regional anesthesia, so that potential emergencies can be managed promptly. Respiratory depression commonly occurs with sedation administered during a regional block; although rare, respiratory paralysis must always be anticipated during spinal, epidural, interscalene, or retrobulbar block. Seizures due to excessively rapid absorption of local anesthetic may cause severe hypoxia and acidosis within minutes, and these seizures require aggressive treatment with oxygen, positive pressure ventilation, and (as soon as possible) induction of paralysis and intubation.[4] Seizures increase ventilatory requirements several fold and simultaneously impair ventilation. Benzodiazepines (or barbiturates) may be administered to stop central seizure activity. However, the possibility of coexisting myocardial depression (particularly with bupivacaine) should be considered, and drugs should be administered cautiously to prevent further myocardial depression. Hypotension and bradycardia occur commonly with spinal or epidural anesthesia. Tachyarrhythmias can be precipitated by hypotension and by epinephrine-containing solutions; this is caused by a direct beta agonist effect on the heart or by a decline in serum potassium that accompanies the

Table 8-1   Resuscitation Equipment for Regional Anesthesia

Equipment	Drugs
Oral airway	Ephedrine, phenylephrine
Self-inflating positive pressure ventilating resuscitation bag and appropriate mask sizes	Epinephrine
Oxygen supply	Atropine
Laryngoscope	Midazolam or diazepam
Endotracheal tubes	Pentothal or methohexital
Suction	Succinylcholine
Cardiac arrest cart	Propranolol, verapamil, or adenosine
	Lidocaine, procainamide, or phenytoin

absorption of epinephrine.[5-6] Both supraventricular and ventricular arrhythmias may occur and require therapy. Supraventricular arrhythmias may be treated with intravenous adenosine 6 mg, verapamil 5 to 10 mg, or beta blocker (propranolol 0.5 mg, or esmolol 500 µg/kg). Ventricular arrhythmias may be treated by intravenous lidocaine 50 mg. If a ventricular arrhythmia occurs when there are already presumably high blood levels of lidocaine (i.e., when lidocaine was used as the primary local anesthetic agent in a dose of 5 to 7 mg/kg), alternative intravenous antiarrhythmics would be preferrable (procainamide 75 mg, or phenytoin 100 mg). If the epinephrine in the local anesthetic solution is the presumed cause of ventricular arrhythmia, cautious use of beta blockers may be the treatment of choice.

Sedation

Sedation is a desirable component of regional anesthesia. Before performing a block, a short-acting opioid (fentanyl, 1 to 2 µg/kg) and an anxiolytic (midazolam, 10 to 20 µg/kg) are effective in minimizing pain and anxiety. Ideally, during injection of local anesthetic, the patient would be sufficiently conscious to express any pain that might accompany intraneural placement of the needle. During surgery, bolus doses of midazolam (in 0.5 to 1.0 mg increments), or infusions of propofol (25 to 75 µg/kg/min) or methohexital (3 mg/kg/hour), work well. Recovery will be most rapid after propofol.[7,8]

Sterility

Sterility should be preserved during regional blocks by utilizing sterile equipment, disinfecting skin with an iodine- or hexachlorophene-containing solution, and preventing contamination of the field and equipment by using sterile drapes.

Equipment and Drugs

Needles

Subarachnoid block

Pencil-point needles (Whitacre, Sprotte) for performing spinal anesthesia lessen the likelihood of postpuncture headache below that seen when 25- to 26-gauge sharp Quincke point needles are used (Fig. 8-1).[9-11] These needles are shaped so that they tend to spread the fibers of the dura rather than cut them, which makes them less likely to cause dural rent, leakage of cerebrospinal fluid, and headache. The aperture for injection is at the side of the distal end of the needle, rather than at the needle tip. It has been conjectured that this configuration may allow the needle to straddle the subarachnoid and epidural spaces; block failure may occur if a portion of the local anesthetic is injected into the epidural space. Both needles may be used with a 20-gauge thin-wall spinal introducer needle, or independently if the shaft of the needle is supported while the needle is advanced. Both Whitacre and Sprotte needles are more costly than a traditional 26-gauge spinal needle (Quincke point). However, a significant reduction in incidence of headache, particularly in young outpatients, justifies their use in the ambulatory population. A 27-gauge Quincke point needle may also convey an equally low incidence of headaches (Table 8-2).[12]

Epidural block

Commonly employed needles for epidural anesthesia include the curved Tuohy or Hustead needle, or the blunt-tip Crawford needle (Fig. 8-1, A). The curved tip of the Tuohy or Hustead needles may lessen the chance of dural puncture, and facilitate threading of the epidural catheter; they are typically preferred for the midline approach. The paramedian approach relies on a perceived loss of resistance as one walks off the edge of the lamina, and the Crawford needle may provide a better feel for contact with the ligamentum flavum without actually puncturing it prematurely. Thin-walled 18-gauge needles permit passage of a 20-gauge epidural catheter.

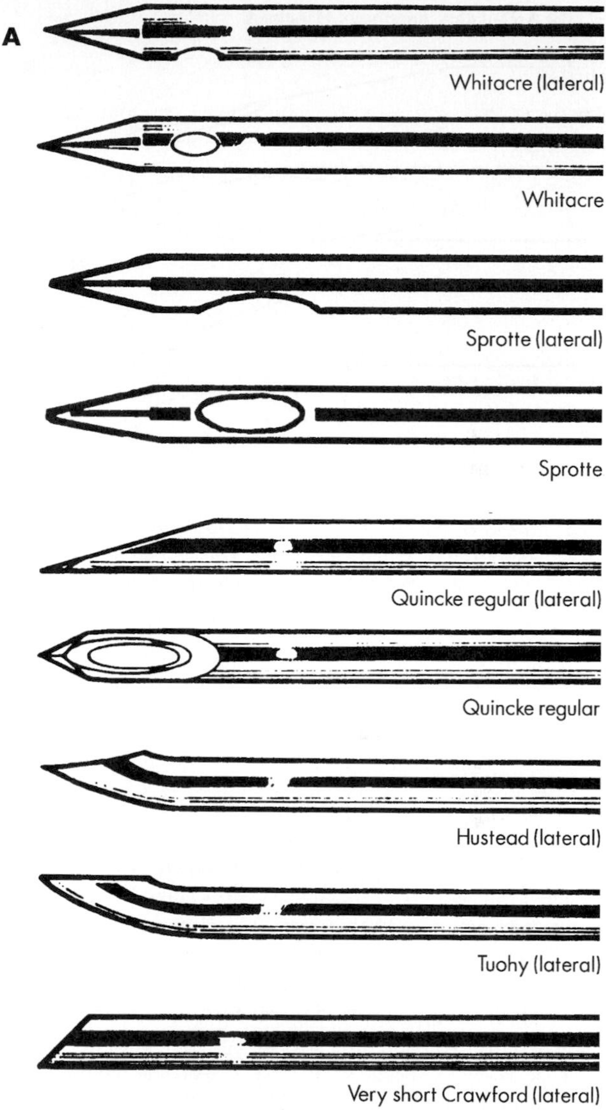

Fig. 8-1 A, Needles recommended for spinal anesthesia (Whitacre or Sprotte) and the sharp Quincke point needle for comparison; and needles recommended for epidural anesthesia (Hustead, Tuohy, or Crawford). (Modified from Mulroy MF: Regional anesthesia: an illustrated procedural guide, Boston, 1989, Little, Brown and Co, p. 59.)

Continued.

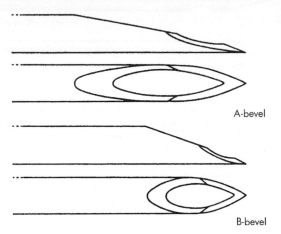

Fig. 8-1, cont'd. B, Sharp A-bevel and intermediate B-bevel needles for nerve blocks. (From Winnie AP: Clinic considerations. In Winnie AP, editor: Plexus anesthesia, vol 1, Philadelphia, 1992, WB Saunders, p. 213.)

A variety of catheters exist, but newer 20-gauge pliable catheters help minimize the risk of dural puncture during insertion.

Regional block

Regional blocks can be performed with 22- and 25-gauge sharp Quincke point needles (A-bevel, 12 degrees), flat-bevel needles (45 degrees), or a variety of intermediate types (B-bevel, 19 degrees)(Fig. 8-1, *B*).[13] Selander's work suggests that sharp cutting needles are more likely to impale and traumatize nerves.[14] Flat-bevel needles may be potentially less traumatic and facilitate identifying fascial sheaths, but they slide less easily through tissues; with the exception of the Crawford tip needle, they are also not readily available for use in epidural anesthesia. The B-bevel nerve-block needles offer a reasonable compromise, enabling identification of fascial sheaths and theoretically making nerve trauma less likely. A third category is the Teflon-coated insulated needle used for performing regional blocks with a nerve stimulator. Disposable sheathed needles that incorporate conductive wiring and a port that can be connected directly to the cathode electrode of a nerve stimulator are commercially available and are most convenient to use.

Table 8-2   Incidence (in Percentage) of Postdural Puncture
Headache in Outpatients

	Incidence (%)				
	Quincke needle		Whitacre needle		Sprotte needle
Age	25-26 g	27 g	25 g	27 g	24 g
All[12,13A, 13B, 13C]	7.1-18	1.7	1-2.5	0.4	4.7
<40[13A, 13B, 13C]	39	1.3	3.3-7	0.6	10

g = gauge

Nerve stimulators

Nerve stimulators are used in regional anesthesia to aid in localizing peripheral nerves. They should be capable of delivering a variable but controllable current, and should provide a visual display of the current delivered. Proximity to a nerve is confirmed by visible twitching of muscle in the distribution of the motor nerve being stimulated. When the nerve stimulator is used in conjunction with an insulated needle, accuracy is enhanced, and visible muscle twitching at a current intensity of 0.5 to 1.0 mA signifies close proximity to a nerve and is predictive of block success.[15] The cathode (negative pole) of the stimulator should be used as the exploring electrode; mistaken use of the anode causes hyperpolarization of the adjacent nerve, and a misleadingly greater stimulus intensity will be required to elicit a muscle twitch.[15,16] Nerve stimulators permit greater accuracy in identifying needle position, which should theoretically result in faster onset and higher success rates, although this has not been conclusively demonstrated. It is particularly useful in a teaching situation, and is considerably less painful for patients than actively seeking parasthesias. It is presumed that blocks performed with a nerve stimulator are less likely to result in nerve injury than do blocks involving active seeking of parasthesias; however, the incidence of neurologic injury using the nerve stimulator to perform peripheral nerve blocks has not yet been reported.[17]

Local anesthetics

The local anesthetic for outpatient surgery must be chosen while considering that after surgery, patients should be fit for discharge within a reasonable time. In general, it is most practical to tailor a regional anesthetic to the usual duration of surgery, recognizing that occasionally block regression may necessitate a brief period of general anesthesia. This can be accomplished by using a variety of local anesthetics, with or without vasopressors, to adjust for presumed duration of surgery.

The maximum recommended doses for a variety of local anesthetics are shown in Table 8-3. Signs and symptoms of local anesthetic toxicity are believed to be similar for most local anesthetics (Fig. 8-2). Bupivacaine may be a notable exception; myocardial depression (toxicity) is observed at relatively low concentration relative to the threshold for central nervous system toxicity. Combinations of local anesthetics (i.e., tetracaine with lidocaine or mepivacaine) to prolong duration but preserve rapid onset may enhance the likelihood of local anesthetic toxicity. In animals, the toxicity of local anesthetics appears to be additive.[18,19] In addition to toxic reactions, allergic reactions to local anesthetics can occur, but are rare with the amide anesthetics.[20] In outpatients, it is prudent to err on the "short side," remembering that the duration of complete recovery (which may determine discharge time) is considerably longer than the duration of surgical anesthesia typically quoted in the literature.

Specific Blocks

Intravenous Regional Anesthesia

Intravenous regional anesthesia is appropriate for short (less than 1 hour) surgical procedures involving the upper extremity. Anesthesia is obtained by injecting the local anesthetic into the vein of a limb that has been exsanguinated with an inflated occlusive tourniquet. The tourniquet also prevents the escape of local anesthetic. Anesthesia results from the drug's direct action at the nerve endings, as well as by its diffusion into nerve trunks.[21] Advantages of intravenous regional anesthesia include that it is easily performed, and it rapidly resolves with tourniquet release. Disadvantages include its limited duration (1 hour), possible local anesthetic toxicity due to inadvertant early tourniquet release, absence of significant postoperative analgesia, poor hemostasis with the double-cuff tourniquet, difficulty in effectively performing the procedure in the obese patient or the patient with open or painful lesions, and typically lower density of block than that of successful nerve block. The technique described here is one

Table 8-3 Physiochemical Properties and Maximum Dose of Selected Local Anesthetic Agents

	Relative lipid solubility	Protein binding (%)	pK	Equieffective concentration	Maximum dose (mg) Plain	Maximum dose (mg) With epinephrine
Esters						
Procaine	0.6	5.8	8.9	2	500	1000 (14 mg/kg)
2-Chloroprocaine	1	-	8.7	2	800	1000 (14 mg/kg)
Tetracaine	80	75.6	8.5	0.25	-	200 (2 mg/kg)
Amides						
Lidocaine	2.9	64.3	7.7	1	300	500 (7 mg/kg)
Mepivacaine	0.8	77.5	7.6	1	400	550 (7 mg/kg)
Prilocaine	0.8	55	7.7	1	500	900 (7 mg/kg)
Bupivacaine	27.5	95.6	8.1	0.25	175	225 (3 mg/kg)

Adapted from Mulroy MF: Regional anesthesia: an illustrated procedural guide, Boston, 1989, Little, Brown and Co., pp. 3, 14.

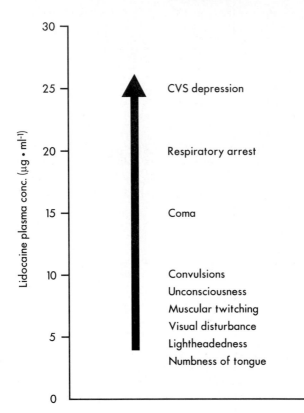

TOXIC EFFECTS

Fig. **8-2** Progressive signs and symptoms of local anesthetic toxicity related to increasing concentrations of lidocaine in blood. (From Carpenter RI, Mackey DC, Barash PG et al: Local anesthetics. In Barash PG, editor: Clinical anesthesia, Philadelphia, 1989, JB Lippincott, pp. 526-9.)

commonly employed for regional anesthesia of the upper limb. Although it may be modified to provide anesthesia of the lower extremity, the volumes of local anesthetic required for the lower limb (75 to 100 ml) may pose a serious hazard if inadvertant tourniquet release occurs.

Position

The patient is placed in the supine position with the arm abducted on a support.

Intravenous catheter

An 18- to 20-gauge catheter is inserted into a vein on the dorsum of the hand or wrist, and is capped with a heparin lock. After aspirating blood to confirm its correct position, the catheter is secured.

Exsanguination

A double-cuffed tourniquet is wrapped about the upper arm and the cuff tubing is connected to a pressure generator set to deliver a cuff pressure of 250 mm Hg (or approximately twice the systolic blood pressure). The patient makes a tight fist around a roll of gauze, the arm is elevated, and an Eshmarch bandage is wrapped tightly about the arm in an overlapping, circumferential manner, beginning at the hand and ending at the tourniquet. The distal and then the proximal cuff are inflated sequentially, forcing blood out from under the tourniquet proximally. Local anesthesia is injected as noted below. The distal cuff is then deflated to permit local anesthetic penetrating under it. When the Eshmarch is removed, the arm should have a cadaveric appearance with absent pulses.

Local anesthetic

Slowly (over more than 90 seconds) 50 ml of 0.5% lidocaine (or 0.5% prilocaine) is injected through the catheter, which should cause venous distension with no evidence of infiltration at the catheter tip. Numbness occurs within 5 minutes, and motor block within 15 minutes.

Tourniquet pain

Pain may occur after 30 to 40 minutes, and is treated by first inflating the distal cuff, then deflating the proximal cuff.

Tourniquet deflation

At termination of surgery, the tourniquet is deflated for 5 to 10 seconds and then immediately reinflated; this sequence is repeated two or three times at 1- to 2-minute intervals. This is intended to release residual local anesthetic in small boluses to permit time for redistribution of a bolus before the next bolus is released.

Potential problems

1. Hemostasis may be poor when a double-cuff tourniquet is used because the individual cuff width is thinner than that of a traditional single cuff, and pressure is less well transmitted to vessels in the arm. Use of higher cuff pressures (300 mm Hg), and attention to detail during limb exsanguination may reduce bleeding in the surgical field. In obese subjects, it may be wise to select a different technique because of difficulties in obtaining a tight fit of the tourniquet.

2. Pain and restlessness that occur in some patients can be alleviated by small amounts of opioid, by sedation, or by a combination of opioid and sedative. In some patients, the density of block may simply be inadequate, and general anesthesia may be required. This block is best applied for soft tissue procedures in which the surgical stimulus is less than that when there is bony involvement.

3. Local anesthetic toxicity can be minimized by confirming the absence of pulses before injection, by injecting the local anesthetic slowly, by administering it into distal rather than proximal veins (thus preventing high pressures and leakage of local anesthetic during injection), and by ensuring that the cuff is deflated for only a few seconds at a time at the end of surgery. After very short procedures (less than 20 minutes), particular care should be exercised and length of time between successive deflations lengthened. The relationship of tourniquet time to local anesthetic blood level upon tourniquet release (Fig. 8-3)[22] predicts relatively high blood levels with release in less than 20 minutes. When 0.5% lidocaine (1.5 mg/kg) is used for intravenous regional anesthesia, minor central nervous system toxicity has been reported to occur in 2% to 10% of patients, and major toxicity (seizures) in 0% to 3% of patients. A number of deaths attributed to myocardial toxicity have been reported following use of bupivacaine for intravenous regional anesthesia, and, therefore, its use is not recommended.[23] Prilocaine offers perhaps the least likelihood of systemic toxicity because of its short plasma half life. Methemoglobinemia, a possible but rarely significant clinical problem with prilocaine, may be treated with intravenous methylene blue, 1 to 5 mg/kg. Prilocaine may be contraindicated when reduced oxygen-carrying capacity of the blood might be poorly

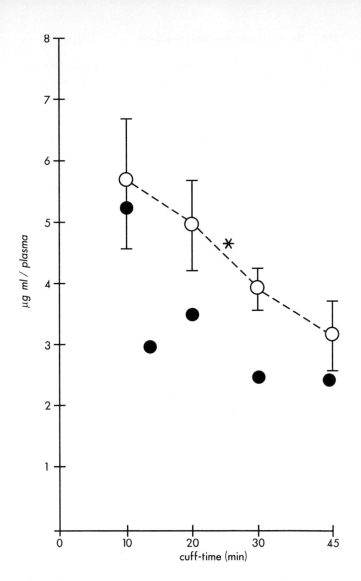

Fig. 8-3 Intravenous regional anesthesia: Relationship between cuff time and arterial plasma level of lidocaine measured at 1 minute after cuff release. *Open circles,* mean data ± SD, 1% solution; *closed circles,* individual data; 0.5% solution; *, difference significant at p < .05. (From Tucker GT, Boas RA: Pharmacokinetic aspects of intravenous regional anesthesia. Anesthesiology 1971; 34:538-49.)

tolerated (i.e., ischemic coronary or cerebrovascular disease, hypoxemia due to underlying lung disease, severe anemia).

Upper Extremity Nerve Blocks

There is a variety of nerve blocks for achieving regional anesthesia of the upper extremity. Typically, supraclavicular, interscalene, and axillary brachial plexus blocks provide adequate anesthesia of the hand. However, the possibility of undetected pneumothorax with a supraclavicular block (0.5% to 6% incidence)[24] makes this an unwise choice in outpatients. Interscalene blocks have particular utility for surgery of the upper arm or shoulder, but they are associated with a relatively slow onset of anesthesia of the hand, and possibly with total sparing of the medial portion of the hand and upper arm. The axillary brachial plexus block produces excellent anesthesia for surgery of the hand, forearm, and elbow. Although the musculocutaneous nerve is occasionally spared, it is relatively easy to anesthetize this nerve specifically while performing the block.

Anatomy of the brachial plexus

The brachial plexus arises from the anterior primary divisions of the fifth cervical through first thoracic nerves (C-5, C-6, C-7, C-8, T-1). After emerging from the intervertebral foramina, the nerves pass laterally, behind the vertebral artery, run through troughs in the cervical transverse processes, and descend over the first rib and under the clavicle to reach the axilla. Above the first rib, they fuse to form superior (C5-C6), middle (C-7), and inferior (C-5, T-1) trunks. As they approach the clavicle, they divide to form divisions, reunite to form cords, and finally emerge in the axilla as individual peripheral nerves (Fig. 8-4). The interscalene block is performed at the level of the roots where the nerves are aligned vertically between the anterior and middle scalene muscles. The axillary block is performed in the axilla where the median nerve lies anterolateral, the ulnar nerve medial, and the radial nerve posteromedial to the axillary artery (Figs. 8-5 and 8-6). The axillary nerve diverges from the axillary sheath at a high level and is not anesthetized by an axillary block. The musculocutaneous nerve leaves the axillary sheath at a slightly lower level and enters the substance of the coracobrachialis muscle. It is occasionally spared with an axillary block.

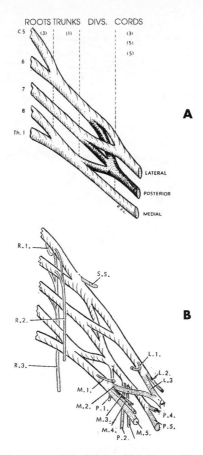

Fig. 8-4 **A,** Formation of the left brachial plexus. The nerves of the brachial plexus are the anterior primary rami of the spinal nerves, C5 to T1. **B,** Branches of the brachial plexus. Branches of roots: *R.1.,* dorsal scapular n.; *R.2.,* n. to subclavius; *R.3.,* long thoracic n. Branches of upper trunk: *S.S.,* suprascapular n. Branches of lateral cord: *L.1.,* lateral pectoral; *L.2.,* musculocutaneous n.; *L.3.,* lateral root of median n. Branches of medial cord: *M.1.,* medial pectoral; *M.2.,* medial root of median n.; *M.3.,* medial cutaneous n. of arm. Branches of posterior cord: *P.1.,* upper subscapular; *P.2.,* thoracodorsal n.; *P.3.,* lower subscapular; *P.4.,* axillary n.; *P.5.,* radial n. (From Last RJ: Anatomy, regional and applied, London, 1972, Churchill Livingstone, pp. 96-7.)

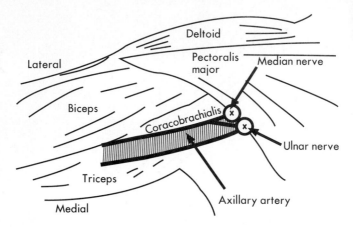

Fig. 8-5 Surface markings for axillary brachial plexus block. The median nerve is located anterolateral to the axillary artery (*X*), and the ulnar nerve medial to the artery (*X*).

Local anesthetics

A variety of local anesthetics (or local anesthetic combinations) may be employed for peripheral nerve blocks of the upper extremity (Table 8-4). Lidocaine or mepivacaine are generally recommended for short outpatient procedures. Tetracaine (0.1% to 0.2%) may be added to 1% lidocaine or mepivicaine ("supercaine") to lengthen the duration of anesthesia to 4 to 6 hours when desired. The prolonged duration of motor block achieved with bupivacaine is typically considered unpleasant and inconvenient by most outpatients, and, therefore, bupivacaine is not recommended. However, in selected instances when outpatients desire prolonged analgesia, bupivacaine 0.375% will provide anesthesia of approximately 10 to 11 hours duration. Patients with persistent motor block can be discharged with the arm secured in a sling, but they must be appropriately cautioned about the potential for injury with a numb, paralyzed extremity. Although it is common practice in some institutions to combine 0.75% bupivacaine with 2% lidocaine to attain rapid onset and prolonged duration of anesthesia, it is important to recognize that toxicities of these two agents appear to be additive. Simultaneous use of

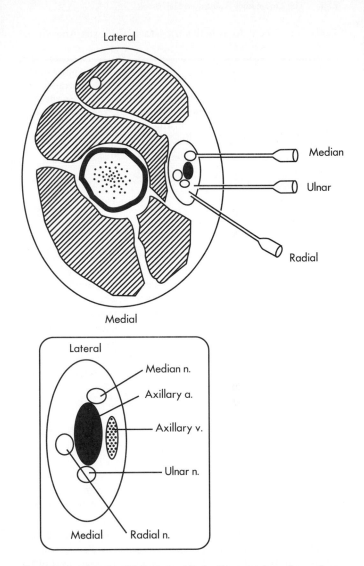

Fig. 8-6 Axillary brachial plexus block. Cross-section of arm demonstrating the position of the nerves relative to the axillary artery, and the direction of the needle required to contact the median, ulnar, and radial nerves.

Table 8-4   Local Anesthetics for Brachial Plexus Anesthesia
in Outpatients

Drug	Concentration (%)	Maximum dose (mg/kg) (with epinephrine)	Approximate duration of surgical anesthesia (hours)
Lidocaine	1-1.5	7	1.5-3
Mepivacaine	1-1.5	7	2-4
Lidocaine/			
mepivacaine	1	< 7	
plus tetracaine	0.1-0.2	< 1.5	4-6
Bupivacaine	0.375	3	10-11

maximum allowable doses of both drugs enhances the likelihood
of toxicity. When local anesthetic solutions are deposited in close
proximity to nerves, there is little evidence that speed of onset of
lidocaine-bupivacaine combinations is appreciably faster than that
of bupivacaine alone. The use of local anesthetic combinations
remains somewhat controversial, and the questionable benefits
must be weighed against the enhanced risks of toxicity. The
relative safety of adding low doses of tetracaine (40 to 50 mg) to
1% lidocaine (or mepivacaine) solutions has been somewhat better
substantiated in the literature.

Axillary block

The patient should be supine with the arm abducted 90 degrees.

Surface landmarks

Surface landmarks include the axillary artery, biceps muscle,
coracobrachialis muscle, X overlying the median nerve (just
lateral to the artery) and ulnar nerve (just medial to the artery)
(Figs. 8-5 and 8-6).

Median nerve: An insulated needle is inserted through a local
anesthetic skin wheal at the X overlying the median nerve, and
advanced proximally at a 45-degree angle to the long axis of the
arm, until the needle is felt to "pop" through the axillary sheath.
It is advanced until a flexor twitch occurs in the hand, or until a
parasthesia is evident on the lateral side of the hand. If a twitch is
not elicited, the needle is partially withdrawn and redirected in a

progressively more lateral or medial direction until a twitch is elicited. The needle is then pivoted at the skin in a mediolateral direction across the path of the nerve, until a maximal twitch is obtained (the "best angle"). Maintaining this angle, the needle is advanced until the twitch just begins to fade (the "best depth"). The needle is then aspirated to ensure it is not in a vessel, and 15 to 25 ml of local anesthetic is injected. The stimulator is initially set to deliver a current of 2.0 to 2.5 mA to facilitate a coarse, hasty search for the nerve. Subsequently, the amperage is reduced until a twitch can be obtained at a stimulus intensity of 0.5 mA or less, which signifies that the tip of the needle is very close to the nerve.

Ulnar nerve: A similar technique is utilized for the ulnar nerve. The needle tip is inserted at the *X* overlying the ulnar nerve and directed toward the medial side of the artery. When a flexion twitch of the fingers is elicited (or when a parasthesia occurs in the fifth digit), the needle is pivoted to obtain the best angle, advanced to the best depth, and 15 to 25 ml of local anesthetic is injected.

Radial nerve: This nerve can be blocked by advancing the needle further after injecting the ulnar nerve. The needle is directed from the *X* on the medial side of the artery, toward the posterior aspect of the artery. (Occasionally it may be more easily located from the lateral side of the vessel.) Any extensor motion of the hand, wrist, or elbow signifies a radial nerve twitch. After optimizing angle and depth, 5 to 15 ml of local anesthetic is injected.

The order in which nerves are injected can be varied so that nerves innervating the site of incision are blocked first with the greatest volume of solution. Some clinicians advocate a single-injection technique in which all local anesthetic is injected with the first twitch (or parasthesia) as a means of reducing the possibility of puncture-induced nerve injury. However, Thompson has demonstrated the existence of fascial compartments that may retard the spread of local anesthetic throughout the axillary sheath, and has suggested that selective blocking of individual nerves is more likely to produce complete anesthesia.[25] The relative importance of such fascial barriers has been questioned by Partridge, who has demonstrated rapid diffusion of methylene blue dye throughout the plexus when injected directly into the axillary sheath of cadavers.[26] It is likely that a variety of techniques, if perfected, will provide adequate anesthesia in a majority of cases.[27] The distribution of anesthesia with an axillary block is shown in Fig. 8-7. The medial aspect of the upper arm may not be

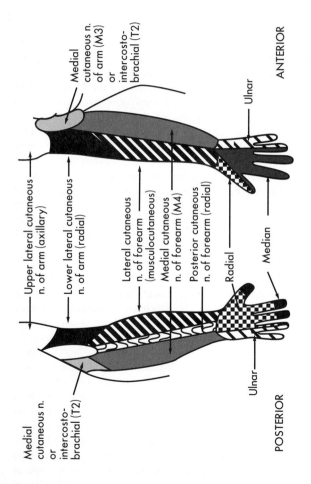

Medial cutaneous n. of arm (M3) or intercosto-brachial (T2)

Upper lateral cutaneous n. of arm (axillary)

Lower lateral cutaneous n. of arm (radial)

Lateral cutaneous n. of forearm (musculocutaneous)

Medial cutaneous n. of forearm (M4)

Posterior cutaneous n. of forearm (radial)

Radial

Median

Ulnar

ANTERIOR

Medial cutaneous n. or intercosto-brachial (T2)

Ulnar

POSTERIOR

Fig. 8-7 Anesthetic distribution of axillary block. (See text for details.)

anesthetized if it is innervated by the intercostobrachial nerve (T-2), which is not part of the brachial plexus. This nerve can be anesthetized by creating a wheal of local anesthetic along the medial aspect of the upper arm high in the axilla. In many individuals, this area is primarily innervated by the medial cutaneous n. of the arm which is part of the brachial plexus, and can be anesthetized by an axillary block. Motor block may be tested as follows: *Median n.*: opposition of the thumb (opponens pollicus); *ulnar n*: abduction of the fingers from the midline (dorsal interossei); *radial n.*: extension at the elbow, or wrist (extensors); *musculocutaneous n.*: flexion at the elbow (biceps brachialis and coracobrachialis muscles). Potential complications include local anesthetic toxicity, hematoma, and nerve injury (0.3% to 2.8%).[14,28]

Musculocutaneous nerve: Failure to achieve adequate anesthesia of the musculocutaneous nerve is the most common problem with the axillary brachial plexus block. To facilitate anesthetizing this nerve during axillary block, proximal spread of local anesthetic up the axillary sheath is promoted by always injecting anesthetic in a cephalad direction, by ensuring the the arm is not abducted to greater than 90 degrees during the block, and by returning the arm to the patient's side immediately after the block to prevent compression of the axillary sheath by the head of the humerus. Manual pressure can also be exerted just distal to the point of injection to promote proximal spread.

Alternatively, specific injections of local anesthetic directed at the musculocutaneous nerve may increase the anesthesia success and speed of onset. In the axilla, the nerve is located within the coracobrachialis muscle, which in turn is located just lateral to the axillary artery, medial to the biceps muscle (Fig. 8-8). An insulated needle is introduced just lateral to the artery (at the X overlying the median nerve) and advanced toward the lateral side of the humerus. When it contacts bone, the needle is partially withdrawn and redirected just lateral to the humerus (toward the tip of the shoulder) until a twitch is obtained (flexion at the elbow). The angle and depth of the needle are optimized, and 5 to 10 ml of local anesthetic injected. Alternatively, blind injections may be made in the same area from the depth of the humerus up to skin, injecting the solution as the needle is gradually withdrawn.

Transarterial approach: A transarterial approach to brachial plexus block consists of injecting 15 to 25 ml of local anesthetic

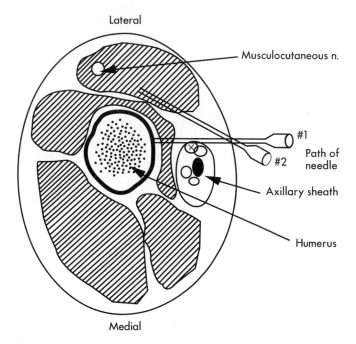

Fig. 8-8 Musculocutaneous nerve. Cross-section of the arm at the axilla demonstrating the position of the musculocutaneous nerve within the coracobrachialis muscle lateral to the axillary sheath and the humerus. The needle is first directed toward the humerus (path 1) and then redirected laterally (path 2) to locate the musculocutaneous nerve in the coracobrachialis muscle.

anterior and posterior to the axillary artery, aspirating blood to signify needle position. Hematoma formation can occur and can occasionally result in pain or a nerve compression syndrome.

Nerve blocks at the elbow

Nerve blocks at the elbow or wrist may be used for hand surgery (if an upper arm tourniquet is not required) or as a means of block retrieval for a brachial plexus block that is incomplete in the distribution of one or more nerves. The description that follows may be performed blindly using a 25-gauge 1½-inch needle, or with the aid of a stimulator and an insulated needle.

Median nerve: The median nerve, located just medial to the biceps tendon and the brachial artery at the elbow, is blocked by injecting 5 to 7 ml of local anesthetic just medial to the brachial artery. Using a stimulator, flexion of the digits can be observed (Fig. 8-9).

Ulnar nerve: The ulnar nerve, which can be easily palpated in the groove on the medial aspect of the distal end of the humerus (between the trochlea and medial epicondyle), is blocked by injecting 5 to 7 ml of local anesthetic in the vicinity of the nerve; this can be confirmed by observing twitching of the fingers (Fig. 8-10).

Radial nerve: The radial nerve, which runs inferolaterally in the spiral groove around the posterior aspect of the humerus, is blocked as it lies on the lateral aspect of the lower humerus (Fig. 8-11). A needle is inserted perpendicular to the skin approximately 6 to 7 cm above the lateral epicondyle on the lateral aspect of the arm, and advanced until bone is contacted. Local anesthetic (2 to 3 ml) is injected just above the bone, the needle is then redirected to contact bone 1 to 2 cm proximal and distal to the initial point of contact, and repeat injections made at these locations. A wall of anesthesia through which the nerve must pass is thus created. Using the nerve stimulator, extensor motions of wrist or fingers signifies proximity to the radial nerve.

Musculocutaneous nerve: The musculocutaneous nerve is located on the anterolateral side of the elbow, just lateral to the biceps tendon, 1 to 2 cm superficial to the humerus. A needle is introduced at the elbow crease, just lateral to the biceps tendon; it is advanced to the humerus and then withdrawn 1 to 2 cm, and 5 to 7 ml of local anesthetic is injected as the needle is withdrawn toward the skin. Using a stimulator, flexion at the elbow signifies proximity to the nerve.

Nerve blocks at the wrist

Median nerve: The median nerve is located just lateral to the palmaris longus tendon (the most prominent flexor tendon at the anterior surface of the wrist) and medial to the tendon of the flexor carpi radialis (palpable just lateral to the palmaris longus when the wrist is flexed). A needle is inserted at the wrist crease approximately 1 to 2 cm deep, and 3 to 5 ml of local anesthetic is deposited beneath the flexor retinaculum (Fig. 8-9).

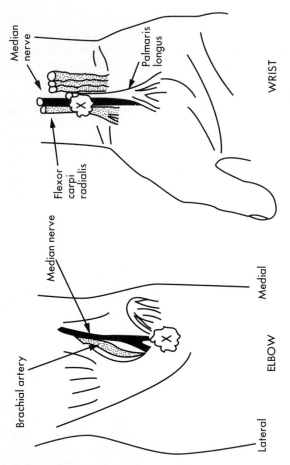

Fig. 8-9 Median nerve block at the elbow or wrist. At the elbow, the nerve is medial to the brachial artery. At the wrist, it lies between the palmaris longus and flexor carpi radialis. (Adapted from Moore DC: Regional block, ed 4, Springfield, Ill, 1979, Charles C. Thomas, pp. 257-74.)

Ulnar nerve: The ulnar nerve lies just medial to the ulnar artery. At the wrist, it divides into dorsal and ventral branches; the ventral branch is located just medial to the ulnar a., while the dorsal branches circles round the medial aspect of the wrist to innervate the dorsolateral aspect of the hand. A needle is inserted at the level of the ulnar styloid just medial to the ulnar artery, and 3 to 5 ml of local anesthetic injected. A subcutaneous wheal of local anesthetic is then created, from the point of the original injection, circumferentially around the medial aspect of the wrist to the midpoint of the dorsal aspect of the wrist. This anesthetizes the branches of the nerve that deviate proximally from the main nerve and provide sensory innervation to the dorsomedial aspect of the hand (see Fig. 8-10).

Radial nerve: The radial nerve lies just lateral to the radial artery on the anterior surface of the wrist. It gives rise to a dorsal branch that runs laterally to supply the dorsolateral aspect of the hand. For this block, 3 to 5 ml of local anesthetic is injected just lateral to the radial artery, and a subcutaneous wheal of local anesthetic is created beginning at the radial pulse and extending laterally around the wrist to the midpoint of the wrist posteriorly (see Fig. 8-11).

Digital nerve blocks

Digital nerves are located at the 2, 5, 7, and 10 o'clock positions relative to the metacarpal bones when viewed in cross-section. A circumferential wheal of local anesthetic is created at the base of the finger, taking care to encompass nerves at each of these locations. Vasoconstrictors are *not* employed with digital blocks because of the proximity of the nerves to terminal branches of digital vessels.

Interscalene brachial plexus block

The patient should be supine with the back elevated at a 10- to 20-degree angle.

Surface landmarks
Surface landmarks include the sternocleidomastoid muscle; anterior and middle scalene muscles; interscalene groove; cricoid cartilage, and a line drawn laterally and horizontally from the cricoid to intersect the interscalene groove laterally; *X* at the junction of the horizontal line (in previous landmark) and the interscalene groove (Fig. 8-12).

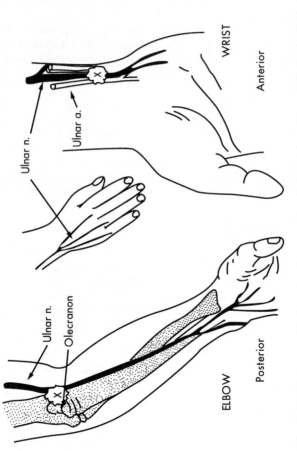

Fig. 8-10 Ulnar nerve block at the elbow or wrist. (Adapted from Moore DC: Regional block, ed 4, Springfield, Ill, 1979, Charles C. Thomas, pp. 257-74.)

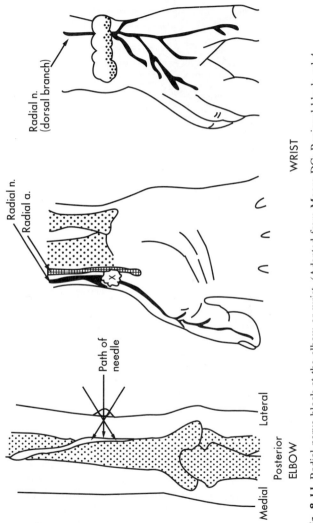

Fig. 8-11 Radial nerve block at the elbow or wrist. (Adapted from Moore DC: Regional block, ed 4, Springfield, Ill, 1979, Charles C. Thomas, pp. 257-74).

Radial n. (dorsal branch)

Radial n.
Radial a.

Path of needle

Medial

Posterior
ELBOW

Lateral

WRIST

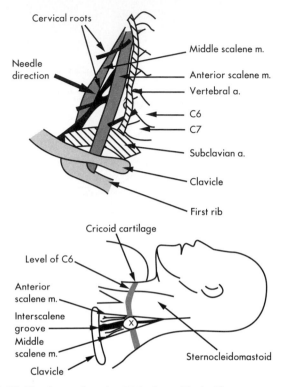

Fig. 8-12 The interscalene brachial plexus block. The nerve roots emerge from between the anterior and middle scalene muscles in the interscalene groove. The cricoid cartilage is identified and a line projected laterally from it to the interscalene groove. A needle is inserted at the junction of this line with the interscalene groove, and directed perpendicular (and slightly caudad) to skin to locate the plexus.

Technique

A 1½- or 2-inch needle is inserted at the *X* perpendicular to skin in all planes (directed slightly caudad to avoid puncture of the vertebral artery), and then advanced until a twitch is obtained (flexion at the elbow) or until bone is contacted. If one fails to obtain a twitch, one should redirect the needle anteriorly (or posteriorly) across the path of the nerve roots. Twitches obtained in other muscle groups may not be predictive of adequate

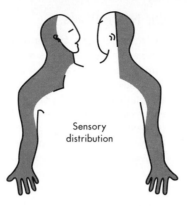

Sensory
distribution

Fig. 8-13 The interscalene brachial plexus block. Sensory distribution of anesthesia. When combined with superficial cervical plexus block, a "cape of anesthesia" is obtained.

anesthesia of the shoulder; if surgery involves the hand, stimulation of the muscles of the hand would be acceptable. The needle is adjusted to obtain the best angle and depth, and after aspirating to ensure that the needle is not in a vessel, a test dose of 1 to 2 ml is injected. If no symptoms of central nervous system toxicity occur, 30 to 40 ml of local anesthetic is injected incrementally. To anesthetize the superficial cervical plexus, a local anesthetic wheal is created beginning at the midpoint of the posterior border of the sternocleidomastoid muscle, and injecting 2 to 3 cm inferiorly, and superiorly, along the posterior border of that muscle.

The interscalene block provides good anesthesia for shoulder surgery and usually provides adequate anesthesia for hand surgery, although the medial aspect of the hand or arm may be spared or anesthesia here may be slow in onset (Fig. 8-13).

Specific complications

Specific complications of this block include occasional vertebral artery injection (central nervous system toxicity), paralysis of recurrent laryngeal (2% to 3%) and phrenic (greater than 6%) nerves, and unilateral Horner's syndrome (18%).[29-31] Rarely, cervical epidural[32] or spinal anesthesia[33] may occur if local anesthetic is injected into a dural cuff, or pneumothorax may occur if the needle is directed too far inferiorly.[29]

Lower Extremity Nerve Blocks

Anesthesia for foot or ankle surgery can conveniently be achieved by nerve blocks at the ankle. Typically, this requires the surgeon to operate without a thigh tourniquet (although a tourniquet may be tolerated for short periods without anesthesia under the cuff). As an alternative to a thigh tourniquet, hemostasis can be achieved by an Eshmarch bandage wrapped about the foot, beginning distally and ending just above the ankle, which is then unwrapped about the forefoot to permit surgery. Ankle blocks impose the least postoperative impairment of function (i.e., ability to walk or mobilize on crutches) and are useful for outpatient procedures exclusively confined to the foot. Nerve blocks at the knee will cause foot drop due to peroneal nerve involvement, making mobilization more difficult. Similarly, sciatic or femoral nerve blocks at the hip make mobilization extremely difficult until motor block has resolved. Additionally, resolution of sciatic and femoral nerve blocks is relatively slow and unpredictable, even with lidocaine. Their routine use in ambulatory patients is not recommended when delays in mobilization and discharge represent a significant disadvantage.

Anatomy (Figs. 8-14 to 8-16)

The sciatic nerve emerges from the greater sciatic notch and descends distally in the thigh, becoming more superficial between the biceps femoris and semitendinous tendons at the apex of the popliteal fossa, where it divides into tibial and common peroneal nerves. The tibial nerve continues distally through the popliteal fossa, and emerges with the posterior tibial artery, medially at the ankle behind the medial malleolus. The common peroneal nerve encircles the head of the fibula laterally, and then divides into deep and superficial peroneal nerves. The deep peroneal nerve crosses the anterior surface of the ankle just lateral to the dorsalis pedis artery, between the extensor hallucis longus tendon and extensor digitorum longus. It provides motor innervation to the extensor digitorum longus and brevis (which can be "twitched" with a nerve stimulator), and sensory innervation of the skin on the dorsum of the foot between the first and second toes. The superficial peroneal nerve arborizes over, and provides sensory innervation of the anteriomedial surface of the foot. The sural nerve arises from branches of the tibial and common peroneal nerves in the popliteal fossa and proceeds distally to the ankle, where it lies between the lateral malleolus and the Achilles

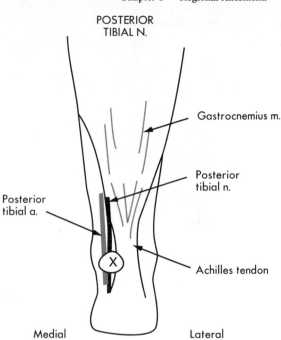

Fig. 8-14 Ankle block. The anatomical position and site of nerve block is illustrated for the posterior tibial n. (See text for further explanation.)

tendon. It provides sensation to the lateral surface of the foot. The anteromedial surface of the foot is innervated by the saphenous nerve, a purely sensory distal continuation of the femoral nerve that emerges medially from behind the medial condyle of the tibia at the knee, and then descends anteromedially with the saphenous vein to reach the ankle just anterior to the medial malleolus.

Ankle block

The patient should be supine, with a bump under the contralateral hip.

Local anesthetics

Absorption of local anesthetic after an ankle block is slow, and local anesthetic concentrations in blood are relatively low.[34]

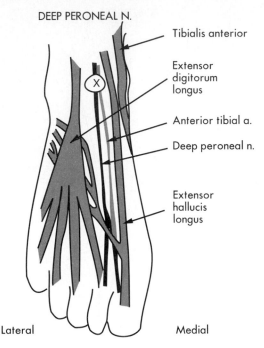

DEEP PERONEAL N.

Tibialis anterior

Extensor digitorum longus

Anterior tibial a.

Deep peroneal n.

Extensor hallucis longus

Lateral   Medial

Fig. 8-15 Ankle block. The anatomical position and site of nerve block is illustrated for the deep peroneal n. (See text for further explanation.)

Therefore, vasopressors for limiting local anesthetic blood levels are unnecessary and potentially hazardous because of the proximity to terminal vessels supplying the digits of the foot. Bupivacaine 0.5% provides anesthesia approximately 8 to 12 hours in duration and is ideal for providing postoperative pain relief. Motor block does not significantly interfere with the ability to walk on crutches. Alternatively, 1% to 1.5% lidocaine or mepivacaine alone will provide anesthesia 2 to 4 hours in duration, and in combination with tetracaine, anesthesia up to 4 to 6 hours.

Landmarks
A line is drawn around the ankle at the level of the malleoli. On that line, the position of the posterior tibial artery (behind the medial malleolus) and the deep peroneal nerve are indicated by an X.

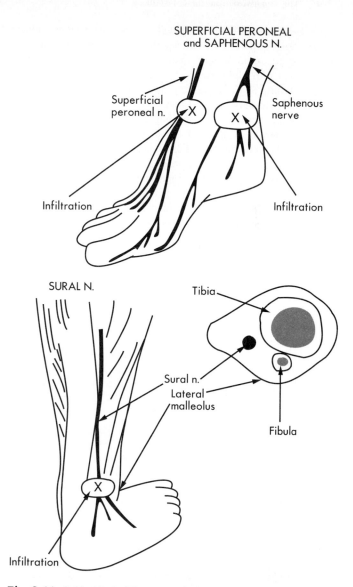

Fig. 8-16 Ankle block. The anatomical position and site of nerve blocks are illustrated for the superficial peroneal n., saphenous n., and the sural n. (See text for further explanation.)

The deep peroneal nerve is midway between the extensor hallucis longus tendon (palpated while dorsiflexing the great toe) and the extensor digitorum longus (palpated while the second, third, fourth, and fifth digits are dorsiflexed without flexing the great toe). It is just lateral to the dorsalis pedis artery, which cannot always be palpated (Figs. 8-14 and 8-15).

Posterior tibial nerve: Standing at the foot of the bed, an insulated needle is inserted through a skin wheal at the *X* overlying the tibial artery, and directed proximally (parallel to and at a 45-degree angle to the long axis of the leg) toward the posterior aspect of the artery (with current adjusted to 1.5 mA) until a twitch of the great toe is elicited. If a twitch is not initially obtained, a coarse search across the path of the nerve is made until a twitch is observed. The needle is then pivoted at the skin across the path of the nerve to obtain the best angle (where the twitch is strongest), then advanced to the best depth (where the twitch just begins to fade). The current should be reduced until a twitch is detectable at 0.5 mA or less. Then 5 to 7 ml of local anesthetic *without* epinephrine is injected (see Fig. 8-14).

Peroneal nerve: An insulated needle is inserted through a skin wheal at the *X* overlying the deep peroneal nerve, and then is directed slightly cephalad until a twitch is elicited (twitching of the extensor digitorum brevis or longus on the anterolateral aspect of the foot). If no twitch is initially obtained, a search laterally (or medially) is performed until one is identified. The best angle and depth are ascertained, and 5 to 7 ml of local anesthetic injected. Alternatively, local anesthetic can be injected just lateral to the dorsalis pedis artery (see Fig. 8-15).

Superficial peroneal, saphenous, and sural nerves: These nerves are blocked by creating a subcutaneous wheal of local anesthetic around the ankle from the medial malleolus to the mid-point of the ankle (saphenous nerve), from the midpoint to the lateral malleolus (superficial peroneal nerve) and from the lateral malleolus to the Achilles tendon (sural nerve) using a 25-gauge 1½-inch Quincke needle. An additional injection is performed for the sural nerve as follows: A needle is inserted midway between the lateral malleolus and the Achilles tendon, directed slightly cephalad until the tibia is contacted, and withdrawn two thirds of the distance; 3 to 4 ml of local anesthetic *without* epinephrine is then injected. Local anesthetic without vasopressors are used because of the proximity to terminal digital vessels (see Fig. 8-16).

Distribution of anesthesia with an ankle block is shown in Fig. 8-17.

Spinal and Lumbar Epidural Anesthesia

Spinal anesthesia provides excellent anesthesia for outpatient surgery involving the lower extremities, pelvis, groin, and lower abdomen, and for urologic surgery by the transurethral approach. Although lumbar epidural anesthesia can often be equally well applied, it is less reliable in achieving satisfactory anesthesia of the sacral segments (feet, perineum, vagina, bladder, perianal area). Additional advantages of spinal over epidural anesthesia for outpatients are that it is technically easier and more rapidly performed, has a faster onset, has a higher success rate, is less likely to be associated with intravascular injection and systemic toxicity, and has a lesser incidence of postanesthesia back pain. Disadvantages of spinal anesthesia include the inability to modify the duration of block once the anesthetic has been injected, and the somewhat greater incidence of postpuncture headache. Bromage quotes an acceptable incidence of wet taps of 0.5% with lumbar epidurals, and suggests that approximately 70% to 80% of patients with wet taps will develop a postpuncture headache.[35] With the currently

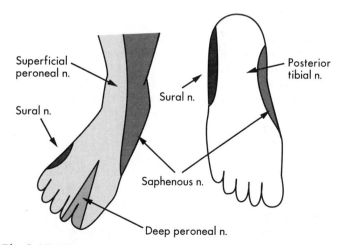

Fig. 8-17 Sensory distribution of five nerves blocked at the ankle: posterior tibial n., deep peroneal n., superficial peroneal n., saphenous n., and sural n.

available pencil-point spinal needles, the incidence of headache in outpatients has dropped significantly (see Table 8-2). Spinal anesthesia (when performed with the same local anesthetic) typically requires a slightly longer recovery time than epidural anesthesia in outpatients. Both spinal and epidural blocks can cause urinary retention that may require bladder catheterization. Intrathecal and epidural opiates have been used in outpatients; however, the lack of controlled studies and the potential for delayed respiratory depression have restricted its uses.

Anatomy (Fig. 8-18)

Spinal and epidural blocks are typically performed at the L3-L4, or L4-5 (occasionally L2-3) space. The spinal cord ends at the level of the L-1 or L-2 vertebra in approximately 90% of people. Below that level, lumbar and sacral nerves (cauda equina) float freely in spinal fluid, devoid of neural sheaths (no dural covering) and are easily penetrated by local anesthetics. The spinal subarachnoid space is bounded by the arachnoid, and the dura mater; external to the dura lies the epidural space, which is covered by the ligamentum flavum. The walls of the spinal canal consist of the vertebral bodies anteriorly, the vertebral pedicles laterally, and the laminae and spine posteriorly. Between vertebral bodies is a diamond-shaped space protected only by the ligamentum flavum. It is here that the spinal subarachnoid space or epidural space is entered. Anatomical structures encountered by a needle during midline spinal puncture include skin, subcutaneous tissue, posterior spinal ligament, interspinous ligament, ligamentum flavum, and dura-arachnoid. With a paramedian approach, the needle passes directly from subcutaneous tissue into muscle, and then the ligamentum flavum.

The epidural space contains loose connective tissue and a vascular plexus. The subdural space (between the arachnoid and the dura) is largely a potential space that contains a thin layer of fluid. It is possible to cannulate the subdural space inadvertently; injection of local anesthetic there will cause anesthesia. Because of the small volume of the subdural space, spread of anesthetic will be exaggerated, and a high block will result if this occurs during attempted epidural block. The shape of the lumbar spine influences the spread of local anesthetic. In the supine position, the highest point of the lumbar curve occurs at approximately L3-4

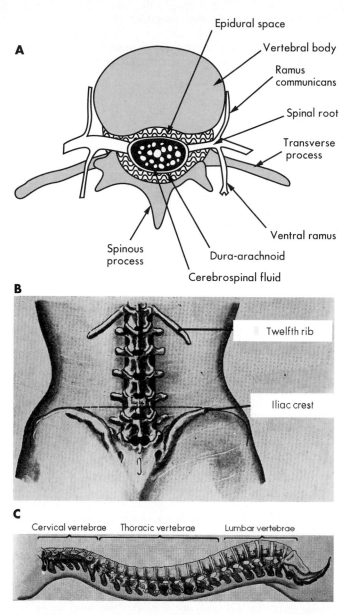

Fig. 8-18 A, Anatomy of spinal column, subarachnoid, and epidural spaces. **B** and **C,** Anatomy of the spinal column. (**B** and **C,** adapted from Moore DC: Regional block, ed 4, Springfield, Ill, 1979, Charles C. Thomas, pp. 341-69.)

(Fig. 8-18,*C*). Thus, hyperbaric spinal anesthetic solutions injected at this level will tend to spread cephalad as well as caudad.

Midline spinal block

The patient should be in the lateral position with neck, back, hips, and knees flexed.

Local anesthetics

Appropriate doses and duration of local anesthetics recommended for outpatient spinal anesthesia are shown in Table 8-5. In general, 0.1 to 0.2 mg of epinephrine (or 2 to 5 mg of phenylephrine) prolongs block duration by approximately 40% to 50%. Tetracaine is not recommended for outpatients because of unduly prolonged recovery times (up to 6 hours). Block height is affected primarily by the mass (mg dose) of drug, the volume in which it is injected, the baricity of the solution, and the position of the patient. Although patient height, age, and weight are of lesser importance, exaggerated spread may occur with short stature, old age, or obesity.

Procaine for spinal anesthesia is available in single-dose vials as a 10% solution containing the antioxidant sodium bisulfite (Novocaine). It is recommended that it be diluted with equal volumes of 10% dextrose to obtain a 5% hyperbaric solution. Hyperbaric spinal bupivacaine is available as a 0.75% solution in 8% dextrose and can be injected undiluted. Hyperbaric "spinal lidocaine" is available as a 5% solution in 7.5% dextrose and can be injected undiluted, or, alternatively, it may be diluted with an equal volume of 10% dextrose to obtain a 2.5% hyperbaric solution. On rare occasions, lidocaine may cause transient but reversible lower extremity pain that resolves over the course of a few days. The pain has not been associated with demonstrable neurologic abnormalities, and it appears to resolve without therapy other than analgesics.[36,37] Dilution of the local anesthetic with equal volumes of dextrose might lessen the likelihood of this occurrence.

Landmarks (Fig. 8-18, *B*)

Landmarks include the iliac crests, L-4 and L-5 spinous processes (and/or L-3 spinous process). A line is drawn that crosses the midline at the level of the superior edge of the iliac crests. This line will cross the midline at the level of the L-4 spinous process, or the L4-5 space. The L-4 and L-5 (and L-3, if desired) spinous processes are thus identified and marked.

Lumbar puncture (Fig. 8-19)

Through a wheal of local anesthetic, a spinal needle is inserted into the midline between the L-4 and L-5 spinous processes (or between the L-3 and L-4 spines), and directed anteriorly and slightly cephalad (10 to 20 degrees cephalad to a line perpendicular to skin) between the spinous processes, until cerebrospinal fluid (CSF) is encountered. The bevel of the needle should be positioned so that it is parallel to the fibers of the dura.[38] The stylette is removed to check for CSF at frequent intervals after the needle is felt to have pierced the ligamentum flavum (signified by a slight loss of resistence). If repeated bony contact is encountered, the clinician should attempt the puncture one space above or below, or consider a paramedian approach.

Local anesthetic

The anesthetic may be injected when CSF can be aspirated with the needle rotated in at least two quadrants (Table 8-5). The upper level of anesthesia to pinprick should be ascertained frequently, and blocks that appear too low should be treated by placing the patient in the Trendelenberg position.

Fluids and vasopressors

Fluids and vasopressors should be administered as required to maintain a satisfactory level of blood pressure and heart rate (5 to 10 mg of ephedrine or 50 to 100 µg of phenylephrine for hypotension; 0.4 to 0.8 mg of atropine for bradycardia).

Table 8-5   Local Anesthetics Recommended for Hyperbaric Spinal Anesthesia in Outpatients

Drug	Concentration (%)	Dose* (mg)	Approximate duration† of surgical anesthesia (mins)	
			plain	with epinephrine
Procaine	10	75-100	45-90	120
Lidocaine	5	50-75	90-120	120-135
Bupivacaine	0.75	12-18	90-150	180

* Dose for T2-T10 block.
† Until T-10 regression.

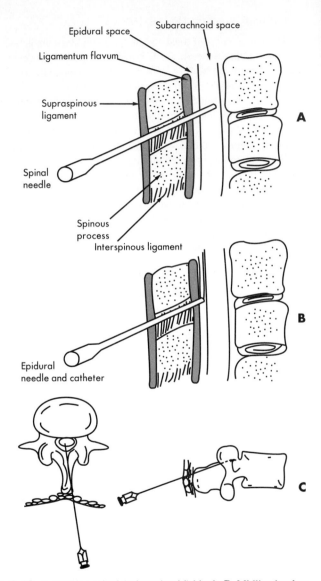

Fig. 8-19 A, Midline spinal (subarachnoid) block. **B,** Midline lumbar epidural block. **C,** Cross-section depicting needle direction with paramedian approach.

Paramedian approach

An *X* is made 1.5 cm lateral to the midline, opposite but approximately 0.5 to 1 cm posterior to the anterior end of the spine of the vertebral body below the space to be entered (Fig. 8-19,*C*). A needle is inserted perpendicular to skin and advanced until it comes to rest on the lamina of the vertebral body. The needle is then directed slightly medially, and walked cephalad "off" the lamina in a few successive steps. "Walking off the lamina" along the base of the spine is particularly useful when landmarks are indistinct. If it is directed too far medially, the needle will cross the midline and hit the lamina on the opposite side; if it is too far laterally, the needle may be walked along articular facets and fail to drop off the bone, or drop off laterally into the paraspinous muscle. Failure to obtain CSF should alert one to malposition of the needle, and landmarks should be reassessed.

Spinal anesthesia in the sitting position

In obese or lordotic patients, the sitting position facilitates identification of the midline and the opening of the intervertebral spaces. The patient should sit on the side of an operating table with feet supported, and hunch forward, forcing their back into a convex shape. After identifying the usual landmarks, a 3½- or 5-inch spinal needle is inserted and advanced until bone or CSF is contacted. It may be helpful to first identify the tip of the spine above with a 22-gauge spinal needle, leave this in place as a marker needle, and then insert and advance a second spinal needle to obtain CSF. If repeated bony contact occurs, a puncture may be made 1.5 to 2.0 cm lateral to the intervertebral space, and an attempt made to enter the subarachnoid space using a more lateral approach. The size of the opening to the subarachnoid space is larger when approached laterally, a point that can be verified by examining a skeleton.

Continuous spinal anesthesia

There has been some interest in continuous spinal anesthesia for outpatients based on a report by Denny et al.[39] of a relatively low incidence of postspinal headache after insertion of a 20-gauge catheter through an 18-gauge epidural needle inserted into the subarachnoid space (less than 1% of patients with mean age of

63 years). These researchers have hypothesized that continuous catheters incite an inflammatory response at the site of dural puncture that facilitates sealing of the puncture site when the catheter is removed. However, other recent studies[40,41] suggest the incidence of headache is typically considerably higher (6% to 50%) when an 18-gauge epidural needle is used to permit placement of a 20-gauge spinal catheter. Although the use of microcatheters in conjunction with smaller-gauge spinal needles may lessen the incidence of headache, the microcatheters have been fraught with additional problems relating to in vivo fracturing of catheters, and possible neurotoxicity due to pooling of relatively large amounts of local anesthetic at the catheter tip. There is little current evidence that continuous spinal anesthesia offers any advantage in the outpatient population, particularly when compared with the low incidence of postpuncture headache attainable with 27-gauge spinal needles.

Midline lumbar epidural anesthesia

The patient is positioned and landmarks identified as for midline spinal anesthesia. An 18-gauge Tuohy needle, attached to a control syringe containing sterile saline, is inserted at the X overlying the L4-5 space, and advanced with the nondominant hand, while constant pressure is maintained on the plunger of the syringe with the opposite hand (Fig. 8-19, B). The needle is advanced until a sudden release is felt as the ligamentum flavum is punctured. Saline acts to tent the dura away from the tip of the needle and thus prevents inadvertant dural puncture. The bevel of the needle is rotated so that it points in a cephalad direction, an epidural catheter is threaded through the needle 2 to 3 cm past the tip, the Tuohy needle is withdrawn, the catheter is secured with a clear sterile dressing, and the proximal end is taped at the patient's shoulder.

After aspirating to ensure the absence of blood or CSF, a test dose (3 ml of a local anesthetic solution containing 1:200,000 epinephrine) is injected, and the effect on heart rate and blood pressure over the succeeding minute noted. A heart rate increase in excess of 20 beats/min suggests an intravascular injection, and the catheter should be replaced.[42] Similarly, the onset of significant anesthesia of more than two or three segments within 5 minutes of injection suggests that the catheter may be in the subarachnoid space or (occasionally) subdural space. In either instance, satisfactory anesthesia may be obtained, but the dose of anesthetic should be altered to accommodate the presumed site of the catheter. A 3 ml test dose of 2% lidocaine will typically produce a T6-T10 spinal block. The effect of local anesthetic in the subdural space is somewhat more unpredictable, but based on the effect of the original test dose, one may inject further local anesthetic in small boluses and gauge further injections based on the reponse obtained.

If the effects of the test dose are satisfactory, sufficient local anesthetic is injected to achieve the required level of block. A somewhat simplified approach is to assume that 1.0 ml per segment is required for a patient aged 50 years, to assume equal cephalad and caudad spread, to calculate the volume required, and then to make a correction for age (e.g., at age 80 years, 0.5 ml per segment is required, and the dose should be reduced by 50%; at age 20 years, 1.5 ml per segment is required, and the dose should be increased by 50%) (Fig. 8-20).[43] It is prudent to reduce the total volume by 10% to 30% for short or very obese patients. In a

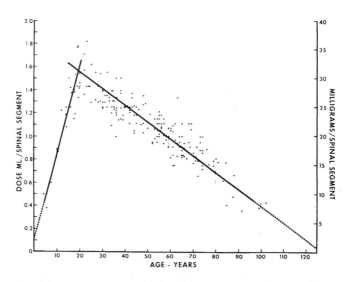

Fig. 8-20 Volume requirements (in ml) of lidocaine 2% with epinephrine 1:200,000 versus age, in 210 surgical patients in supine position. (From Bromage PR: Aging and epidural dose requirements. Br J Anaesth 1969; 41:1016.)

50-year-old patient of average height requiring a T-7 block, the calculated volume (excluding the test dose) with a catheter tip at L-2 would be approximately 8 ml for cephalad spread to T-7, plus 8 ml (assuming equal caudad spread) for a total of 16 ml of local anesthetic solution. For a very short patient (5 feet or less), or a very obese patient, the dose might be reduced by $0.3 \times 16 = 4.8$ ml, to a total volume of 11 ml. If the resultant block is too low, additional 5 ml increments of local anesthetic can be injected at 5- to 10-minute intervals until the desired level is attained.

Reinjections can be made as follows: one half of the initial volume may be given if injected after one half of the predicted minimum duration of the block has elapsed; or two thirds of the initial volume may be given if injected after two thirds of the predicted minimum duration of the block has elapsed.

The local anesthetic solutions recommended are shown in Table 8-6. Chloroprocaine may be preferable for very short procedures because it sometimes permits more rapid recovery and discharge.[44,45] However, backache has been described after epidural injection of chloroprocaine that appears to be dose related, and in general, volumes in excess of 20 ml should be avoided to prevent this problem.[46] This type of backache is typically present as soon as the block recedes and is described as being a deep, aching, burning pain that varies in severity from mild to severe.

Table 8-6   Local Anesthetics Recommended for Lumbar Epidural Anesthesia in Outpatients*

Drug	Concentration (%)	Typical volume (ml)	Approximate duration of surgical anesthesia (minutes)
2-Chloro- procaine	2.0-3.0	18-24	30-60
Lidocaine	1.5-2.0	18-24	60-90
Mepivacaine	1.5-2.0	18-24	90-120
Prilocaine	2.0-3.0	18-24	90-120

*The doses suggested are predicated on using epinephrine-containing solutions of local anesthetic (1:200,000). If plain solutions are injected (no epinephrine), blood levels achieved may be higher, and consideration must be given to injecting the lesser volumes or concentrations of local anesthetic.

Adapted from Ramsey D, Thompson GE: The case for regional anesthesia for adult outpatient surgery. Anesth Clin North Am 1987; 5:97-111.

Paramedian epidural

This block is best performed using an 18-gauge Crawford (or Hustead) needle, which facilitates identification of the ligamentum flavum before to entering the epidural space. The patient is prepared and landmarks drawn as for a paramedian spinal. A Crawford needle is inserted through a skin wheal at the X 1.5 cm lateral to the anterior end of the spine below the space to be entered. The needle is advanced perpendicular to the skin, with the bevel parallel to the fibers of the dura, until the lamina is contacted, then redirected in a slightly medial and cephalad direction until the lamina is again contacted. This step is repeated two or three times until the needle is felt to pass just beyond the superior edge of the lamina and to engage in the ligamentum flavum (Fig. 8-19). A control syringe containing sterile saline is then connected to the Crawford needle, and the needle is advanced while maintaining steady pressure on the plunger of the syringe until a sudden release is felt as the needle punctures the ligamentum flavum and enters the epidural space. An epidural catheter is then inserted in the usual manner, and local anesthetic is injected after appropriate testing of the catheter as for a midline epidural.

Recovery from spinal and epidural anesthesia

Recovery from central neuraxis blocks should initially be performed in a fully equipped recovery unit (phase I recovery) with regular monitoring of vital signs and oxygen saturation. When the block has receded to an L-1 level or below, residual hemodynamic effects of the block are minimal, and patients can be transferred to a phase II recovery unit. We recommend that blocks be totally resolved before discharge to ensure that bowel and bladder control are regained. It is also prudent to ensure that patients void before discharge. Discharge before that time exposes patients to the risk of urinary retention, overdistension of the bladder, and symptoms of hypotonic bladder that may persist for weeks. Catheterization of bladder with specific instruction regarding symptoms of urinary retention may permit discharge of select patients following central neural blockade. A more complete discussion of recovery following regional anesthesia is found in Chapter 12.

Complications and side effects of spinal/epidural anesthesia

Relatively common side effects that occur during spinal or epidural anesthesia include hypotension, bradycardia due to sympathetic nervous system blockade, and occasional nausea or vomiting.[47,48] Inadvertant injection of large volumes of local anesthetic into the subarachnoid space during epidural block or excessive spread of anesthesia during spinal anesthesia may cause a high spinal blockade ("total spinal") with severe hypotension and respiratory paralysis. Postpuncture headache occurs in 0.4% to 7% of patients after spinal anesthesia with Whitacre needles and slightly higher with Sprotte needles (see Table 8-2) and in 0.5% to 1% of patients after epidural anesthesia. Backache is reported in 10% to 50% of patients after spinal and epidural anesthesia. Rarely, subarachnoid and subdural hematomas (manifested by failure of a block to recede appropriately) have occurred; these require emergent decompression to prevent permanent neurologic deficit. Spinal and epidural blocks are contraindicated in patients with known or suspected coagulation abnormalities. Epidural abscess or meningitis can occur; however, infection is exceedingly rare if sterile technique and sterile solutions are employed.

Caudal Anesthesia

The resolution of caudal anesthesia in adults is relatively slow, and caudal anesthesia has a higher failure rate than spinal and epidural anesthesia. For these reasons, it is not advocated for routine anesthesia in adult outpatients, even though it is not associated with postpuncture headache. In children, it is useful for postoperative analgesia after surgery of the groin, genital area, or lower extremities. The following technique is therefore designed for use in young children (less than 5 years old) and is most easily instituted while the child is anesthetized or heavily sedated.[49] It may then be used as part of the anesthetic technique for surgery, with heavy sedation or general anesthesia superimposed to ensure a quiet child. It is particularly useful for hernia repairs, hydrocelectomy, circumcision, hypospadius repair, and muscle biopsies.

Anatomy (Fig. 8-21)

The anatomy of the caudal space in children is similar to that in adults with a few exceptions. In children, termination of the

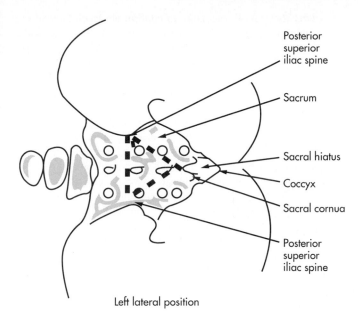

Left lateral position

Fig. 8-21 Anatomy of the sacrum (left lateral position) demonstrating the position of the sacral hiatus between the sacral cornua (the unfused spinous process of the S-5 vertebra), where the needle is inserted during caudal block. The posterior superior iliac spines form an equilateral triangle with the sacral hiatus.

subarachnoid space occurs more caudally (i.e., at the S2-3 or S3-4 space, rather than at the S1-2 as in adults). The absolute distance from the sacral hiatus to the spinal subarachnoid space is only about 1 inch; therefore, it is therefore relatively easily penetrated. The posterior sacrococcygeal ligament is relatively easily located between the sacral prominences (the unfused posterior laminae of the S-5) and gives a firm "pop" when penetrated.

Technique

The child is placed in the lateral position with knees and hips flexed. The sacral prominences are identified and an *X* made at the sacral hiatus. A 21- or 23-gauge butterfly needle at a 60-degree angle is inserted into the skin and advanced until it pops through the sacrococcygeal ligament and contacts the ventral surface of the sacral canal. After aspirating to confirm absence of blood or spinal fluid, local anesthetic (0.125% to 0.25% bupivacaine, with or without epinephrine 1:200,000) is injected, and the needle is withdrawn. (Because the total injected dose is relatively small and test doses are not very reliable, test doses are generally not advocated.) Dose of local anesthetics can be calculated using the formula of Takasaki,[50] which is 0.056 ml/kg/segment to be blocked, or alternatively, 0.75-1.0 ml/kg to produce a T11-T4 block.[51] The latter appears to be more reliable and predictive of block success.[49] Analgesia typically persists for 4 to 6 hours; incomplete muscle paralysis occurs with more concentrated (0.25% to 0.5%) solutions. Analgesia appears to be equally effective and of similar duration, regardless of concentration (0.125% to 0.5%) utilized. Epinephrine prolongs the duration of block by approximately 30 minutes.[49] Children are subsequently allowed to recover from the effects of general anesthesia (or heavy sedation) in a conventional manner. In selected instances, they may be discharged while sensory and motor effects of the block persist, if they are in the company of a responsible adult. Parents must be given appropriate instructions about the anticipated duration of the block, the need to protect blocked extremities, and the need to begin oral (or rectal) analgesic drug therapy when the child first begins to experience pain. Because young children have a relative predominance of vagal control over cardiovascular function (i.e., they have little resting sympathetic tone), the effects of sympathetic nervous system blockade are minimal, permitting safe discharge while the block is still in effect.[51] Urinary retention after caudal block in children has not been a problem, and voiding before discharge is unnecessary. It is prudent, however, to caution parents that failure to void within 6 to 8 hours after discharge should be a cause for concern, and should prompt them to seek consultation with their surgeon or anesthesiologist.

Iliohypogastric and Ilioinguinal Nerve Blocks

Ilioinguinal and iliohypogastric nerve blocks, using 0.5% bupivacaine (with or without epinephrine, 1:200,000), can be advantageously employed for perioperative analgesia in children or adults undergoing orchiopexy or hernia repairs in the groin. These two nerves are branches of the anterior primary rami of L-1 that encircle the trunk and provide sensation to the lower anterior abdominal wall. They lie on the surface of the quadratus lumborum, then pass through the transverse abdominis muscle, and travel in the neurovascular plane beneath the internal oblique muscle, which they perforate above the anterior superior iliac spine. They then course inferomedially between the external and internal oblique muscles on the anterior abdominal wall. The iliohypogastric nerve pierces the aponeurosis of the external oblique muscle just above the superficial inguinal ring, and this nerve provides sensory innervation of the skin over the lower part of the rectus abdominis. The ilioinguinal nerve enters the spermatic cord and supplies the anterior one third of the scrotum, the root of the penis, and the upper and medial part of the groin. The two nerves are blocked just medial to the anterior superior iliac spine and lateral to the rectus abdominis as they lie between or within the oblique muscles of the abdomen (Fig. 8-22).

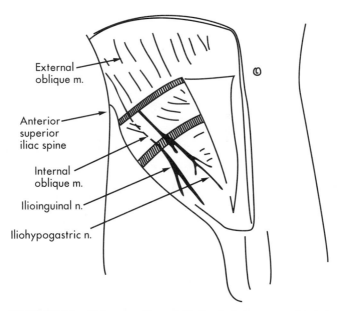

Fig. 8-22 The iliohypogastric and ilioinguinal nerves are located approximately 2.5 cm (adults) or 1.0 cm (children) medial to the anterior superior iliac spine, typically between the external and internal oblique muscles (or deep to, or within the internal oblique muscle).

In adults, a 2- to 3-inch needle is inserted at a point 2.5 cm medial to the anterior superior iliac spine on a line drawn between the latter bony prominence and the umbilicus. (In children, the needle is inserted approximately 1 cm medial to this bony landmark.) The needle is directed inferolaterally and inferomedially, and local anesthetic is then infiltrated throughout the muscles of the lower anterior abdominal wall (Fig. 8-23). Anesthesia of the groin region should persist for 6 to 12 hours, and minimal supplementation by analgesics should be required with a successful block.Although the combination of ilioinguinal and hypogastric nerve block provides good analgesia after groin surgery, it alone is not adequate for surgical anesthesia. The latter also requires genitofemoral nerve block and local infiltration of the incision line. This typically is performed by the surgeon when the intent is to perform surgery under local anesthesia alone.

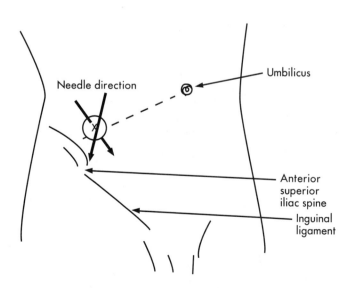

Fig. 8-23 Iliohypogastric and ilioinguinal nerve blocks. Local anesthetic is infiltrated inferolaterally towards the iliac spine, and medially towards the rectus sheath, into the internal and external oblique muscles.

Regional Anesthesia of the Eye

Regional anesthesia of the eye is most commonly employed for cataract surgery, but may also be utilized for procedures involving the cornea or retina. It is appropriate for subjects who are able to lie still with minimal sedation, and for subjects who can communicate with operating room personnel during the procedure. Very anxious, deaf, or retarded patients, or patients with language problems, may be better managed with a general anesthetic. Regional anesthesia of the eye is most often performed using a combination of a facial nerve block to prevent contraction of the extraocular muscles (orbicularis oculi), and a retrobulbar block to achieve anesthesia and akinesia of the eye. The retrobulbar block ablates sensation of the eye by anesthetizing the ophthalmic division of the fifth (trigeminal) cranial nerve and prevents movement of the globe by anesthetizing the third and sixth cranial nerves. Typically, the optic nerve is not blocked during retrobulbar anesthesia because it is ensheathed by a cuff of dura that extends from the cranial cavity into the orbit.

Nerve block

The facial nerve can be blocked at its site of exit from the skull (Nadbath block); in this case, all components of the nerve will be temporarily paralyzed (Fig. 8-24). Occasionally, the vagus or glossopharyngeal nerve may also be paralyzed, which may cause hoarseness and a choking sensation. Alternatively, the facial nerve can be blocked distally, inferiorly, and superiorly to the eye (VanLint block); this block does not paralyze the nonocular nerve components, but it is moderately painful and causes bruising and swelling of the eyelid (Fig. 8-24).[52]

Retrobulbar block

With the eye relaxed and gazing straight ahead, a 23- or 25-gauge needle, only 1½ inches long, is inserted inferior to the eye, and through the skin at the junction of the medial and lateral thirds of the eye (Fig. 8-25). It should be inserted sufficiently inferior to the eye to pass just beneath the globe as it is advanced directly posteriorly. After passing the equator of the globe, the needle is angled approximately 30 degrees superiorly and slightly medially, so that it penetrates the muscular cone of the eye. After aspirating to ensure that the needle is not in a vessel, 3 to 4 ml of local anesthetic is injected slowly, and the needle removed. Gentle

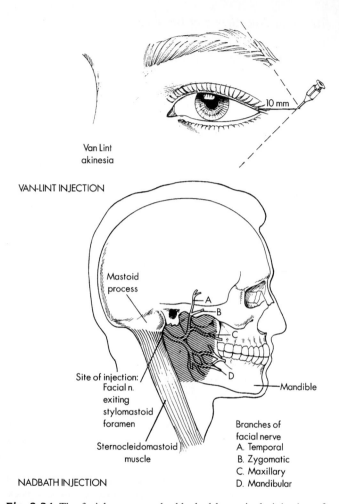

Van Lint
akinesia

VAN-LINT INJECTION

Mastoid
process

A. Temporal
B. Zygomatic
C. Maxillary
D. Mandibular

Site of injection:
Facial n.
exiting
stylomastoid
foramen

Mandible

Branches of
facial nerve
A. Temporal
B. Zygomatic
C. Maxillary
D. Mandibular

Sternocleidomastoid
muscle

NADBATH INJECTION

Fig. 8-24 The facial nerve can be blocked by a single injection of
3 ml of local anesthetic at the site of exit of the nerve from the
stylomastoid foramen of the skull (Nadbath technique), just anterior to
the mastoid process and posterior to the ramus of the mandible using
a 3/8-inch 23- to 25-gauge needle, or by infiltration of local anesthetic
along the superior and inferior orbital ridges (VanLint block) using a
1⅝-inch 25-gauge needle. (From Spigelman AV, Lindquist TD, Lindstrom RL: Anesthesia in ocular surgery. In Lindquist TD, Lindstrom
RL, editors: Ophthalmic surgery looseleaf and update service, Chicago, 1990, Year Book Medical Publishers, pp. 1-8.)

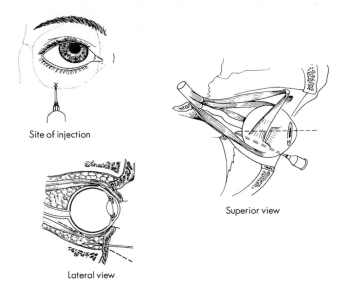

Site of injection

Superior view

Lateral view

Fig. 8-25 Retrobulbar block is performed inferior to the globe, at the junction of the middle and lateral thirds of the eye. A 23-gauge 1.5-inch needle is directed posteriorly and slightly inferiorly beneath the globe until it passes the equator of the eye, then it is angled superomedially to pass into the muscular cone to a depth of 1 to 1.25 inches. Three to four milliliters of local anesthetic is injected after gentle aspiration to prevent intravascular injection. (From Hersh PS: Ophthalmic surgical procedures, Boston, 1988, Little, Brown and Co, p. 21; and Spigelman AV, Lindquist TD, Lindstrom RL: Anesthesia in ocular surgery. In Lindquist TD, Lindstrom RL, editors: Ophthalmic surgery looseleaf and update service, Chicago, 1990, Year Book Medical Publishers, pp. 1-8.)

pressure is maintained over the closed eye for 5 minutes to facilitate the spread of anesthetic throughout the orbit and to minimize the volume of the orbital contents. The block may be performed with 0.5% to 0.75% bupivacaine, or with a mixture of 0.75% bupivacaine and 2% lidocaine. Hyaluronidase is included in the mixture to promote tissue diffusion. Complications of this block include retrobulbar hemorrhage (0.5%),[53] perforation of the globe (rare),[54] and optic nerve injury (rare).[55] Retrobulbar hemorrhage, which can be due to arterial or venous bleeding, usually manifests as subconjunctival hemorrhage and can result in

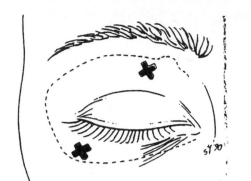

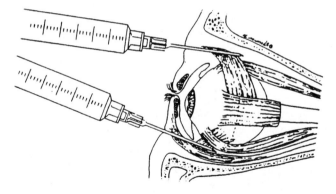

Fig. 8-26 The technique of peribulbar block. The needle is inserted at the supraorbital notch and advanced 1 inch (away from the globe slightly), and 4 to 6 ml of local anesthetic with hyaluronidase is injected. A second puncture is made at the inferior orbital notch, the needle is advanced 1 inch (directed slightly away from the globe), and 4 to 6 ml of local anesthetic with hyaluronidase is injected outside of the muscular cone. Local anesthetic diffuses gradually out of the orbit to anesthetize the orbicularis oculi, and within the orbit to block the third and sixth cranial nerves, and the three branches (frontal, nasociliary, and lacrimal) of the ophthalmic division of the trigeminal nerve. (From Ahmad S, Ahmad A, Benzon HT: Clinical experience with the peribulbar block for ophthalmolgic surgery. Regional Anesthesia 1993; 18:184-8.)

proptosis and increased intraocular pressure. Most often, surgery must be delayed or cancelled, and surgical releasing incisions may be required. Full recovery almost always ensues.[53] Perforation of the globe and optic nerve injury can cause permanent vision loss. Subarachnoid or subdural injection of local anesthetic occur rarely, but are possible when the injection penetrates the sheath surrounding the optic nerve. Retrograde spread of anesthetic has resulted in complications such as transient respiratory paralysis, contralateral visual abnormalities, hypotension, bradycardia, and a variety of cranial nerve palsies.[56,57] Some clinicians advocate an alternative technique, the peribulbar block, as being less likely to cause retrobulbar hemorrhage. The globe can be perforated. Local anesthetic is injected outside the muscular cone (Fig. 8-26). The needle is placed inferior to the eye at the same site as that for retrobulbar injection; however, it is only inserted just past the equator of the orbital globe so that the muscle cone is not penetrated. The landmarks for the superior injection are 0.5 to 1 cm inferior to the superior orbital notch. Approximately three-quarters of the length of the needle is advanced posteriorly. If it meets any resistance, the needle should be withdrawn and redirected. Retrobulbar needles or 25- or 27-gauge needles (1½ inch long) can be used, taking care to avoid neural injury. Aspiration for fluid or blood before injecting the local anesthetic is essential. The peribulbar technique does not require separate injections to anesthetize the orbital divisions of the facial nerve.[58] Large volumes (5 to 10 ml) are required, and the onset of anesthesia is longer. A Honan's balloon, or a pressure cuff inflated to 30 cm H_2O, may be applied to the eye to accelerate diffusion of the local anesthetic and to reduce periocular pressure.

Summary

The success of regional anesthesia as an alternative to general anesthesia for outpatient surgery lies in proper patient selection and appropriate choice of technique. The ability to provide total operative site anesthesia without obtunding mental function or airway reflexes, reducing emesis, and minimizing postoperative pain makes regional anesthesia particularly attractive for outpatient surgery. With appropriate local anesthetics, patients may actually recover faster than they would with general anesthesia. In fact, after peripheral nerve bocks, patients may bypass phase 1 recovery and be mobilized immediately after surgery. The monitoring and resuscitative equipment necessary for general anesthesia is required for regional anesthesia. Although sedation may be an adjunct to a regional technique, the fastest recoveries are associated with absence of long-acting sedative-hypnotics. Spinal anesthesia using pencil-point needles or 26- and 27-gauge Quincke point needles is gaining acceptance, because it reduces the incidence of postdural puncture headache. Appropriate dosing of local anesthetics will reduce toxicity and decrease the duration of action. Peripheral upper extremity blocks, including axillary blocks, interscalene blocks, and intravenous regional anesthesia, are particularly useful for ambulatory surgery. The anatomical landmarks for lower extremity ankle blocks are discussed. Infiltration with long-acting local anesthetics provide prolonged duration of analgesia; however, consideration must be given to ambulating patients after lower extremity blocks. Patients with central neural axis blocks (spinal, epidural) should be placed in a fully equipped recovery unit and transferred to phase 2 recovery when the block has receded to L-1 level or below, and when the residual effects of the block are minimal. Before discharge, patients should ambulate without any orthostatic blood pressure changes; their bowel and bladder control must be regained; and they should void. Common side effects of spinal or epidural anesthetics include hypotension, bradycardia, and the results of inadvertent injection of large volumes of local anesthetic into the subarachnoid space. Postpuncture headache may occur with varying incidence following spinal anesthesia (depending on needle type), and in 0.5% to 1.0% of patients following epidural anesthesia. After spinal and epidural anesthesia, 10% to 50% of patients experience backache. In children, caudal anesthesia may be easily induced using concentrations of anesthetics that provide perioperative anesthesia and analgesia without interfering with voiding or ambulation. Miscellaneous techniques discussed include iliohypogastric and ilioinguinal blocks and ophthalmic anesthesia.

References

1. Allen HW, Mulroy MF, Fundis K, Carpenter RL: Regional versus propofol general anesthesia for outpatient hand surgery. Anesthesiology 1993; 79:A1.

2. D'Alessio J, Freitas D, Rosenblum M, Shea K: Is general anesthesia superior to interscalene block for shoulder surgery? Anesth Analg 1993; 76:S67.

3. Maurer P, Greek R, Torjman M et al: Is regional anesthesia more efficient than general anesthesia for shoulder surgery? Regional Anesthesia 1993; 18:3.

4. Moore DC, Crawford RD, Scurlock JE: Severe hypoxia and acidosis following local anesthetic-induced convulsions. Anesthesiology 1980; 53:259-60.

5. Hahn RG: Decrease in serum potassium concentration during epidural anaesthesia. Acta Anaesthesiol Scand 1987; 31:680-3.

6. Brown MJ, Brown DC, Murphy MB: Hypokalemia from beta$_2$-receptor stimulation by circulating epinephrine. New Engl J Med 1983; 309:1414-9.

7. White PF, Negus JB: Sedative infusions during local and regional anesthesia: a comparision of midazolam and propofol. J Clin Anesth 1991; 3:32-9.

8. Urquhart ML, White PF: Comparison of sedative infusions during regional anesthesia: methohexital, etomidate and midazolam. Anesth Analg 1989; 68:249-54.

9. Mayer DC, Quance D, Weeks SK: Headache after spinal anesthesia for cesarean section: a comparison of the 27-gauge Quincke and 24-gauge Sprotte needles. Anesth Analg 1992; 75:377-80.

10. Buettner J, Wresch K, Klose R: Postdural puncture headache: comparison of 25-gauge Whitacre and Quincke needles. Regional Anesthesia 1993; 18:66-9.

11. Devcic A, Sprung J, Patel S et al: A PDPH in obstetric anesthesia: comparison of 24-gauge Sprotte and 25-gauge Quincke needles and effect of subarachnoid administration of fentanyl. Regional Anesthesia 1993; 18:222-5.

12. Kang S, Lee Y, Graf J et al: Comparison of 25-g Whitacre, 27-g Quincke needles for spinal anesthesia. Anesthesiology 1993; 79:A33.

13A. Winnie AP: Clinical considerations. In Winnie AP, editor: Plexus anesthesia, vol I, Philadelphia, 1993, WB Saunders, p. 213.

13B. Broome JA, Schapiro HM: Post-dural puncture headache rate using Sprotte vs. Whitacre spinal needle. Anesth Analg 1993; 76:A28.

13C. Clarke GA, Power KJ: Spinal anaesthesia for day case surgery. Ann R Coll Surg Engl 1988; 70:144-6.

14. Selander D, Edshage S, Wolff T: Paresthesiae or no paresthesiae? Acta Anaesth Scand 1979; 23:27-33.

15. Pither CE, Raj PP, Ford DJ: The use of peripheral nerve stimulators for regional anesthesia. Regional Anesthesia 1985; 1049-58.

16. Tulchinsky A, Weller RS, Rosenblum M, Gross JB: Nerve stimulator polarity and brachial plexus block. Anesth Analg 1993; 77:100-3.

17. Brown AR: Unassisted peripheral nerve blocks. Regional Anesthesia 1993; 18:137-8.

18. Spiegel DA, Dexter F, Warner DS et al: Central nervous system toxicity of local anesthetic mixtures in the rat. Anesth Analg 1992; 75:922-8.

19. Moore DC, Bridenbaugh LD, Bridenbaugh PO et al: Does compounding of local anesthetic agents increase their toxicity in humans? Anesth Analg 1972; 51:579-85.

20. Adriani J, Coffman VD, Naraghi M: The allergenicity of lidocaine and other amides and related local anesthetics. Anesthesiology Rev 1986; 13:30-6.

21. Rosenberg PH: Intravenous regional anesthesia: nerve block by multiple mechanisms. Regional Anesthesia 1993; 18:1-5.

22. Tucker GT, Boas RA: Pharmacokinetic aspects of intravenous regional anesthesia. Anesthesiology 1971; 34:538-49.

23. Heath ML: Deaths after intravenous regional anaesthesia. Br Med J 1982; 285:913-4.

24. Brown DK, Cahill DR, Bridenbaugh SD: Supraclavicular nerve block: anatomic analysis of a method to prevent pneumothorax. Anesth Analg 1993; 76:530-4.

25. Thompson GE, Rorie DK: Functional anatomy of the brachial plexus sheaths. Anesthesiology 1983; 59:117-22.

26. Partridge BL, Katz J, Benirschke K: Functional anatomy of the brachial plexus sheath: implications for anesthesia. Anesthesiology 1987; 66:743-7.

27. Goldberg ME, Gregg C, Larijani GE et al: A comparison of three methods of axillary approach to brachial plexus blockade for upper extremity surgery. Anesthesiology 1987; 66:814-6.

28. Winchell SW, Wolfe R: The incidence of neuropathy following upper extremity nerve blocks. Regional Anesthesia 1985; 10:12-5.

29. Ward ME: The interscalene approach to the brachial plexus. Anaesthesia 1974; 29:147-57.

30. Wildsmith JAW, Tucker GT, Cooper S et al: Plasma concentrations of local anaesthetics after interscalene brachial plexus block. Br J Anaesth 1977; 49:461-6.

31. Kayerker UM, Dick MM: Phrenic nerve paralysis following interscalene brachial plexus block. Anesth Analg 1983; 62:536-7.

32. Scammell SJ: Inadvertent epidural anaesthesia as a complication of interscalene brachial plexus block. Anaesth Intens Care 1979; 7:56-7.

33. Edde RR, Deutsch S: Cardiac arrest after interscalene brachial-plexus block. Anesth Analg 1977; 56:446-7.

34. Mineo R, Sharrock NE: Venous levels of lidocaine and bupivacaine after midtarsal ankle block. Regional Anesthesia 1992; 17:47-9.

35. Bromage PR: Identification of the epidural space. In Bromage PR, editor: Epidural analgesia, Philadelphia, 1978, WB Saunders, pp. 208-10.

36. Schneider M, Ettlin T, Kaufmann M et al: Transient neurologic toxicity after hyperbaric subarachnoid anesthesia with 5% lidocaine. Anesth Analg 1993; 76:1154-7.

37. DeJong RH: Last round for a "heavyweight"? Anesth Analg 1994; 78:3-4.

38. Mihic DN: Postspinal headache and relationship of needle bevel to longitudinal dural fibers. Regional Anesthesia 1985; 10:76-81.

39. Denny N, Masters R, Pearson D et al: Post dural puncture headache after continuous spinal anesthesia. Anesth Analg 1987; 66:791-4.

40. Gold BS, Bogetz MS, Orkin FK, Drasner K: Continuous spinal anesthesia for ambulatory surgery patients. Anesthesiology 1989; 71(suppl): A-722.

41. Norris MC, Leighton BL: Continuous spinal anesthesia after unintentional dural puncture in parturients. Regional Anesthesia 1990; 15:285-7.

42. Moore DC, Batra MS: The components of an effective test dose prior to epidural block. Anesthesiology 1981; 55:693-6.

43. Bromage PR: Ageing and epidural dose requirements. Br J Anaesth 1969; 41:1016-24.

44. Kopacz DJ, Mulroy MF: Chloroprocaine and lidocaine decrease hospital stay and admission rate after outpatient epidural anesthesia. Regional Anesthesia 1990; 15:19-25.

45. Neal JM, Deck JJ, Lewis MA, Kopacz DJ: A double-blind comparison of epidural 2-chloroprocaine vs. lidocaine for outpatient knee arthroscopy. Anesthesiology 1993; 79:A12.

46. Stevens RA, Urmey WF, Urquhart BL, Kao T: Back pain after epidural anesthesia with chloroprocaine. Anesthesiology 1993; 78:492-7.

47. Bonica JJ, Kennedy WF, Ward RJ, Tolas AJ: A comparison of the effects of high subarachnoid and epidural anesthesia. Acta Anaesth Scand 1966 (Suppl); 23:429-36.

48. Caplan RA, Ward RJ, Posner K, Cheney FW: Unexpected cardiac arrest during spinal anesthesia: a closed claims analysis of predisposing factors. Anesthesiology 1988; 68:5-11.

49. Broadman L: Regional anesthesia in children. 1992 IARS review course lectures. Anesth Analg 1992; 4:68-74.

50. Takasaki M, Dohi S, Kawabata Y, Takahashi T: Dosage of lidocaine for caudal anesthesia in infants and children. Anesthesiology 1977; 47:527-33.

51. Dalens B, Hasnaoui A: Caudal anesthesia in pediatric surgery: success rate and adverse effects in 750 consecutive patients. Anesth Analg 1989; 68:83-9.

52. Spigelman AV, Lindquist TD, Lindstrom RL: Anesthesia in ocular surgery. In Lindquist TD, Lindstrom RL, editors: Ophthalmic surgery looseleaf and update service, Chicago, 1990, Year Book Medical Publishers, pp. 1-8.

53. Edge KR, Nicoll JMV: Retrobulbar hemorrhage after 12,500 retrobulbar blocks. Anesth Analg 1993; 76:1019-22.

54. Zaturansky B, Hyams S: Perforation of the globe during the injection of local anesthesia. Ophthalmic Surg 1987; 18:585-8.

55. Pautler SE, Grizzard WS, Thompson LN, Wing G: Blindness from retrobulbar injection into the optic nerve. Ophthalmic Surg 1986; 17:334-7.

56. Javitt JC, Addiego R, Friedberg HL et al: Brain stem anesthesia after retrobulbar block. Ophthalmology 1987; 94:718-24.

57. Wittpenn JR, Rapoza P, Sternberg P et al: Respiratory arrest following retrobulbar anesthesia. Ophthalmology 1986; 93:867-70.

58. Ahmad S, Ahmad A, Benzon HT: Clinical experience with the peribulbar block for ophthalmologic surgery. Regional Anesthesia 1993; 18:184-8.

Sedation Techniques

9

Carolyn P. Greenberg and Hernando De Soto

Conscious sedation techniques encompass the use of sedatives, tranquilizers, analgesics, and subanesthetic concentrations of inhalational anesthetics alone or in combination to supplement local or regional anesthesia (Box 9-1). These classes of drugs, when combined, confer three essential components of conscious sedation: amnesia, anxiolysis, and analgesia.[1-5] The concept of conscious sedation originated in the domain of office-based dentistry and oral surgery. With the development of newer, short-acting pharmacologic agents and of noninvasive monitoring, conscious sedation techniques have been adapted for use by anesthesiologists and other medical practitioners for both surgical and diagnostic procedures. It has been estimated that at least 10% to 30% of anesthesia cases involve sedation techniques, and many of these are provided for outpatients by anesthesiologists as monitored anesthesia care (MAC).[2]

Goals

The goal of outpatient sedation is to provide a balance between patient comfort and patient safety, while preventing cardiovascular or respiratory compromise, or delay in recovery (Box 9-2). The technique of sedation is as much an art as a science. Experience and sensitivity are required to achieve just the right amount. Component drugs are primarily administered intraoperatively via the intravenous route; however, one or more drugs may also be administered as premedication via the oral, intramuscular,

---

Box 9-1 Classification of Agents Used for Sedation Techniques

---

Barbiturates

Thiopental
Methohexital

Tranquilizers

Diazepam
Midazolam
Droperidol

Other Intravenous Sedative Agents

Propofol
Ketamine
Etomidate

Narcotics

Fentanyl
Alfentanil
Sufentanil

Narcotic Agonist/Antagonists

Butorphanol
Nalbuphine

Inhalational Agents

Nitrous oxide
Potent inhalational agents

---

transmucosal, or rectal routes. The drugs are all central nervous system depressants and, depending on dose, can induce a state anywhere on the continuum from relaxation to unconsciousness (Fig. 9-1). Drugs in combination exert additive effects that may ultimately cause suppression of reflexes, airway obstruction, and especially, respiratory depression. For conscious sedation, the objective is to promote quiescence, analgesia, and tolerance for administration of local anesthetic or regional block. Sedation facilitates acceptance of local or regional anesthesia by blunting sensations such as pressure, movement, traction, position change, or awareness of noise and activity in the environment.[6]

Box 9-2 *Goals of Sedation*

To guard the patient's safety and welfare

To minimize physical discomfort or pain

To minimize negative psychologic responses to treatment by providing analgesia, and to maximize the potential for amnesia

To control behavior

To return the patient to a state in which safe discharge as determined by recognized criteria is possible

---

Adapted from the American Academy of Pediatrics. Pediatrics 1992; 89:1110-5.

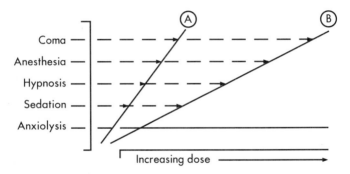

Fig. 9-1 Spectrum of central nervous activity. Sedative-hypnotic compounds produce a dose-dependent spectrum of CNS depression. In this schematic, drug *A* might represent a barbituate whereas drug *B* might represent a benzodiazepine. (Adapted from White PF: Pharmacologic and clinical aspects of preoperative medication. Anesth Analg, 1968; 65:963.)

Patient and Procedure Selection

The success of the sedation technique depends on factors related to the patient, the surgeon, and the procedure. Sedation is ideal for patients who fear general anesthesia, who refuse it, or who are at higher risk because of age or underlying medical conditions. It must be used with caution, however, for impaired, unwilling, or anxious patients, or for those who are fearful of pain or of being aware during the procedure. A patient with hypertension, coronary artery disease, or obesity may be more difficult to manage with sedation, which may result in a situation less under control than that seen with general anesthesia. Tachycardia or hypertension can occur secondary to anxiety, inadequate analgesia, cardiovascular or hormonal response to noxious stimuli, and exogenous epinephrine in the local anesthetic solution. Oxygen desaturation has been reported in unsedated patients having local anesthesia alone for oral surgery; this is caused by breath holding due to fear or pain.[7] The surgeon must feel comfortable about operating on a patient who is awake, and must be capable of working in a gentle but expeditious manner.

The outpatient procedures that are amenable to management with conscious sedation are numerous and represent various specialties: orthopedics, plastics, gynecology, urology, otolaryngology, ophthalmology, general surgery, and dental and oral surgery. Many diagnostic cardiologic, gastrointestinal, and radiologic procedures can also be performed with these techniques. Frequently performed procedures involving sedation techniques include arthroscopy, upper extremity surgery, dilatation and curettage, in vitro fertilization, rhytidectomy, rhinoplasty, blepharoplasty, superficial skin procedures, breast and other biopsies, cataract extraction, cystoscopy, insertion of lines and shunts, herniorraphy, bronchoscopy, dental extractions, and gastrointestinal endoscopy.[8]

Preparation

Preoperative and postoperative medical and administrative requirements for patients receiving conscious sedation should be the same as those for general or regional anesthesia. History, physical examination, airway assessment, and appropriate laboratory tests should be performed. Fasting guidelines should be enforced, and an escort should be available. Since conscious sedation implies safety, and since the point of transformation of conscious to unconscious sedation (general anesthesia) cannot always be predicted, the extent of preparation and care for conscious sedation should be identical to that for general anesthesia.[9]

Psychological preparation of the patient is particularly important. At least 85% of patients anticipating surgery are said to be anxious or afraid. Patients undergoing ambulatory surgery may even be more concerned about their anesthesia than surgery, since surgery is usually minor. McCleane determined that 50% to 60% of patients feared intraoperative awareness, postoperative pain, and nausea and vomiting.[10A] Patients also may fear the wait to go into the operating room, loss of control, loss of consciousness, injury, or even death. Although considered trivial, the gas mask and the intravenous needle may worry some patients. A realistic and informative personal interview in which expectations can be defined is more useful in allaying anxiety than premedication. The ambulatory surgery facility should offer pleasant physical surroundings and ambiance with helpful and supportive staff.

During the procedure, it is very important for the anesthesiologist to maintain verbal contact with the patient, provide reassurance, warn of events, and assess nonverbal patient response.[8] The anesthesiologist can influence patient perception, cooperation, and satisfaction. In fact, 85% of patients preferred local anesthesia with sedation over local anesthesia alone for oral surgery. The degree of satisfaction was proportional to the extent of sedation.[2]

Definition

The term *conscious sedation* was first used by Bennett to describe intravenous supplementation of local and regional anesthesia, with minimal depression of consciousness (Table 9-1).[11] McCarthy more specifically describes a minimally depressed level of consciousness that retains the patient's ability to independently and continuously maintain the airway and respond to physical stimulation and verbal command (Table 9-2).[12] During conscious sedation, somnolence or basal narcosis should not be produced and the cardiovascular, respiratory, and reflex functions should remain intact. Scamman described the three key elements of conscious sedation as: (1) sedation without risk, which requires communication with the patient, monitoring, and equipment available for emergency resuscitation; (2) relief from anxiety, presence of amnesia, and reduction of unpleasant stimuli (noise, cold) in the surroundings; and (3) relief from pain, achieved by the administration of local anesthetics and narcotics.[13] *Deep sedation* or *unconscious sedation* is defined by the American Academy of Pediatrics (AAP) as a state of depressed consciousness or

Table 9-1   Conscious versus Unconscious Sedation

Conscious sedation	Unconscious sedation
Mood altered	Patient unconscious
Patient conscious	Patient unconscious
Patient cooperative	No patient cooperation

Protective reflexes active and intact	Protective reflexes obtunded
	    Airway may become obstructed
	    Respiratory: hypoxia, hypercapnia
	    Cardiovascular: hypotension, hypertension bradycardia, tachycardia

Vital signs stable	Vital signs labile
Analgesia may be present; regional/local analgesia required	Pain eliminated centrally; regional analgesia not required
Recovery room stay not prolonged	Recovery room stay prolonged or admission required
Risk of complications low	Risk of complications high
Postoperative complications infrequent	Postoperative complications frequent
Difficult or mentally incompetent patient may not be manageable	May be required to manage mentally incompetent patient

Adapted from Bennett CR: Conscious sedation in dental practice, ed 2, St Louis, 1978, Mosby, p. 22; and Kallar SR: Conscious sedation in ambulatory surgery. Anesth Rev 1990; 17:45.

unconsciousness from which a patient cannot be easily aroused, accompanied by partial or complete loss of protective reflexes, including ability to independently maintain a patent airway, and unresponsiveness to physical stimulation or verbal command.[14]

***Table* 9-2** Proposed Definitions of Analgesia and Sedation by the American Dental Association Council on Dental Education

Analgesia	Diminution or elimination of pain in the conscious patient
Local anesthesia	Elimination of sensations, especially pain, in one part of the body by the topical application or regional injection of a drug
Conscious sedation	Minimally depressed level of consciousness that retains the patient's ability to independently and continuously maintain an airway and respond appropriately to physical stimulation and verbal command, produced by a pharmacologic or nonpharmacologic method, or a combination
General anesthesia or deep sedation	Controlled state of depressed consciousness or unconsciousness, accompanied by partial or complete loss of protective reflexes, including the ability to independently maintain an airway and respond purposefully to physical stimulation or verbal command, produced by a pharmacologic or nonpharmacologic method, or a combination

Adapted from McCarthy FM, Solomon AL, Jastak J et al: Conscious sedation: benefits and risks. J Am Dental Assoc 1984; 109:546; and Kallar SR: Conscious sedation in ambulatory surgery. Anesth Rev 1990; 17:45.

This state is not dissimilar to a description of general anesthesia. Drugs and techniques should include a margin of safety to render unintended loss of consciousness unlikely.

Sedation scores have been developed to measure degree of sedation qualitatively or quantitatively. The following is a scale modified from White.[15]

1. Awake and alert
2. Awake but drowsy
3. Dozing, easily arousable to command

4. Sleeping, and only arousable to physical stimulation
5. Asleep, unarousable, unresponsive to stimuli

Administration

The ideal intravenous drug for conscious sedation would possess several desirable characteristics (Box 9-3). In pharmacologic terms, a small volume of distribution, short elimination half life, and rapid clearance are desirable features.[1-5,9] Midazolam, fentanyl, alfentanil, propofol, and methohexital are the drugs most commonly used for conscious sedation during ambulatory surgery. The tranquilizer is usually administered first, followed by the narcotic, and finally by the sedative hypnotic. Drugs may be administered by bolus or by infusion. The initial dose is determined by clinical judgment, depending on the length of the procedure and the patient's weight, physical condition, anxiety level, and drug history. Drugs for conscious sedation must be carefully titrated according to patient response. The endpoint will vary depending on the particular patient and surgical situation. Combinations of drugs, including premedication, lead to more

---

Box 9-3 The Ideal Drug for Intravenous Sedation

Water soluble, nonirritating, stable
Rapid onset
Specific, identifiable, and readily titratable effect
Short, reliable duration of action
Ease of administration
Absence of cardiovascular or respiratory depressant effects
No hypersensitivity reactions
Non–organ dependent elimination
Absence of toxicity
Pharmacokinetic independence of altered physiology
Rapid recovery
Favorable cost-benefit ratio

Adapted from White PF: Clinical uses of intravenous infusions and analgesic infusions. Anesth Analg 1989; 68:161; and Twersky RS: The pharmacology of anesthetics used for ambulatory surgery. In American Society of Anesthesiologists: Annual refresher courses, Philadelphia, 1993, JB Lippincott, p. 159.

profound sedation. Continuous infusion requires frequent readjustment based on clinical effect. The anesthesiologist must correctly identify the presence of pain or agitation and its etiology in order to determine appropriate treatment. Pain is best treated by local anesthetics and intravenous analgesics. Anxiety is best treated by intravenous benzodiazepines. Failure to distinguish inadequate analgesia from inadequate sedation may result in agitation or respiratory depression if the situation is inappropriately treated by hypnotic or anxiolytic drugs. Improper administration of an opioid is equally dangerous and is likely to produce unconsciousness, respiratory depression, and hypoxia. If patients are excessively sedated, the advantage of conscious sedation is lost and recovery time may exceed that for general anesthesia.

Monitoring

Central nervous system, cardiovascular, and respiratory monitoring are necessary to ensure patient safety during conscious sedation. Monitoring refines the administration of anesthesia by providing information to assess the effectiveness of drugs and to detect adverse effects. Monitoring should be performed by qualified personnel apart from those performing the surgical procedure. According to the American Society of Anesthesiologist (ASA) guidelines, during conscious sedation or monitored anesthesia care (MAC), specific parameters should be monitored (Box 9-4).[16] Vital signs, presence of end tidal CO_2, O_2 saturation, drugs administered, dosages, and interventions undertaken should be recorded. A precordial stethoscope is useful for monitoring cardiac and respiratory status. Supplementary oxygen should be administered routinely via nasal prongs or mask. Capnography can be accomplished by inserting the gas sampling tube via an adaptor into the nasal prong and connecting it to a gas analyzer.[3] Nasal prongs that incorporate the capnographic connection are also commercially available. Cardiovascular monitoring may detect changes in heart rate or blood pressure secondary to cardiovascular depression, inadequate sedation, or arrhythmia. Cardiovascular monitoring also serves as an indirect index of hypercarbia or hypoxia. Initially, heart rate and blood pressure may increase due to sympathetic stimulation, but eventually bradycardia supervenes. In infants and children, bradycardia may be the initial sign

---

Box 9-4 *American Society of Anesthesiologists Standards for Basic Anesthetic Monitoring in Monitored Anesthesia Care*

Standard I

Qualified anesthesia personnel shall be present in the room throughout the conduct of all general anesthetics, regional anesthetics, and monitored anesthesia care.

Standard II

During all anesthetics, the patient's oxygenation, ventilation, circulation, and temperature shall be continually evaluated.

Oxygenation

Blood oxygenation: During all anesthetics, a quantitative method of assessing oxygenation, such as pulse oximetry, shall be employed. Adequate illumination and exposure of the patient is necessary to assess color.

Ventilation

During regional anesthesia and monitored anesthesia care, the adequacy of ventilation shall be evaluated, at least by continual observation of qualitative clinical signs.

Circulation

Every patient receiving anesthesia shall have the ECG continuously displayed from the beginning of anesthesia until preparing to leave the anesthetizing location.

Every patient receiving anesthesia shall have arterial blood pressure and heart rate determined and evaluated at least every 5 minutes.

Temperature

There shall be readily available a means to continuously measure the patient's temperature.

Adapted from American Society of Anesthesiologists: Standards for basic anesthetic monitoring, 1986, Park Ridge, Ill, 1994, ASA, p. 735. A copy of the full text can be obtained from ASA, 520 N. Northwest Highway, Park Ridge, IL 60068-2573.

---

of hypoxia. Since desaturation cannot be detected visually until oxygenation is dangerously impaired, use of a pulse oximeter and supplemental oxygen should be routine. Monitoring of ECG, blood pressure, respiratory rate, and pulse oximetry should be continued into the postoperative period.[3]

Safety

How safe is conscious sedation? There are numerous reports in the literature and in the media of adverse cardiovascular and respiratory events associated with sedation techniques.[1,3-5] Some of these reflect its performance in remote areas by individuals lacking monitoring or emergency equipment, or lacking skill in airway management or resuscitation. Even for the anesthesiologist, security and predictability are not always assured with conscious sedation techniques. Transient if not profound hypoxemia has the potential to occur frequently. In Campbell's study, normal volunteers who received 100 µg of fentanyl and 10 mg of diazepam, pO_2 was reduced by 30 torr and pCO_2 increased by 7 torr.[17] Bailey studied the effects of 0.05 mg/kg of midazolam alone, 2 µg/kg of fentanyl alone, and a combination in normal volunteers. Midazolam alone did not produce hypoxia or apnea. Fentanyl alone produced hypoxia (less than 90% saturation) in 50% of patients, but not apnea. The combination of midazolam plus fentanyl produced hypoxia in 92% of patients, and apnea or obstruction in 50%.[18] Patients expected to be most susceptible to the effects of these medications are the elderly, the obese, and those with cardiac, respiratory, renal, or hepatic disease.[4,5] According to the Food and Drug Administration (FDA) data, midazolam has been implicated in at least 80 deaths during gastrointestinal endoscopy, which have occurred mainly in the absence of monitoring or an anesthesiologist.[19] Respiratory events were responsible for 78% of the incidents; in 57% of cases, patients had received a sedative and an opioid. Kallar reported 8000 cases of conscious sedation over a 9-year period at the Medical College of Virginia in which there were no deaths or serious complications. Transient hypoxemia (less than 90% saturation) occurred in 28% of patients; this was often associated with management by less experienced anesthesia personnel, but it was easily corrected by supplemental oxygen.[4] Adverse cardiorespiratory events during sedation techniques in pediatric patients were attributed to inattention to dose, rate of drug administration, age of patient, and past medical history.[20] At risk are newborns and patients with altered mental status, hemodynamic instability, history of apnea, ventilatory disorder, or airway problem. Yaster reported a cardiac arrest in a 14-month-old 13 kg infant associated with midazolam and fentanyl intravenous sedation for bone marrow aspiration in the prone position. He advised that when administering intravenous sedation,

Table 9-3 Complications and Anesthetic Technique

Technique	No. of patients	No. of complications	Incidence
Local only	10,169	38	1/268
Local and sedation	10,229	96	1/106
General	61,299	513	1/120
Regional	1936	7	1/277

From FASA Special Study 1, 1986. Courtesy of the Federated Ambulatory Surgery Association, Alexandria, Va.

the physician must anticipate, recognize, and be capable of treating life-threatening adverse drug effects. Intraoperative and postoperative monitoring should be performed by a qualified individual.

Mortality and morbidity may occur more frequently with sedation techniques than with general anesthesia; this is due to drug reactions, airway events (e.g., obstruction, aspiration, bronchospasm), or cardiovascular events related to hypertension and arrhythmia.[1,3-5] In a 1984 Federated Ambulatory Surgery Association (FASA) study of 87,000 patients in 40 freestanding ambulatory surgery centers, the complication rate was 1/106 with local anesthesia plus sedation, compared to 1/120 for general anesthesia, 1/268 for local only, and 1/277 for regional anesthesia (Table 9-3).[21] Not all anesthetics were administered by anesthesiologists. Campbell reported a mortality rate of 1/314,000 for MAC versus 1/324,000 for general anesthesia in dentistry.[22] In a recent study by Cohen of 100,000 anesthetics, MAC morbidity was 208/10,000, higher than that of other modes of anesthesia.[23] Closed claims analysis has identified several cardiac arrests related to sedation accompanying spinal anesthesia in healthy patients. Inadequate ventilation was the most common anesthesia mishap identified by closed claims analysis,[24] and it is estimated that 69% of such mishaps can be prevented. Future studies are needed to evaluate recovery and long-term outcome after local/intravenous sedation versus general anesthesia for outpatient surgery.

Standards of Care

Standards of care and guidelines for conscious sedation techniques or MAC have been established by various organizations such as the American Dental Association (ADA), AAP, ASA, and Joint

Commission on Accreditation of Healthcare Organizations (JCAHO). The role and responsibility of the anesthesiologist in delivering conscious sedation, now termed monitored anesthesia care (MAC), as originally defined by the American Society of Anesthesiologists was to provide a service to the patient; to control nonsurgical aspects of medical care, including monitoring of vital signs; and to remain available to administer anesthetics or deliver other medical care. In 1989, The ASA House of Delegates expanded its definition of services for MAC to include preanesthesia examination and evaluation; prescription of anesthesia care; personal participation in or medical direction of the entire plan of care; continuous physical presence of the anesthesiologists, resident, or CRNA; and proximate presence or availability of the anesthesiologist for diagnosis and treatment of emergencies. It was stated further that all institutional regulations are to be observed and usual services provided, including noninvasive cardiovascular and respiratory monitoring, oxygen administration when indicated, and intravenous administration of sedatives, tranquilizers, antiemetics, narcotics, other analgesics, beta blockers, vasopressors, bronchodilators, antihypertensives, or other pharmacologic treatment.[25] The same level of care is required for MAC as for general or regional anesthesia. Since 1988, JCAHO standards have been in effect when patients receive sedation. The 1994 JCAHO hospital manual in the section on surgery and anesthesia services that deals with operative and other invasive procedures states that standards apply "when any patient, in any setting, receives, for any purpose, by any route [general, spinal, or regional anesthesia] or sedation (with or without analgesia) for which there is a reasonable expectation that in the manner used, the sedation/analgesia will result in the loss of protective reflexes."[26]

Discharge Policies

The ASA has established standards for the postanesthesia period that apply to patients who receive monitored anesthesia care (Box 9-5).[27] All patients who have received sedation should be recovered in a postanesthesia care unit (PACU) or comparable facility attended by personnel competent to assess recovery. Discharge criteria to be met are equivalent to those for general anesthesia, and include stable vital signs; orientation; mobilization

Box 9-5 *American Society of Anesthesiologists Standards for Postanesthesia Care in Monitored Anesthesia Care*

Standard I

All patients who have received general anesthesia, regional anesthesia, or monitored anesthesia care shall receive appropriate postanesthesia management. A postanesthesia care unit (PACU) or an area which provides equivalent postanesthesia care shall be available to receive patients after surgery and anesthesia. All patients who receive anesthesia shall be admitted to the PACU except by specific order of the anesthesiologist responsible for the patient's care.

Standard II

A patient transported to the PACU shall be accompanied by a member of the anesthesia care team who is knowledgeable about the patient's condition. The patient shall be continually evaluated and treated during transport with monitoring and support appropriate to the patient's condition.

Standard III

Upon arrival in the PACU, the patient shall be re-evaluated and a verbal report provided to the responsible PACU nurse by the member of the anesthesia care team who accompanies the patient.

Standard IV

The patient's condition shall be evaluated continually in the PACU.

1. The patient shall be observed and monitored by methods appropriate to the patient's medical condition. Particular attention should be given to monitoring oxygenation, ventilation, circulation and temperature. During recovery from all anesthetics, a quantitative method of assessing oxygenation such as pulse oximetry shall be employed in the initial phase of recovery.

Continued.

Box 9-5 *American Society of Anesthesiolgists—cont'd*

2. An accurate written report of the PACU period shall be maintained.
3. General medical supervision and coordination of patient care in the PACU should be the responsibility of an anesthesiologist.
4. There shall be a policy to assure the availability in the facility of a physician capable of managing complications and providing cardiopulmonary resuscitation for patients in the PACU.

Standard V

A physician is responsible for the discharge of the patient from the postanesthesia care unit.
1. When discharge criteria are used, they must be approved by the Department of Anesthesiology and the medical staff.
2. In the absence of the physician responsible for the discharge, the PACU nurse shall determine that the patient meets the discharge criteria. The name of the physician accepting responsibility for discharge shall be noted on the record.

Adapted from American Society of Anesthesiologist: Standards for Postanesthesia Care, 1988, Park Ridge, Ill, 1994, ASA, p. 737. A copy of the full text can be obtained from ASA, 520 N. Northwest Highway, Park Ridge, IL 60068-2573.

and absence of significant pain, nausea, or bleeding.[1,3,9] A responsible escort must be present, and verbal or written discharge instructions should be given. Information should be provided regarding activity level and emergency access. Patients should be cautioned not to drive, consume alcohol, operate machinery, or make important decisions for 12 to 24 hours (see Chapter 12 for specific discharge instructions).

Drugs and Sedation Techniques

The dosages and pharmacologic characteristics of drugs used for conscious sedation are outlined in Tables 9-4 and 9-5.

Table 9-4   Dosages of Drugs for Conscious Sedation

Drug	Loading dose (μg/kg)	Maintenance infusion rate (μg/kg/min)	Plasma drug level
Thiopental	1000-3000	100-300	4-8 μg/ml
Methohexital	250-1000	10-50	2-5 mg/ml
Diazepam	50-150		
Midazolam	25-100	0.25-1	40-100 ng/ml
Droperidol	5-17		
Propofol	250-1000	10-50	1-2 μg/ml
Ketamine	500-1000	10-20	0.1-1 μg/ml
Etomidate	100-200	7-14	100-300 ng/ml
Fentanyl	1-3	0.01-0.03	1-2 ng/ml
Alfentanil	10-25	0.25-1	25-75 ng/ml
Sufentanil	0.1-0.5	.005-.01	0.02-0.2 ng/ml
Butorphanol	0.01-0.03		
Nalbuphine	0.07-0.2		

Adapted from Fragen RJ, editor: Drug infusions in anesthesiology, New York, 1991, Raven Press; and Twersky RS: The pharmacology of anesthetics used for ambulatory surgery. In American Society of Anesthesiologists: Annual refresher courses, vol 21, Philadelphia, 1993, JB Lippincott, pp. 159-75; and Glass PSA, Jacobs JR, Reeves JG: Intravenous drug delivery system. In Miller R, editor: Anesthesia, ed 4, New York, 1994, Churchill Livingstone, pp. 389-410.

Barbiturates

Thiopental

Thiopental is the most familiar barbiturate used in anesthetic practice.[28,29] Its fat solubility and large volume of distribution prolong its elimination half life to 10 to 12 hours. A bolus of 2.6 mg/kg produces 120 seconds of sleep.[30] After 5 minutes, patients are able to ambulate and converse. Larger doses have a more prolonged effect. The drug has profound hemodynamic effects and produces respiratory depression, including apnea. Other respiratory phenomena are cough and laryngospasm. Mild pain and flushing may occur on injection; tissues may be irritated with extravasation; or thiopental may precipitate in the presence of other injected drugs because of its alkalinity. The advantages of

Table 9-5 Pharmacologic Characteristics of Agents Used for Sedation Techniques

Drug	V_d (l/kg)	Cl (ml/kg/min)	$t_{1/2}\alpha$ (minutes)	$t_{1/2}\beta$ (hours)	Protein binding (%)
Thiopental	2.3	3.4	2-4	12.0	83
Methohexital	2.2	10.9	5-6	3.9	73
Diazepam	1.1	0.4		46.5	98
Midazolam	1.1	7.5	7-15	2.7	94
Propofol	2.8	59.4	2-4	0.9	97
Ketamine	3.1	19.1	11-17	3.1	12
Etomidate	2.5	17.9	2-4	2.9	77
Fentanyl	3.2-5.9	11-21	1.4-1.7	3.1-4.4	79-87
Alfentanil	0.5-1	5-7.9	1-3.5	1.2-1.7	89-92
Sufentanil	2.8	13	1.4	2.7	92.5

$V_d \equiv$ = volume of distribution
Cl = clearance
$t_{1/2}\alpha$ = distribution half life
$t_{1/2}\beta$ = elimination half life
Adapted from Fragen RJ, editor: Drug infusions in anesthesiology, New York, 1991, Raven Press; and Twersky RS: The pharmacology of anesthetics used for ambulatory surgery. In American Society of Anesthesiologists: Annual refresher courses, Philadelphia, 1993, JB Lippincott, pp. 159-75.

thiopental are low cost and infrequent nausea and vomiting. Thiopental lacks analgesic properties, and may cause excitement and disorientation when analgesia is not provided by other means. Because its therapeutic index is lower than that of the benzodiazepines and because it is highly susceptible to drug interactions, thiopental has no real role in ambulatory surgery sedation.

Methohexital

Methohexital is an oxybarbiturate more potent than thiopental. Its redistribution half life and volume of distribution are similar to those of thiopental. Rapid clearance, three to four times faster than that of thiopental, and shorter elimination half life, 1.5 to 4 hours, result in more rapid recovery especially with cumulative doses.[28,29] After an 0.88 mg/kg bolus dose, sleep lasted 2.5 minutes.[30] Side effects, such as involuntary movement and pain on injection, sometimes occur. The characteristics and incidence of respiratory and cardiovascular depression are similar to that produced by thiopental. When methohexital is combined with narcotics or tranquilizers, its depressant effects are prolonged. Following 5 to 15 mg of diazepam with 5 to 10 mg of methohexital, recovery of perception or cognition required more than 3 hours. Compared with thiopental, patients emerge more quickly, and are less sedated and more clearheaded.[31] Following 1 mg/kg of methohexital, recovery based on tests of coordination occurred within 30 to 60 minutes; following 2 mg/kg, in 45 to 90 minutes. Following 2.5 mg/kg of thiopental, recovery occurred in 30 to 75 minutes, while following 5 mg/kg of thiopental, recovery did not occur until 100 to 200 minutes.

Tranquilizers

Diazepam

Diazepam, a lipid-soluble benzodiazepine first used as a component of conscious sedation, produces sedation, amnesia, and anxiolysis within 2 to 3 minutes of intravenous injection.[28,29,32] It should be titrated to effect by 2.5 mg increments administered every 2 to 3 minutes. Respiratory and cardiovascular depression from diazepam alone are minimal; however, when diazepam is combined with opioids or other centrally acting drugs, its depressant effects are potentiated. A diazepam dose of 0.14 mg/kg depressed ventilatory response to carbon dioxide, increased dead space to tidal volume ratio, and produced an elevation in CO_2 lasting 25 to 30 minutes.[33] Diazepam is used in conjunction with local or regional anesthesia to produce amnesia, both for the local injection itself and for the surgical procedure. It also increases the seizure threshold of the local anesthetic. A diazepam dose of 5 to 10 mg produced anterograde amnesia lasting 30 minutes in 50% to 90% of patients.[34] Pain and phlebitis may result from solvent-induced venous irritation. Lack of analgesic properties may contribute to restlessness in the presence of inadequate analgesia.

Although acute recovery occurs within 90 minutes, its elimination half life of 24 to 48 hours, its enterohepatic recirculation, and its metabolically active metabolites may prolong effects. Clearance is delayed by cimetidine. Cognitive and motor skill recovery are slower after diazepam than that after methohexital or halothane general anesthesia. Coordination and reaction time remained abnormal for 6 hours after a 0.15 mg/kg dose.[35] Following a 0.30 to

0.45 mg/kg dose, impaired coordination and deficiency in driving skills were present for 10 hours; when combined with narcotics, these effects persisted for 24 hours.[35] Because of the development of shorter-acting, equally effective alternatives, the use of diazepam for ambulatory anesthesia has diminished.

Midazolam

Midazolam is a newer water-soluble benzodiazepine, which is two to four times more potent than diazepam. It produces comparable or superior sedation, amnesia, and anxiolysis, which are usually less prolonged. The redistribution and elimination half lives of midazolam are shorter than those of diazepam, and its metabolites have no significant pharmacologic activity. The drug is administered intravenously in 1 to 2 mg increments over 2 to 3 minutes, and onset occurs in 1 to 2 minutes. In contrast to diazepam, midazolam does not produce pain on injection. Large doses may result in prolonged drowsiness and impairment of motor skills. Interpatient variability is great, and some patients may be extremely sensitive. In elderly patients or in patients with chronic disease, elimination is slower and the dose should be reduced. Effects are synergistic with narcotics for sedation and amnesia. When combined with thiopental, fentanyl, alfentanil, or propofol, the dose of midazolam should be reduced by 25% to 30%. Midazolam is very selective for amnesia, the amnestic dose being one tenth of the hypnotic dose.[36] A 5 mg dose produced amnesia lasting 20 minutes in 90% of patients.[37] Midazolam depresses the slope of the CO_2 response curve, and decreases the ventilatory response to hypoxia. Apnea is the most frequently reported adverse reaction. Respiratory depression is proportional to depression of mental status. In patients receiving 0.10 to 0.15 mg/kg of midazolam for sedation, 40% to 50% became transiently unconscious or apneic, and drowsiness lasted for 2 hours.[38]

When midazolam was first introduced, there were reports of deaths from airway obstruction, apnea, and hypoxia mainly in older patients with concomitant cardiovascular or respiratory disease. The package insert now contains warnings about the necessity of appropriate monitoring, ability to manage the airway, and availability of emergency resuscitation equipment. Studies have shown that after midazolam sedation, motor function recovered in 30 minutes, amnesia in 40 minutes, and ability to ambulate in 75 minutes, but drowsiness persisted for 2 hours.[39,40] In a study comparing various drugs for regional anesthesia supplementation, at 2 hours 80% of patients were awake following midazolam, while only 67% of patients were awake following diazepam.[41,42] Midazolam produced greater amnesia and less pain on injection than propofol.[15] For outpatient oral surgery in patients sedated with 0.1 mg/kg of midazolam, onset was more rapid, amnesia more profound, and postoperative drowsiness was less than that seen with diazepam; however, recovery time was the same.[43] The duration of the amnestic effect equaled the duration of sedation. Following bronchoscopy under local anesthesia, immediate clinical recovery (standing, walking), and performance on several psychomotor tests repeatedly performed, were similar after premedication with diazepam or midazolam.[44]

Droperidol

Droperidol is a butyrophenone capable of producing sedation and detachment with minimal amnesia.[45] When combined with a narcotic, it produces an anesthetic state called neuroleptanalgesia. The fixed combination of droperidol and fentanyl (innovar) is not ideal for sedation because it contains a relative excess of the longer-lasting droperidol. While the distribution half life for the drug is only 10 minutes, its elimination half life is 2.3 hours. The recommended doses for sedation are 2.5 to 10 mg. Increased doses result in excess and prolonged sedation, extrapyramidal symptoms, dysphoria, restlessness, and hypotension. Droperidol alone produces minimal respiratory depression. It has a significant antiemetic effect and may be used in small doses (0.625 to 1.25 mg) in adults as prophylaxis for or treatment of postoperative emesis. Kortilla found that after a 5 mg intravenous dose, clinical recovery occurred in 25 minutes, but drowsiness, impaired coordination, and attention deficit persisted for 10 hours in 50% of patients.[46]

Other Intravenous Agents

Propofol

Propofol is a unique sedative hypnotic of the alkyl phenol class. It is a highly lipid-soluble drug stabilized in an aqueous oil emulsion at a concentration of 10 mg/ml. To retain its stability, the emulsion should not be diluted below 2 mg/ml. Its rapid onset, distribution, and clearance are ideally suited for outpatient sedation and anesthesia. Its elimination half life of 1 to 3 hours is considerably shorter than that of methohexital (6 to 8 hours) or thiopental (10 to 12 hours). Clearance is in excess of hepatic blood flow. On induction, 1.5 to 2.5 mg/kg produces sleep in less than 60 seconds, and awakening occurs in 4 to 8 minutes. For intravenous sedation, an initial bolus dose of 0.5 mg/kg or an initial infusion dose of 100 to 150 µg/kg/min should be given over 3 to 5 minutes. Maintenance bolus increments of 10 to 20 mg, or an infusion rate of 25 to 75 µg/kg/min (1.5-4.5 mg/kg/hr), is recommended.[47]

The drug should be given more slowly and doses should be reduced by at least 20% in elderly, debilitated, or ASA class 3 patients to prevent depression of blood pressure, heart rate, and respiration. Hypotension and apnea frequently occur. Cardiovascular and respiratory effects are potentiated by narcotics. Facilities and personnel capable of maintaining the airway and providing artificial ventilation and circulatory resuscitation should be immediately available. Pain on injection is due to irritation of the venous wall and release of mediators (kinogens). The pain is less noticeable when the intravenous catheter is inserted in a larger vein of the arm and when the drug is injected rapidly. Gehan[48] found that lidocaine 0.1 mg/kg preceding or combined with the propofol reduced the incidence of pain from 40% to 5% to 15%. Other side effects include occasional trunk erythema, involuntary movements, or hiccups. Recovery following propofol is spectacular, with sedation and lightheadedness disappearing within a few minutes and prompt return of psychomotor function. Resedation does not occur, and nausea and vomiting are infrequent.

The Centers for Disease Control (CDC) has reported postsurgical infections and hyperthermic reactions that were associated with propofol.[49] The lipid emulsion is an excellent culture medium for bacteria. Sterile handling and immediate single-patient use after preparation are the current FDA and manufacturer recommendations. The drug should be discarded if not administered within 6 hours after opening. The use of a stopcock as a loading port to refill syringes on syringe pumps is controversial because it may promote contamination.[50] The sideport must always be recapped and the refill syringe discarded after each use.

Oei-Lim et al.[51] recommended propofol in subanesthetic doses (5 to 6 mg/kg/hr) as an alternative to nitrous oxide for conscious sedation in mentally handicapped patients with epilepsy undergoing dental procedures. In nonepileptic patients, a smaller dose

(3.5 mg/kg/hr) was required. There were no hemodynamic or respiratory changes in either group, but close supervision of airway and respiration was maintained. The level of sedation should not exceed easy arousability to command. Zacny et al.[52] studied the effect of subanesthetic doses of propofol on mood and psychomotor cognitive performance in the following dose ranges in volunteers: low, 0.08 mg/kg followed by 0.5 mg/kg/hr; moderate, 0.16 mg/kg, then 1 mg/kg/hr; high, 0.3 mg/kg followed by 2 mg/kg/hr. In all groups, mood returned to baseline by 1 hour. Psychomotor impairment and anterograde amnesia occurred only with the high dose. They concluded that propofol is well suited for ambulatory use and does not produce dysphoria.

Ketamine

Ketamine is a phencyclidine derivative that produces a dissociative state, characterized by catalepsy, catatonia, sedation, hypnosis, amnesia, and analgesia. Ketamine is effective within 30 to 60 seconds of intravenous injection. Nystagmus, detachment, and extraneous movements are commonly observed. Ketamine maintains ventilatory response to CO_2 and promotes bronchodilation. Its cardiovascular and sympathetic nervous system stimulant effects produce increases in blood pressure, heart rate, and peripheral vascular resistance. Intracranial and intraocular pressures are increased. The drug is not recommended for use in eye surgery or for patients with coronary disease or hypertension. Although upper airway reflexes may be heightened, protection against aspiration is not assured. Vomiting and increased production of secretions may be expected.

Emergence reactions are common. Delirium, hallucinations, and bad dreams occur in 40% of patients.[53] Benzodiazepines, such as midazolam, are most effective in blunting this response. A ketamine dose of 2 mg/kg, administered before injection of local anesthesia for nerve block, produces unconsciousness lasting 15 minutes, but complete recovery may be delayed. Dizziness, incoordination, and blurred vision may persist. Quiet recovery is recommended, as opposed to the usual "stir up" routine for ambulatory surgery patients. Of plastic surgery patients given 0.4 to 0.5 mg/kg of ketamine, 87% experienced amnesia without unpleasant memories, while 8.5% reported unpleasant memories and lack of analgesia.[54] Ketamine resulted in less alertness, increased incidence of headache, dizziness, bad dreams, and nausea and vomiting compared with thiopental. Benzodiazepines and droperidol, when given to treat these side effects, extended recovery time. For lithotripsy, midazolam 0.4 mg/kg followed by ketamine 25 µg/kg/min was associated with cardiorespiratory stability; however, patients moved during the procedure and exhibited side effects, and recovery time was prolonged when compared with that of propofol or alfentanil.[55]

Etomidate

Etomidate is a water-soluble imidazole compound. Peak effect occurs in 1 minute. The main advantage of etomidate is hemodynamic stability. Respiratory depression is moderate. Etomidate does not provide analgesia. Pain on injection occurs in 50% of patients and involuntary movements in 70%. These side effects can be diminished by prior administration of opioid or benzodiazepine. Etomidate is also associated with a high incidence of nausea, vomiting, and emergence excitement. Even a single dose may produce prolonged adrenocortical suppression. Persistence of sedation and depression of psychomotor function is greater with etomidate than with methohexital, but less than with thiopental.[56] This drug has no advantage as a component of conscious sedation for ambulatory surgery.

Narcotics

Fentanyl

Fentanyl, a phenylpiperidine derivative, is the most widely used narcotic for ambulatory anesthesia. It produces analgesia, drowsiness, sedation, and euphoria, but not amnesia. The drug is injected in 25 to 50 µg increments at 1 to 2 minute intervals to a usual loading dose of 1 to 3 µg/kg. Its onset is within 5 minutes, its peak is at 10 minutes, and its effect lasts 45 to 60 minutes. Over time, progressive saturation of inactive tissue sites leads to increased duration of analgesia and respiratory depression. Its elimination half life is 3 to 6 hours, which is prolonged in the elderly because of reduced clearance.[57,58]

Although peak respiratory effect is at 30 minutes, respiratory depression comparable with that produced by morphine may last as long as 4 hours. Shift in the ventilatory response curve to CO_2, increase in end tidal and pCO_2, decrease in pO_2, and depression of hypoxic ventilatory drive occur. These effects occur with narcotic doses too small to alter consciousness. They are heightened during sleep or when external stimuli are reduced, and may be seen in the PACU and even beyond. The effects are greater with fentanyl than alfentanil, which is more titratable, or sufentanil, which has greater opioid receptor affinity. When fentanyl is combined with benzodiazepines, the incidence and degree of hypoxemia, hypercarbia, and apnea increases. Effects may be delayed or persistent due to reabsorption of drug from the gastrointestinal tract or from peripheral sites.

Fentanyl produces vagally mediated bradycardia, emesis, and chest wall rigidity. The rigidity may be blunted by pretreatment with a small dose of muscle relaxant. The nausea and vomiting may be treated with various antiemetics such as droperidol, metoclopramide, or ondansetron. Fentanyl is not associated with histamine release. Based on psychomotor tests, Korttila found that patients who had received 100 µg of fentanyl were ready for discharge in 1 to 2 hours, but psychomotor impairment of driving skills lasted for at least 2 hours. After receiving 200 µg, they were discharge ready in 2 hours, but impaired for up to 8 hours.[59]

Alfentanil

Alfentanil is the most short-acting narcotic currently available. It is one fifth as potent, and its duration one third that of fentanyl. While sedation and euphoria may be more profound, respiratory depression is briefer. In unionized form at physiological pH, alfentanil has a rapid onset and redistribution. Its low lipid solubility, high protein binding and small volume of distribution make it available for rapid elimination, within 1 to 2 hours. It is cumulative only after prolonged administration or large doses. Clearance is decreased in the obese, in the elderly, in patients with liver disease, and in the presence of erythromycin.[47,57,58]

Following a bolus or infusion loading dose of 5 to 10 µg/kg, onset is within 1 to 2 minutes, and duration is 20 minutes. The drug is conveniently administered via syringe pump, and titrated to effect as are volatile anesthetics. Major variability in patient response is attributed to differences in distribution and clearance. For ease of bolus administration, the dose of drug may be diluted according to the following formula (Paul H. Hertz, M.D., personal communication):

1. ml of alfentanil = 0.1 × patient weight (kg)
2. Dilute to a final volume of 10 ml for a final concentration of 5 µg/kg/ml.

For a 70 kg patient, 7 ml of alfentanil would be drawn into a 10 ml syringe and diluted to 10 ml with intravenous fluid.

Scamman compared fentanyl 1.3 to 3 µg/kg with alfentanil 7.5 to 15 µg/kg for sedation for otolaryngological procedures. Respiratory depression was more prolonged with fentanyl (30 to 80 minutes) than with alfentanil (10 to 40 minutes). The fentanyl-to-alfentanil respiratory depression ratio was 13:1 based on CO_2 response curves. In these doses, memory was not specifically impaired, but there was decreased alertness and attention.[60] White compared fentanyl and alfentanil by bolus and infusion technique for general anesthesia. He found that patients who had received alfentanil were more awake, oriented, and ambulatory. The incidence of respiratory depression was 20% to 52% for patients who had received fentanyl, and 4% to 12% for those who had received alfentanil.[61] Alfentanil produces vagally mediated bradycardia and, occasionally, hypotension. Side effects include rigidity involving the chest and larynx, and nausea and vomiting. Delayed respiratory depression has been reported following alfentanil administration in general anesthesia. Krane speculated that this might be explained by a large dose, increased plasma level, increased potency, patient variability in pharmacokinetics, gastric trapping, or interactions with other drugs.[62]

Sufentanil

Sufentanil, a thiamyl analog of fentanyl, is the most potent opioid currently in use. It is approximately 5 to 10 times more potent than fentanyl, and has a more rapid onset and a slightly shorter elimination half life. Compared with fentanyl, it is more fat soluble and more highly protein bound, and it has a smaller volume of distribution. Initial dose for sedation is 0.1 to 0.5 µg/kg. Its respiratory depressant effect is considered less than that of fentanyl, and it has increased analgesic and amnesic properties. Other than bradycardia, cardiovascular side effects are minimal. Sufentanil is effective in blunting cardiovascular effects such as hypertension and tachycardia due to noxious stimuli.

Although its rapid onset and slightly shorter elimination half life (compared with those of fentanyl) might suggest desirability for use in ambulatory surgery, sufentanil has not attained popularity, because of cost and the frequent occurrence of chest wall rigidity. Its potency presents a potential danger and mandates dilution if used for sedation techniques. Fentanyl and alfentanil are safer and more convenient for this purpose.

Narcotic Agonist/Antagonists

Butorphanol and nalbuphine

Butorphanol and nalbuphine are agonist/antagonist drugs with κ (kappa) receptor agonism and μ (mu) receptor antagonism. Compared with that seen with other narcotics, respiratory depression is minimal and is limited by a ceiling effect. Additional advantages are a lower incidence of nausea and vomiting and nondependence. However, these drugs lack the efficacy of pure agonists. They can antagonize respiratory depressant effects of opioids while maintaining analgesia. Butorphanol is five times as potent as morphine, with similar prolonged duration of action, and less dysphoria. Onset occurs within 2 minutes, but duration may be 3 to 4 hours. Elimination half life is 2.5 to 3.5 hours. Butorphanol may increase blood pressure, pulmonary artery pressure, and cardiac output, and may cause nausea and diaphoresis. After a dose of 20 μg/kg given before induction of general anesthesia, recovery time was no different than that following fentanyl 2 μg/kg. When the dose was increased to 40 μg/kg patients experienced nausea and dizziness, and recovery time was prolonged.[63] Limited data is available for use in conscious sedation and is addressed below.

Nalbuphine potency is equal to that of morphine. Sedative doses do not prevent movement with pain. The drug also has a ceiling effect on respiratory depression and has no direct cardiac effects. In a comparison of nalbuphine 300 to 500 μg/kg versus fentanyl 1.5 μg/kg administered before induction of general anesthesia, nalbuphine recovery time was increased because of disorientation, sedation, and anxiety. Bad dreams were experienced by 20% to 30% of patients.[64] When fentanyl 3 μg/kg, butorphanol 60 μg/kg, and nalbuphine 300 μg/kg were compared for balanced anesthesia, fentanyl had the shortest awakening period, and no patients required admission. One patient who had received nalbuphine was admitted. Three patients who had received butorphanol were admitted because of drowsiness. Nausea and vomiting were comparable for all groups.[65]

Although potentially useful for sedation techniques because of their limited respiratory depressant effects, narcotic agonist/antagonist drugs have a prolonged duration of action comparable with that of morphine, and persistence of drowsiness or dizziness, which make them undesirable for ambulatory surgery. Few studies have documented their inclusion in sedation techniques.

Recommended analgesic doses are 1 to 3 mg of butorphanol or 5 to 15 mg of nalbuphine.[9] One study compared sedation with fentanyl (71 µg) and diazepam (4.7 mg) versus nalbuphine (7.3 mg) and methohexital (36 mg) for cataract patients at the time of insertion of retrobulbar block. Of patients who had received nalbuphine and methohexital, 81% were drowsy or unarousable.[66] Another study compared the intravenous use of butorphanol 1 mg or meperidine 50 mg with diazepam 12 to 15 mg for dental extraction. Patients who received butorphanol were better sedated, relaxed, and amnesic; however, they were also more sleepy at time of discharge.[67]

Inhalational Agents

Nitrous oxide

Nitrous oxide was first used for sedation in dentistry. Its rapid uptake and elimination; analgesic effect; absence of cardiovascular and respiratory depression; and sweet, nonpungent odor are desirable characteristics. For sedation, it is usually administered in concentrations of 30% to 50%. Concentrations greater than 30% may produce excitement, nausea, and dizziness.[68] Operating room pollution is a concern. In order for the administered concentration to reach the expired concentration, a tight-fitting, nonrebreathing mask is necessary. The end tidal concentration reaches only 30% of the inspired concentration when a clear rebreathing mask is used. A clear mask allows visualization of secretions or vomitus. Psychomotor impairment is brief. The resultant analgesia is related to patient expectation of pain. Suppression of airway reflexes and aspiration risk are of concern, especially at higher concentrations and in combination with sedative drugs. Nitrous oxide 30% impaired word recall, arithmetic ability, coordination, and driving skills after 1 minute, and this persisted for up to 30 minutes.[69] Nitrous oxide has been implicated in a higher incidence of nausea and vomiting, at least with general anesthesia. The AAP has established guidelines for nitrous oxide sedation, recommending its use only for ASA 1 or 2 patients, in concentrations less than 50%, with oxygen, and without other sedative or narcotic medications. Verbal communication must be maintained throughout, and pulse oximetry is strongly advised.[14]

Potent inhalational agents

Potent inhalational agents have been used in subanesthetic concentrations for sedation.[32,45,68] These agents are delivered by mask or by insufflation, and are characterized by rapid uptake via ventilation and rapid reversibility. Their major use has been for minor surgery on closed space infections. As potent agents, they have the potential for respiratory and cardiovascular depression, coughing, aspiration, and operating room pollution. Halothane is the least irritating of these agents and has bronchodilating properties, but it may induce arrhythmias by sensitizing the myocardium to catecholamines, especially during dental procedures involving local anesthetic with epinephrine. Enflurane is analgesic, amnesic, relatively potent, and insoluble, and promotes rapid recovery. The recommended enflurane concentration for sedation is 0.5%. At 0.2% (approximately 0.1 MAC), enflurane impaired digit memory, reaction time, and manual dexterity. At 0.5% (0.24 MAC), patients were too drowsy for testing and 10% were amnesic.[70] Isoflurane is a pungent agent that can produce headache, dizziness, and respiratory irritation. Rodrigo determined that isoflurane 0.5% in oxygen is better than nitrous oxide/oxygen for conscious sedation for cases lasting up to 50 minutes. Some patients experienced headache or dizziness. Discharge criteria were met in 10 minutes.[71] Desflurane is the least soluble inhalational agent, and is associated with the most rapid uptake and elimination, and negligible metabolism and toxicity. It is also the least potent (MAC 5% to 6%). It is pungent and has produced airway difficulty in pediatric patients. Thus, it is unlikely to be favored for sedation techniques. It tends to stimulate the sympathetic nervous system especially at higher concentrations, which helps maintain blood pressure, heart rate, and cardiac output. Sevoflurane, a promising agent soon to be available for general use in the United States, is reported to provide rapid induction and emergence. When used for general anesthesia, it can result in cardiovascular and respiratory depression. It is nonpungent and may prove more acceptable for sedation purposes than the inhalational agents now used.

Bolus Sedation Techniques

Tranquilizers, opioids, sedative hypnotics, and inhalational agents may be used in various combinations to enhance sedation, amnesia, and analgesia (Table 9-6). Shane was the first to describe a technique of intravenous amnesia that included opioid, anticholinergic, ataractic, and barbiturate in small doses.[71B] Scamman accomplished baseline sedation with benzodiazepine to an endpoint of half-lid or Verril's sign (lid droop), horizontal nystagmus,

Table 9-6   Intravenous Bolus Sedation Techniques

Procedure	Drug
Dental[10B]	Alphaprodine 30 mg, atropine 0.6 mg, hydroxyzine 50 mg, methohexital 30-60 mg
Dental/ENT[13]	Diazepam 10-20 mg, fentanyl 50 µg increments, scopolamine 0.25 mg
Oral surgery[75]	Midazolam 0.12 mg/kg, fentanyl 100 µg
Neuroradiology[72]	Midazolam 2.5-20 mg, fentanyl 50-300 µg *or* Propofol 100-450 mg, fentanyl 50-125 µg
Endoscopy[73]	Diazepam 10 mg, meperidine 50-75 mg
Endoscopy[74]	Midazolam 0.05 mg/kg, alfentanil 5µg/kg
Multiple ambulatory surgery procedures[4]	Midazolam 2-3 mg alfentanil 250-500 µg *or* Fentanyl 50-100 µg, methohexital 20-30 mg *or* Propofol 10-20 mg

or slurred speech; fentanyl was then titrated to an endpoint of sedation with responsiveness, analgesia, or a respiratory rate of 12 breaths per minute. Following the procedure, the patient was able to move to the bed, with complete recovery in 30 minutes. An escort was required and the patient was cautioned not to drive or operate machinery.[13] Allan compared fentanyl and midazolam with fentanyl and propofol titrated to suitable sedation endpoint for neuroradiologic procedures. Mean doses required were fentanyl 91 µg (50 to 300 µg)/midazolam 6.8 mg (2.5 to 20 mg), versus fentanyl 64 µg (50 to 125 µg)/propofol 232 mg (100 to 450 mg). There was little difference in outcome. Hypoxia occurred with both techniques, and the pulse oximeter and supplemental oxygen were useful. CO_2 was slightly elevated (50 torr) and patients were easily arousable.[72] Boldy reported on sedation for endoscopy, comparing diazepam 10 mg alone and diazepam 10 mg plus meperidine 50 to 75 mg. The combination improved sedation and patient cooperation, and reduced retching. There was no difference between the groups in recovery performance tests.[73]

Kallar[4] has described the technique used at Medical College of Virginia for a variety of outpatient surgical procedures on thousands of patients. A 2 to 3 mg dose of midazolam is administered, followed by 250 to 500 µg of alfentanil or 50 to 100 µg of fentanyl, with 20 to 30 mg methohexital or 10 to 20 mg propofol given at the time of local anesthesia or block—to an endpoint of divergent pupils or nystagmus. Additional increments of fentanyl 25 to 50 µg, alfentanil 250 µg, or methohexital 10 to 20 mg are given as needed. With this subanesthetic technique, the patient is still able to obey commands, but does not respond to surroundings.

Combinations of drugs exert synergistic effects, which allows for lower doses of each drug—and thus more rapid recovery. In a study of sedation for outpatient endoscopy, the addition of alfentanil 5 µg/kg to basal midazolam 0.05 mg/kg improved intraoperative conditions and clinical and psychomotor recovery over that seen with midazolam alone. No patient experienced desaturation.[74] Ochs showed that by combining fentanyl 100 µg with midazolam for oral surgery sedation, midazolam dose was reduced from 0.17 mg/kg to 0.12 mg/kg.[75] It is important to titrate combinations carefully in order to prevent airway obstruction, loss of consciousness, and reflex suppression. Vinik showed synergistic interaction of midazolam and alfentanil. Required doses were 21% and 33%, respectively, of the required doses when the drugs were used individually.[36]

Reversal of Sedation

Flumazenil

Flumazenil is a recently introduced specific benzodiazepine antagonist that reverses the central effects of benzodiazepines by competitively inhibiting the GABA receptor. Flumazenil is not an effective antagonist of central nervous system depressants other than benzodiazepines. It possesses no agonist activity and has infrequent side effects such as nausea, anxiety, tremor, and, rarely, seizure, which is associated with withdrawal from chronic benzodiazepine use. Onset after intravenous administration is within 1 minute, and the drug should be titrated in increments of 0.2 mg to a maximum dose of 1 mg.[76] Flumazenil confers increased safety for benzodiazepine use and ensures a more rapid recovery; however, it should not be routinely used for ambulatory surgery patients since reversal of sedation is often incomplete and may be brief. Following the usual doses of flumazenil, sedation and hypnosis are reversed while amnesia and anxiolysis are retained. Some depressant effects of benzodiazepines (e.g., depression of ventilatory response to CO_2 and to hypoxia) may not be completely reversed. This may be particularly true when benzodiazepines have been combined with narcotics.

In studies involving patients undergoing gastrointestinal endoscopy, intravenous administration of 0.4 to 1.0 mg of flumazenil 30 minutes after diazepam or midazolam improved memory, psychomotor performance, and patient perception of alertness; however, at 3.5 hours, there was no difference in these parameters compared with those in patients who had not been reversed.[77] Kestin studied patients who had received spinal anesthesia and were sedated with midazolam, 0.075 mg/kg, midazolam plus flumazenil, and propofol. Psychomotor and cognitive tests were impaired for all groups at 2 hours. Recovery was best in the propofol group. In the group that received flumazenil, after initial but incomplete improvement, performance declined after 1 hour.[78] Since the elimination half life of flumazenil is only 1 hour, while that of midazolam is 2 to 3 hours, and significantly longer, there is potential for resedation. Therefore, premature discharge of ambulatory patients should be avoided, an escort should be present, and driving should be prohibited.[79]

Naloxone

Naloxone is an antagonist used to treat opioid-induced respiratory depression. It is given intravenously in doses of 0.1 to 0.4 mg and should be cautiously titrated. It has a duration of 30 to 45 minutes when given intravenously. Since elimination half time is approximately 60 minutes, renarcotization can occur. Intramuscular administration at twice the intravenous dose, and administration by infusion, produce sustained effect. Reversal of narcosis may cause nausea and vomiting; cardiovascular and sympathetic nervous system stimulation; and pain resulting in tachycardia, hypertension, pulmonary edema, or arrhythmia. When included in sedation techniques for outpatients, narcotics should be carefully titrated to effect, obviating the need for routine reversal. Since the narcotic effect may extend beyond that of naloxone, the patient requires an adequate period of observation and should be discharged in the company of a responsible adult.

Infusion Techniques

Objectives

Infusion techniques have gained in popularity and practice for administration of various sedative-hynotic, narcotic, and tranquilizer drugs, individually or in combination, for general anesthesia as well as for sedation techniques (Table 9-4). Infusion offers an advantage over bolus techniques because a steady state is better achieved, peaks and valleys of anesthetic levels are minimized, and the total amount of drug required to produce anesthesia or sedation is reduced, thereby decreasing recovery time, need for reversal or supplementation, and side effects (Fig. 9-2). Because surgical stress is variable and completion of surgery may be unexpected or early, this mode of delivery is optimal. Less total drug is given because an infusion maintains plasma concentration over time more efficiently than a bolus dose, while hemodynamic stability is maintained.[80,81] The objective is to titrate and maintain the plasma concentration just above the therapeutic threshold, thereby avoiding excess, and allowing the concentration to fall quickly below the threshold at the end of the case. This mode of delivery of intravenous anesthetics is analogous to the delivery of inhalational anesthetics via vaporizer.

Pharmacologic Principles

Administration of drugs according to this scheme requires knowledge of drug pharmacokinetics and pharmacodynamics (Table 9-5). *Pharmacokinetics* relates a drug's movement from the site of administration to the sites of distribution and elimination: what the body does to the drug. *Pharmacodynamics* relates drug concentration to clinical effect: what the drug does to the body. A drug is introduced into the central compartment and then is distributed throughout the total volume of distribution. The central nervous system concentration (representing the primary site of sedative drug effect) will decline over time because of continued distribution and clearance, and this will lead to recovery unless multiple injections or infusions are provided.[81-83]

To achieve a steady state, the plasma level of drug requires 4 to 5 elimination half lives when it is started as a constant rate

A

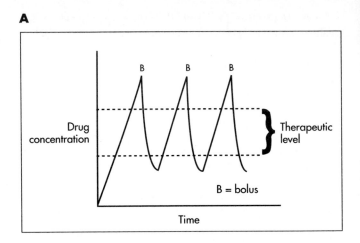

B

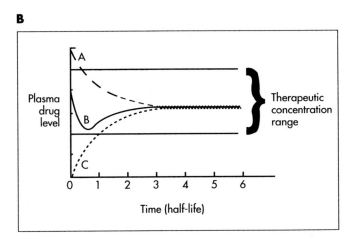

Fig. 9-2 A, Intermittent bolus injections of a drug to maintain anesthesia can lead to excessive levels immediately after the bolus is administered (peaks) and inadequate levels during the interval between bolus injections (valleys). **B,** Simulated drug level curves when a continuing infusion is administered following a "full" loading dose (*A*), a smaller loading dose (*B*), or in the absence of a loading dose (*C*). (Adapted from Pace NA, Victory RA, White PA: Anesthetic infusion techniques—how to do it. J Clin Anesth 1992; 4[Suppl 1]: 45S-52S.)

infusion. Therefore, to reach an effective plasma level quickly, a loading dose (LD) of drug (in μg/kg) is first given via a bolus or priming infusion.[81-83]

$$LD = C_p \times V_d$$

where C_p is the desired plasma concentration in μg/ml, and V_d the volume of distribution in ml/kg. The loading dose is followed by a minimum infusion rate (MIR):

$$MIR = C_p \times Cl$$

where MIR is in μg/kg/min, and Cl is the clearance rate of the drug in ml/kg/min. The plasma concentration (C_p) is determined by the desired pharmacologic effect (analgesia, sedation, hypnosis), the combination of drugs being administered, the nature of the surgery, and individual sensitivity. To reach an effective plasma concentration, the LD should not be too large, too small, or given too rapidly. The smaller the LD, the greater MIR required. The inflow (rate of the infusion) must equal the outflow (redistribution and elimination) to maintain a steady drug level in the blood. Over time the redistribution sites become saturated, the rate of elimination becomes increasingly important, and MIR can be decreased.[81-83] Continuous infusion does not mean constant infusion. In practice, the infusion dosage is varied according to the degree of stimulation and response of the patient (vital signs, movement). If the patient responds to intraoperative stimuli, a small bolus dose and/or increase in rate of infusion are undertaken to increase the plasma level. If the patient does not respond to intraoperative stimuli, the infusion rate is progressively decreased to reach a minimal effective dose.

Although it is useful for the one-compartment model, the concept of half life does not aid in determination of appropriate dosing or plasma drug concentrations for the multicompartment pharmacokinetic/pharmacodynamic model. The relative importance of distribution and elimination at a point in time depends on the degree of equilibration of the drug concentrations in the central and peripheral compartments, and this in turn depends on the dosing regimen, particularly its duration. To predict the rate at which the plasma drug concentration will decrease after terminating infusion, it is preferable to consider the *context-sensitive half time,* which is the time required for the central compartment drug concentration to decrease to 50% (half time) of the desired plasma concentration (C_{pd}) at the point of termination of an infusion regimen designed to maintain a constant plasma concentration *for a specific period of time* (context). This provides an upper limit of the time required for the plasma drug concentration to fall below the threshold for recovery.[84,86] The infusion is terminated before the end of the case as determined by context sensitive half time.[84,85]

Drug concentration in a peripheral compartment with a large clearance and small volume will equilibrate with the central compartment much more rapidly than drug concentration in a peripheral compartment with low clearance and large volume. The former compartment will be a primary determinant of the context-sensitive half time following a brief infusion. A small volume-to-clearance ratio (leading to rapid elimination from the central compartment) or a small clearance ratio (indicating sluggish return of drug from a peripheral compartment) will reduce the plasma drug concentration and shorten the context-sensitive half time, even after long infusions.[86] This explains why using β-elimination half lives results in inaccurate determinations of recovery from intravenous anesthetic infusion.

Administration Devices

Infusions can be administered simply via Buretrol, more efficiently via volumetric or syringe pumps, and very precisely via computer-controlled volumetric pumps (Table 9-7).[87-89] For ambulatory surgery practice, the syringe pump is most practical and convenient. With the syringe pump, a drug can be administered in concentrated form, and the syringe is calibrated for accurate dosing. The pumps are user-friendly and portable, and they mount on an IV pole in the operating room. Many manufacturers have developed syringe pumps, each with particular advantages, disadvantages, and varying capabilities (Figs. 9-3 and 9-4).[87-89] The pumps vary in maximum bolus delivery rate. They can be calibrated to the optimal delivery rate for the particular medication. Rates may be in ml/hr, µg/kg/min, µg/kg/hr, mg/kg/min, or mg/kg/hr. Some pumps can only accommodate a large (60 cc) syringe, while others can accept syringes of many sizes. Air must be evacuated from the syringe. The syringe flange is inserted into a groove on the pump, and the barrel of the syringe is clasped mechanically. Incorrect syringe size or improper insertion can result in error in volume and rate of infusion. The pump should have a built-in gravity free flow protection mechanism to prevent inadvertent bolusing.

Programming may be simplified (preprogrammed) at an optimal delivery rate for a specific drug or require more complex

Table 9-7   Comparison of Techniques Available for
Administration of Intravenous Anesthetic Agents

	Syringe	Buretrol	Volumetric pump	Syringe pump	CACI*
Bolus	+			+	
Infusion		+	+	+	+
Inexpensive	+	+			
Flexible dosing	+	+	+	+	+
Established dosing methods	+	+	+	+	?
Conceptual appeal					+
Convenient instrumentation	+	+	+	+	?
User friendly	+	+	+	+	+
Data provided by device					
Cumulative dose (ml)				+	+
Cumulative dose (mg)				+	+
Cumulative volume (ml)	+	+	+	+	+
Infusion rate			+	+	+
Theoretical plasma level					+
Predictive capability					+
Availability	+	+	+	+	
Accuracy	+	+	+	+	?

*CACI = Computer assisted continuous infusion.
Modified from Reves JG: Automated drug infusion systems in anesthesia. In American Society of Anesthesiologists: Annual refresher courses lectures, Philadelphia, 1990, JB Lippincott, p. 233.

program entry. Bolus and infusion rate are set according to patient weight. The pump must be fully programmed to function. It is always wise to double-check the settings. Some "smart" pumps will sound an alarm or will fail to function if settings are in error. The infusion is begun in the *run* mode. If the pump is to be temporarily stopped or a dosing adjustment made, the pump should be set in the *standby* mode. Once the pump is permanently stopped by turning the power off, the infusion data recorded by the pump and the programming are lost. Pump alarms include

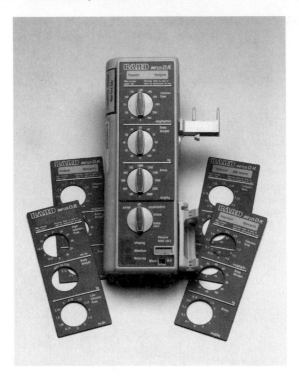

Fig. 9-3 Bard infusOR syringe pump with magnetic labels.

syringe empty, air, low battery, and occlusion—all of which will stop the pump automatically. Other alarms notify regarding incorrect programming or pump malfunction (system error). Alarms can be temporarily bypassed in most pumps. Some pumps have rechargeable batteries lasting 6 to 25 hours depending on infusion rate, some have dry cell batteries. Those with rechargeable batteries may be charged via the power cord while in use. In the future, small, computerized, multichannel, context- sensitive automatic infusion devices for the operating room are expected to be marketed. These improved delivery systems will confer increased control.

Computer Assisted Continuous Infusion

Computer assisted continuous infusion (CACI) is a pharmacokinetic model–driven infusion of intravenous anesthetic drugs based

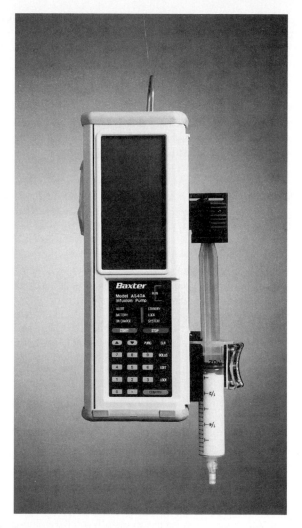

Fig. 9-4 Baxter model AS40A programmable syringe infusion pump.

on mathematically predicted theoretical therapeutic plasma drug concentration.[80,82,87-89] This is in contrast to the present mode of administration based on drug dosage or closed loop control (by measurement). Drug concentration at the effector site determines drug action, not the dose or rate of administration. The infusion is based on a *BET* dosing scheme for drugs exhibiting two compartment kinetics, where *B* represents the bolus to fill the central compartment. This is followed by a constant rate continuous infusion to replace drug lost by elimination (*E*), and transfer (*T*), from the central to the peripheral compartment. Computer assisted continuous infusion requires limited programming; the drug to be infused, patient weight or age, and desired plasma concentration must be entered. Known plasma concentrations for intravenous sedatives are provided in Table 9-4 and plasma levels appropriate to various levels of stimulation in Table 9-8.

As with measurement of concentrations of inhalational agents via gas analyzers, the theoretical plasma concentration is calculated by the pump every 10 to 15 seconds, and the rate is adjusted to maintain the desired concentration. Due to pharmacokinetic and pharmacodynamic variability, predicted drug levels are only an approximation of the actual concentration, (accuracy ± 30%). Therefore, vigilance is necessary and adjustments are required to titrate to clinical effect. Prediction errors occur as a result of patient disease, age, gender, and administration of other drugs that alter pharmacokinetics. By assessing cumulative dosage and predicting decay rate for the plasma level of a drug based on the context-sensitive half time (the time for 50% decrease in plasma concentration of drug), the pump can also determine when an infusion should be discontinued. One problem with infusion systems is determining the endpoint or depth of anesthesia. In the future, establishment of the C_p50, plasma concentration to suppress movement to surgical stimulus in 50% of patients for intravenous drugs, analogous to MAC for inhalational agents, may be useful.

Sedation Infusion Techniques

Infusion techniques have been successfully used for individual drugs or combinations, and for various surgical procedures (Table 9-9). The infusion rates are intended for adults in the normal weight range (60 to 80 kg). The infusion rates should be increased for larger patients and decreased for smaller patients. It is important to check repeatedly that the infusion is running.

Table 9-8 Plasma Drug Concentration Ranges for Various Surgical Stimuli

Drug	Skin incision	Major surgery	Minor surgery	Spontaneous ventilation	Awakening	Sedation or analgesia
Alfentanil (ng/ml)	200-300	250-450	100-300	<200	–	25-75
Fentanyl (ng/ml)	3-6	4-8	2-5	<2	–	1-2
Sufentanil (ng/ml)	0.3-1.5	0.5-2	0.3-1.5	<0.2	–	0.02-0.2
Propofol (μg/ml)	3-5	4-7	3-5	–	1-3	1.0-2.0
Methohexital (mg/ml)	5-10	5-15	5-10	–	1-3	1-3
Thiopental (μg/ml)	7.5-12.5	10-20	10-20	–	4-8	4-8
Etomidate (ng/ml)	400-600	500-1000	300-600	–	200-350	100-300
Midazolam (mg/ml)	–	50-250 (when combined with an opiate)	50-250 (when combined with an opiate)		150-200 (reduced to 20-70 in presence of an opiate)	40-100
Ketamine (μg/ml)	–	–	1-2	–	–	0.1-1

The drug concentrations for skin incision minor and major surgery are combined with 65% to 70% N_2O unless otherwise stated. Effective plasma concentrations may differ markedly depending on premedication and intraoperative drug combinations.

Adapted from Glass PSA, Shafer SL, Jacobs JR, Reves JG: Drug anesthetic delivery system. In Miller R, editor: Anesthesia, ed 4, New York, 1994, Churchill Livingstone, pp. 389-416.

Table 9-9 Intravenous Infusion Sedation Techniques

Procedure	Drug	Bolus	Infusion
Multiple procedures with local/regional anesthesia[15]	Midazolam	3-6 mg	3-14 mg/hr
	Propofol	45-95 mg	80-450 mg/hr
Multiple procedures with local/regional anesthesia[91]	Methohexital	30-90 mg	115-245 mg/hr
	Etomidate	4.5-21 mg	20-44 mg/hr
	Midazolam	2-5 mg	3-12 mg/hr
Ovum retrieval[92]	Mixture of 50 ml propofol (10 mg/ml) plus 4 ml alfentanil (500 μg/ml)	–	2 ml/kg/hr, then 1 ml/kg/hr
Knee arthroscopy[93]	Alfentanil	8 μg/kg	0.75 μg/kg/min
			or
	Propofol	1 mg/kg	50 μg/kg/min
Extracorporeal shock wave lithotripsy[94]	Midazolam	0.05 mg/kg	
	Alfentanil	10 μg/kg	1 μg/kg/min
	or		
	Fentanyl	1.5 μg/kg	
	Propofol	0.5 mg/kg	50 μg/kg/min
Extracorporeal shock wave lithotripsy[55]	Midazolam	4-9 mg	
	Alfentanil	10 μg/kg	0.5-2 μg/kg/min
	or		
	Midazolam	4-14 mg	
	Ketamine	0.4 mg/kg	25-50 μg/kg/min

Continuous infusions are prone to equipment problems, such as leaving the clamps on the line, running out of a drug, placing excessive back pressure in the line, etc. If the infusion stops for more than a few minutes, the patient will awaken during the operation. White and Negus[15] compared infusions of midazolam or propofol during local/regional anesthesia. Midazolam 4.2 ± 1.4 mg or propofol 69 ± 23 mg loading doses were followed by variable rate infusion of midazolam 8.6 ± 5.4 mg/hr or propofol 265 ± 185 mg/hr. Overall quality of intraoperative sedation was similar. With midazolam, pain was less and amnesia greater. With propofol, there was less postoperative sedation, drowsiness, confusion, and amnesia, and more rapid cognitive recovery. Sedation returned to baseline at 30 minutes after propofol and 90 minutes after midazolam. Immediate but not intermediate recovery was more rapid with propofol, and discharge times were similar. Recovery after midazolam sedation was also longer than after methohexital or etomidate. White also described a midazolam/ketamine technique for plastic surgery. Midazolam 0.05 to 0.15 mg/kg was given over 5 minutes, and followed by ketamine 0.5 mg/kg. No patient experienced cardiovascular or respiratory depression.[90]

Urquhart compared three agents for sedation during regional anesthesia. Loading doses were methohexital 59 ± 29 mg, etomidate 12 ± 8 mg, and midazolam 3.7 ± 1.5 mg over 5 to 15 minutes. Then a variable rate infusion was maintained with methohexital 180 ± 65 mg/hr, etomidate 32 ± 12 mg/hr, and midazolam 7.5 ± 4 mg/hr. While amnesia was superior, oxygen saturation of less than 95% was more frequent with midazolam. There was more intraoperative and postoperative sedation and decline in psychomotor test performance following midazolam. Within 10 minutes of discontinuation of infusion, all patients responded. At 30 minutes, 77% of patients were awake, regardless of technique. Discharge times were similar.[91] Sherry described an infusion technique supplementing paracervical block for oocyte retrieval that involved a mixture of 50 ml of propofol (10 mg/ml) and 4 ml alfentanil (500 μg/ml) in the same syringe to yield a final concentration of propofol 9.3 mg/ml and alfentanil 37 ug/ml. The infusion was run at 2 ml/kg/hr then decreased to 1 ml/kg/hr. The surgery lasted 1 hour. The mean maintenance propofol dose was 6.8 mg/kg/hr and alfentanil 27 μg/kg/hr. During the procedure, 60% of patients were rousable to command or mild physical stimulation.[92] Lee studied the combination of alfentanil and propofol in patients undergoing knee arthroscopy. Patients received 8 μg/kg of alfentanil, followed by 1 mg/kg of propofol. Local anesthesia was injected into the knee. Anesthesia was maintained with infusion rates of either propofol 50 μg/kg/min or alfentanil 0.75 μg/kg/min. Small boluses were given if needed, and the infusion rate was progressively decreased. The techniques were entirely comparable with respect to nausea, sedation, pain control, and ultimate discharge.[93]

Finally, Monk compared various infusion and other anesthetic techniques for extracorporal shock wave lithotripsy (ESWL). Midazolam/alfentanil, fentanyl/propofol, and epidural block were compared. Midazolam/alfentanil provided better amnesia (81%) than with fentanyl/propofol (38%), but a greater incidence of transient oxygen desaturation. Fentanyl/propofol was associated with greater intraoperative cardiovascular depression but fewer postoperative side effects. Compared to epidural anesthesia, intravenous anesthesia was associated with shorter preparation times, better mobility of patients to facilitate positioning, no need for postoperative catheterization, shorter recovery times, and no unanticipated admissions.[94] In another study, midazolam/alfentanil infusion was compared with midazolam/ketamine. Ketamine was associated with more cardiorespiratory stability, but it caused increased spontaneous movement that interfered with success of fragmentation, and a high incidence of dreaming and postoperative confusion (31%). With alfentanil, the incidence of desaturation and pruritis were greater, but discharge times were decreased.[55]

In conclusion, infusion techniques are superior to bolus techniques and are facilitated with a "smart" pump. In the future, improved devices and dosing strategies, guidelines for maintenance of the appropriate balance between analgesic and sedative components, and definition of clinical situations in which these techniques can be used to greatest benefit will represent a major advance in sedation practices for ambulatory surgery patients.

Pediatric Sedation Techniques

One of the most challenging situations in the practice of pediatric anesthesia is the provision of conscious sedation. For sedation to be successful, the patient must have a degree of intellectual development so that he or she can understand what is happening and cooperate. The age at which this occurs is unpredictable. Fortunately, several regimens have been devised to safely provide sedation in children. Over the last few years, there has been a significant increase in outpatient diagnostic radiologic studies and minor surgical procedures in pediatric patients. These at times occur in the operating room, but often they may be performed outside the operating room, and are addressed in more detail in Chapter 10. The radiologist needs the patient to lie still for computerized tomography (CT) scans and magnetic resonance imaging (MRI) scans. The gastroenterologist and pulmonologist must have a cooperative and comfortable patient to perform an endoscopy. Finally, the cancer patient at times must undergo repetitive and painful procedures. Consequently, children need some form of distraction, analgesia, or sedation to make these procedures humane and feasible. Over the years, institutions have developed individual guidelines and parameters to assure patient safety. Issues on who should be administering the sedation and what are the best sedation techniques remain controversial.

Recognizing the need for some general directives, the AAP Committee on Drugs recently revised guidelines for monitoring and managing pediatric patients during and after sedation for diagnostic and therapeutic procedures.[14] The goals of sedation in the pediatric patient are shown in Box 9-2.

This section will deal with five basic factors to attain these AAP goals: personnel involved with the sedation, patient preparation, monitoring, drugs, and discharge criteria.

Personnel

Obviously it would be ideal to have anesthesia care providers in charge of administering sedation to children. Unfortunately, this is often not possible because of several reasons, including cost and availability of personnel. So it is important for physicians who are not anesthesiologists, but who are involved in administering sedation, to understand the pharmacology of the medications they are using and to be well acquainted with airway management in children. At least one member of the health care team trained in airway management must be present; this person is responsible for observing and monitoring the patient at all times. Airway monitoring might be the most important factor in assuring the safety of the patient.

> Box 9-6 *Clinical Conditions of Importance in the Preparation of Pediatric Patients for Sedation*
>
> ---
>
> Congenital heart disease (smaller cardiopulmonary reserve)
> Esophageal reflux (unprotected airway)
> Reactive airway disease (sedative medications or contrast media may cause bronchospasm)
> Neurologic disease with increased intracranial pressure (sedative regimens could increase pCo_2 and thus increase ICP)
> Abnormal airway

Patient Preparation

A thorough history and physical examination is warranted, regardless of the location in which the procedure is held. Particular attention should be directed to patients with congenital heart disease, esophageal reflux, neurologic disease (increased intracranial pressure), lung disease (especially reactive airway disease) and patients with abnormal airways (e.g., Pierre Robin or Treacher Collins syndromes).[95] Box 9-6 lists these conditions, which should be as well controlled as possible. Routine fasting guidelines should be applied. Recent evidence suggests that clear fluids given up to 3 hours before surgery does not place the patient at an increased risk of aspiration pneumonitis.[96]

Monitoring

The ideal monitoring conditions have been recommended by the AAP (Box 9-7).[14] These, along with capnography, are readily available if sedation occurs in the operating room. Unfortunately, these conditions may not exist outside the operating room, and it is unlikely that nonanesthesiologists will insist on a fully monitored sedation patient. However, it is a fact that sedation may cause respiratory depression. Because of this potential, the most important monitors are the capnograph, to monitor end-tidal CO_2 and ventilation, and the pulse oximeter, to measure oxygen saturation. Since capnography can be difficult to measure in the awake, sedated patient, the pulse oximeter and an ECG are the two most important and vital monitors, and we feel that they should be

---

Box 9-7 *Suggested Monitoring for Sedation in Pediatric Patients*

Positive pressure oxygen delivery system capable of administering at least 90% O_2
Functional suction
Blood pressure monitoring
Pulse oximeter
Electrocardiogram
Defibrillator
End tidal CO_2

Adapted from American Academy of Pediatrics Committee on Drugs: Guidelines for monitoring and management of pediatric patients during and after sedation for diagnostic and therapeutic procedures. Pediatrics 1992; 89:1110-15.

placed on all pediatric patients undergoing sedation. Irrespective of which way the sedation is administered, all sedated or anesthetized patients should receive supplemental oxygen via mask, nasal cannula, or hose.

Drugs

Tables 9-10 to 9-12 describe the most commonly performed techniques.

Oral Premedication/Sedation

The oral route is one of the most popular routes because of children's fear of needles. A thorough and extensive description of premedication schemes has been made in Chapter 5. Many times, oral premedication is sufficient to safely separate children from parents and to enable them to lie still for very short and quick procedures. For small infants up to 12 months old, we prefer to use chloral hydrate in doses of 25 to 50 mg/kg.[97] Chloral hydrate is a safe drug to use, as long as very high doses are avoided; and it is still the most widely used drug by nonanesthesiologists,[98] although many infants remain asleep for 30 to 45 minutes. The onset of action is generally 30 to 60 minutes.

For older children (more than 1 year old), ketamine and midazolam are good and safe choices. Ketamine produces a dissociative sedation and has been shown to be a safe and

Table 9-10 Oral Sedation Techniques in Children

Drug	Usual dose
Chloral hydrate	25-50 mg/kg (for small infants up to 12 months)
	25-75 mg/kg (for children older than 12 months)
Ketamine	5-10 mg/kg (above 1 year)
Midazolam	0.5-1.0 mg/kg orally
	0.2-0.3 mg/kg intranasally
	(above 1 year)
Fentanyl (Oralet)	5-15 µg/kg transmucosally (for children weighing more than 15 kg)

Table 9-11 Intramuscular Sedation Techniques in Children

Drug	Usual dose
Ketamine	2-5 mg/kg
Midazolam	0.08 mg/kg
Pentobarbital	4-5 mg/kg
	(Injection can
DPT Cocktail	be painful)
Meperidine	2 mg/kg
Promethazine	1 mg/kg
Chlorpromazine	1 mg/kg

predictable drug at doses up to 10 mg/kg.[99] Midazolam is probably the most commonly used drug by anesthesiologists for oral premedication and sedation. In doses of 0.5 to 1.0 mg/kg, it rapidly produces a happy and relaxed child.[100] The onset of action is 15 to 30 minutes. It can also be used safely via the nasal route.[101,102] Finally, the use of oral transmucosal fentanyl (Oralet) has been found to produce adequate sedation at doses of 5 to 15 µg/kg, although its use can result in significant respiratory problems.[103]

It is important to recognize that these techniques may not be enough to provide the necessary sedation, but they will allow to separate the child from the parents. Then the clinician can proceed with an intramuscular, intravenous, or inhalation sedation technique as needed.

Table 9-12   Intravenous Sedation Techniques in Children

Drug	Usual dose
Pentobarbital	2.5 mg/kg; may repeat up to 7.5 mg/kg; watch for apnea
Methohexital	0.5 to 1.0 mg/kg; may repeat as needed; watch for apnea
Midazolam	0.08 mg/kg; may follow with infusion at 0.04 to 0.12 mg/kg/hr
Propofol	1 to 2 mg/kg; may follow with infusion at 4 to 8 mg/kg/hr
Ketamine	0.5 to 1.0 mg/kg; may repeat as needed
Fentanyl	0.5 to 2.0 µg/kg

Intramuscular Sedation

Although most children would rather not receive a needlestick, several techniques of intramuscular (IM) sedation can be very useful and predictable. This form of sedation is useful in children older than 1 year. The most popular drug via this route is ketamine, which is given in doses of 2 to 5 mg/kg.[104] Ketamine is especially useful in very uncooperative or retarded children. It lasts anywhere between 15 and 30 minutes, and has a very short onset time. Midazolam, because of its water solubility and good absorption, is ideal for IM administration[105] in a dose of 0.08 mg/kg. Pentobarbital, at doses of 4 to 5 mg/kg, can also be used, although the injection can be very painful for the child.[106]

An old technique for IM sedation involves the combination of meperidine (2 mg/kg), promethazine (1 mg/kg), and chlorpromazine (1 mg/kg), the so-called DPT cocktail.[107,108] It is still used today, although it has a significant potential for prolonged sedation and respiratory depression.

Intravenous Sedation

Barbiturates, benzodiazepines, propofol, ketamine, and narcotics are the most commonly used drugs for intravenous sedation in the child. This route can be used in children more than 1 year old. It is important to recognize that there is a fine line between sedation and induction of anesthesia with these drugs given intravenously; therefore, monitoring becomes a crucial factor. Pentobarbital is used at doses of 2.5 mg/kg for induction of sedation.[109] It may be supplemented by repeated boluses as needed, up to a total dose of 7.5 mg/kg. Methohexital can be used at doses of 0.5 to 1.0 mg/kg, followed by repeated boluses as needed.[110] Both of these medications should be given slowly, and the patient observed for the possibility of apnea. Midazolam can be given at doses of 0.08 mg/kg.[111] If needed, this injection can be followed by an infusion at a rate of 0.04 to 0.12 mg/kg/hr.

Propofol, one of the new agents, has become very popular for conscious and deep sedation in children.[112] It is used at doses of 1 to 2 mg/kg, followed by an infusion at 4 to 8 mg/kg/hr.

Ketamine, at doses of 0.5 to 1.0 mg/kg followed by repeated boluses as needed, has been shown over the years to be an excellent and predictable drug for intravenous sedation in children.[104]

Finally, fentanyl can be used alone or in combination with the other previously described drugs at doses of 0.5 to 2.0 µg/kg.[113]

These drugs can cause significant respiratory depression, and their usage warrants strict vigilance and monitoring of oxygenation and ventilation.[114] Nevertheless, with proper care and judicious use, these drugs are excellent choices for sedation.

Inhalation Sedation

The most commonly used inhalation agent for sedation in children is nitrous oxide. In our experience, nitrous oxide must be combined with other agents to be effective. It is used in concentrations of 40% to 70%.[115]

Box 9-8 Discharge Criteria After Pediatric Sedation

Conscious patient; responds appropriately
Stable vital signs; minimal nausea or vomiting
Respiratory status showing no significant change from preoperative status
Minimal pain and discomfort
Minimal or no bleeding
No impairment of circulation (e.g., after tourniquet)
No new postprocedure problems that may threaten a safe recovery
Responsible adult to take patient home from the ambulatory unit

Discharge Criteria

After the procedure, the patient should be taken to a recovery area. The child's condition should be as close as possible to baseline before he or she is discharged. Box 9-8 lists suggested recovery area discharge criteria, which are discussed in more detail in Chapters 10 and 12.

Summary

The development of new shorter-acting pharmacological agents has enabled anesthesiologists and medical practitioners both in and outside the operating room to utilize sedation for a wide variety of procedures. The goal of sedation is to provide a balance between patient comfort and safety, and prevention of cardiovascular and respiratory compromise and delay in recovery. Although the majority of the sedatives are administered intravenously, many can be administered orally, intramuscularly, transmucosally, or rectally. There is a dose-dependent potential for central nervous system depression and respiratory depression. The provider must have an understanding of the continuum from relaxation to unconsciousness. Sedation facilitates the acceptance of local and regional anesthesia by blunting sensations such as pressure, movement, traction, position change, and awareness of noise and activity in the operating room. Guidelines for monitoring and equipment needed for use during sedation have been developed by the ASA and by other specialty organizations. Patients receiving sedation should receive the same degree of preoperative and intraoperative vigilance as patients receiving general anesthesia. The existence of a continuum of sedation permits a light level of sedation, or a deeper plane resulting in unconsciousness and loss of protective airway reflexes. Therefore, it is important that the patient be monitored appropriately by qualified personnel. Oxygen must be available for positive pressure ventilation, and monitoring of respiratory function, heart rate, and blood pressure, and the use of pulse oximetry is basic to perioperative monitoring. An appropriate level of postsedation monitoring as well as criteria for discharge should be uniform throughout the facility.

Benzodiazepines, barbiturates, propofol, ketamine, etomidate, and narcotics may be administered by a bolus technique and by continuous infusion technique. The role of nitrous oxide and other inhalational agents, as well as the antagonists flumazenil and naloxone, are discussed. Familiarity with the pharmacokinetics and pharmacodynamics of various drugs allows the anesthesiologist to administer continuous infusion techniques that provide a steady state of sedation in which the difference between the peaks and valleys of anesthetic levels are minimized. Currently, computerized pumps are available that enable the clinician to administer continuous infusions with relative ease. These infusion devices are currently open-loop devices; the anesthesiologists serves to close the loop by inputing the patient's response and altering the infusion rate.

More procedures being conducted on pediatric patients outside the operating room demand high-quality sedation. The same degree of vigilance for perioperative care needs to be maintained. Children may be adequately sedated with premedicant drugs such as ketamine, midazolam, or oral transmucosal fentanyl, avoiding the painful intramuscular or intravenous routes. Doses and recommendations for pediatric sedation are discussed. Regardless of location, the success of sedation in ambulatory patients depends on proper preparation, knowledge of the pharmacology of the various intravenous and inhalational drugs, and adherence to uniform standards.

References

1. Apfelbaum JL, Kallar SK, Wetchler BV: Adult and geriatric patients. In Wetchler BV, editor: Anesthesia for ambulatory surgery, ed 2, Philadelphia, 1985, JB Lippincott, pp. 197-307.
2. White PF, Zelcer J: Monitored anesthesia care—use of adjuvant drugs. In International Anesthesia Research Society: Review course lectures, Baltimore, 1991, Williams & Wilkins, pp. 130-4.
3. Zelcer J, White PF: Monitored anesthesia care. In White PF, editor: Outpatient anesthesia, New York, 1990, Churchill Livingstone, pp. 243-62.
4. Kallar SK: Conscious sedation in ambulatory surgery. Anesth Rev 1990; 17(Suppl 2): 45-51.

5. Kallar SK: Conscious sedation in ambulatory surgery. Anesth Rev 1991; 18(Suppl 1): 9-12.

6. Philip BK: Local anesthesia and sedation techniques. In White PF, editor: Outpatient anesthesia, New York, 1990 Churchill Livingstone, pp. 263-91.

7. Gravenstein N, Paulus DA, Dawlick MF et al: Pulse oximetry monitoring during oral surgery outpatient procedures. Anesthesiology 1986; 65:A167.

8. Wetchler BV: Outpatient anesthesia. In Barash PB, Cullen BF, Stoelting RK, editors: Clinical anesthesia, ed 2, Philadelphia, 1992, JB Lippincott, pp. 1389-416.

9. Epstein BS, Wurm SB: Opioids for monitored anesthesia care. In Estafanous FG, editor: Opioids in anesthesia, Boston, 1991, Butterworth-Heinemann, pp. 179-207.

10A. McCleane GJ: The nature of pre-operative anxiety. Anaesthesia 1990; 45:153-5.

10B. Shane SM: Conscious sedation for ambulatory surgery, Baltimore, 1983, University Park Press, pp. 1-11.

11. Bennett CR: The spectrum of pain control. In Conscious sedation in dental practice, ed 2, St Louis, 1978, Mosby, pp. 10-23.

12. McCarthy FM, Soloman AL, Jastak JT et al: Conscious sedation: benefits and risks. J Am Dental Assoc 1984; 109:545-57.

13. Scamman FL, Klein SL, Chio WW: Conscious sedation for procedures under local or topical anesthesia. Ann Otol Rhinol Laryngol 1985; 94:21-4.

14. American Academy of Pediatrics Committee on Drugs: Guidelines for monitoring and management of pediatric patients during and after sedation for diagnostic and therapeutic procedures. Pediatrics 1992; 89:1110-5.

15. White PF, Negus JB: Sedative infusions during local and regional anesthesia: a comparison of midazolam and propofol. J Clin Anesth 1991; 3:32-9.

16. American Society of Anesthesiologists: Standards for basic intraoperative monitoring. In ASA directory of members, Park Ridge, Ill, 1994, ASA, p. 735.

17. Campbell RL, Dionne RA, Gregg JM: Respiratory effects of fentanyl, diazepam, and methohexital. J Oral Surg 1979; 37:355-9.

18. Bailey PL, Pace NL, Ashburn MA et al: Frequent hypoxemia and apnea after sedation with midazolam and fentanyl. Anesthesiology 1990; 73:826-30.

19. Food and Drug Administration: Warning re-emphasized in midazolam labeling. FDA Drug Bulletin 1986; 27:5.

20. Yaster M, Nichols DG, Deshpandr JK et al: Midazolam-fentanyl intravenous sedation in children: case report of respiratory arrest. Pediatrics 1990; 86:463-7.

21. Natof HE: Federated Ambulatory Surgery Association: Special study 1, Alexandria, Va, 1986, Federated Ambulatory Surgery Association.

22. Campbell RL: Prevention of complications associated with intravenous sedation and general anesthesia. J Oral Maxillofac Surg 1986; 44:289-301.

23. Cohen MM, Duncan PG, Tate RB: Does anesthesia contribute to operative mortality? JAMA 1988; 260:2859-63.

24. Caplan RA, Ward RJ, Posner K et al: Unexpected cardiac arrest during spinal anesthesia: a closed claims analysis of predisposing factors. Anesthesiology 1988; 68:5-11.

25. American Society of Anesthesiologists: Position on monitored anesthesia care. In ASA directory of members, Park Ridge, Ill, 1994, ASA, pp. 768-9.

26. Joint Commission on Accreditation of Healthcare Organizations: Surgical and anesthesia services. In Accreditation Manual for Hospitals 1994, Oakbrook Terrace, Ill, 1994, JACHO, pp. 19-21.

27. American Society of Anesthesiologists: Standard for postanesthesia care. In ASA directory of members, Park Ridge, Ill, 1994, ASA, pp. 737-8.

28. Fragen RJ: General anesthesia. In White PF, editor: Outpatient anesthesia, New York, 1990, Churchill Livingstone, pp. 313-41.

29. Fragen RJ, Avram MJ: Nonopioid intravenous anesthetics. In Barash PG, Cullen BF, Stoelting RK, editors: Clinical anesthesia, ed 2, Philadelphia, 1992, JB Lippincott, pp. 385-412.

30. Elliott CJR, Green R, Howells TH et al: Recovery after intravenous barbiturate anesthesia. Lancet 1962; 1:68.

31. Vickers MD: The measurement of recovery from anesthesia. Br J Anaesth 1965; 37:296-302.

32. Philip BK, Covino BG: Local and regional anesthesia. In Wetchler BV, editor: Anesthesia for ambulatory surgery, ed 2, Philadelphia, 1985, JB Lippincott, pp. 309-74.

33. Gross JB, Smith L, Smith TC: Time course of ventilatory response to carbon dioxide after intravenous diazepam. Anesthesiology 1982; 57:18-21.

34. Korttila K, Mattila MI, Linnolla M: Prolonged recovery after diazepam sedation. The influence of food, charcoal ingestion and injection rate on the effects of intravenous diazepam. Br J Anaesth 1976; 48:333-40.

35. Korttila K, Linnolla M: Recovery and skills related to driving after intravenous sedation: dose response relationship with diazepam. Br J Anaesth 1975; 47:457-63.

36. Vinik HR, Bradley EL, Kissin I: Midazolam-alfentanil synergism for anesthetic induction in patients. Anesth Analg 1989; 69:312-7.

37. Dundee JW, Wilson DB: Amnesic action of midazolam. Anaesthesia 1980; 35:459-61.

38. Forster A, Gardaz JB, Suter PM et al: Respiratory depression by midazolam and diazepam. Anesthesiology 1980; 53:494-9.

39. Dundee JW, Samuel IO, Toner W et al: Midazolam: a water-soluble benzodiazepine. Anaesthesia 1980; 35:454-8.

40. Gamble JAS, Kawar P, Dundee JW et al: Evaluation of midazolam as an intravenous induction agent. Anaesthesia 1981; 36:868-73.

41. Dixon J, Power SI, Grundy EM et al: Sedation for local anesthesia. Comparison of intravenous midazolam and diazepam. Anesthesia 1984; 39:372-6.

42. McClure JH, Brown DT, Wildsmith JAW: Comparison of the intravenous administration of midazolam and diazepam as sedation during spinal anesthesia. Br J Anaesth 1983; 55:1089-93.

43. Skelly AM, Boscoe MJ, Dawling S et al: A comparison of diazepam and midazolam as sedatives for minor oral surgery. Eur J Anaesthesol 1984; 1:253-67.

44. Driessin JJ, Smets MJW, Goey LS et al: Comparison of diazepam and midazolam as sedatives for minor oral premedicants for bronchoscopy under local anesthesia. Acta Anaesth Belg 1982; 33:99-103.

45. Philip BK: Supplemental medication for ambulatory procedures under regional anesthesia. Anesth Analg 1985; 64:1117-25.

46. Korttila K, Linnolla M: Skills related recovery after intravenous diazepam, flunitrazepam or droperidol. Br J Anaesth 1974; 46: 961-9.

47. Twersky RS: The pharmacology of anesthetics used for ambulatory surgery. In American Society of Anesthesiologists: Annual refresher course lectures, Philadelphia, 1993, JB Lippincott, pp. 159-75.

48. Gehan G, Karoubi P, Quinet F et al: Optimal dose of lidocaine for preventing pain on injection of propofol. Br J Anaesth 1991; 66: 324-6.

49. Centers for Disease Control: Postsurgical infections associated with an extrinsically contaminated intravenous anesthetic agent: California, Illinois, Maine, and Michigan, 1990. MMWR 1990; 39:426-33.

50. O'Flynn RP, Siler JN: A "loading port" for syringe infusion pumps (letter). Anesth Analg 1991; 72:407-8.

51. Oei-Lim VL, Kalkman CJ, Bourvy-Berends ECM et al: A comparison of the effects of propofol and nitrous oxide on the electroencephalogram in epileptic patients during conscious sedation for dental procedures. Anesth Analg 1992; 75:708-14.

52. Zacny JP, Lichtor JL, Coalson DW et al: Subjective and psychomotor effects of subanesthetic doses of propofol in healthy volunteers. Anesthesiology 1992; 76:696-702.

53. White PF, Way WL, Trenor AJ: Ketamine—its pharmacology and therapeutic uses. Anesthesiology 1982; 56:119-36.

54. Vinnick CA: An intravenous dissociation technique for outpatient plastic surgery: tranquility in the office surgical facility. Plastic Reconstr Surg 1981; 67:799-805.

55. Monk TG, Rater JM, White PF: Comparison of alfentanil and ketamine infusions in combination with midazolam for outpatient lithotripsy. Anesth Analg 1991; 74:1023-8.

56. White PF: Continuous infusions of thiopental, methohexital or etomidate as adjuvants to nitrous oxide for outpatient anesthesia. Anesth Analg 1984; 63:282.

57. Murphy MR: Opioids. In Barash PG, Cullen BF, Stoelting RK, editors: Clinical anesthesia, ed 2, Philadelphia, 1992, JB Lippincott, pp. 413-38.

58. Kallar SK, Jones GW: Opioids and same-day surgery. In Estafanous FG, editor: Opioids in anesthesia, Boston, 1991, Butterworth-Heinemann, pp. 139 -50.

59. Korttila K: Recovery and driving after brief anesthesia. Anaesthetist 1981; 30:377-82.

60. Scamman FL, Ghoneim MM, Korttila K et al: Ventilatory and mental effects of alfentanil and fentanyl. Acta Anaesthesiol Scand 1984; 28: 63-7.

61. White PF, Coe V, Shafer A et al: Comparison of alfentanil with fentanyl for outpatient anesthesia. Anesthesiology 1986; 64:99-106.

62. Krane BD, Kreutz JM, Johnson DL et al: Alfentanil and delayed respiratory depression: case studies and review. Anesth Analg 1990; 70:557-61.

63. Wetchler BV, Alexander CP, Shariff MSY et al: A comparison of recovery in patients receiving fentanyl vs. those receiving butorphanol. J Clin Anesth 1989; 1:339-43.

64. Garfield JM, Garfield FB, Philip B et al: A comparison of clinical and psychologic effects of fentanyl and nalbuphine in ambulatory surgical patients. Anesth Analg 1987; 66:1303-7.

65. Fine J, Finestone SC: A comparative study of the side effects of butorphanol, nalbuphine and fentanyl. Anesth Rev 1981; 8:13-7.

66. Gilbert J, Holt JE, Johnston J et al: Intravenous sedation for cataract surgery. Anaesthesia 1987; 42:1063-9.

67. Zallan RD, Cobetto GA, Bohmfalk C et al: Butorphanol/diazepam compared to meperidine/diazepam for sedation in oral, maxillofacial surgery: a double blind evaluation. Oral Surgery 1987; 64: 395-401.

68. Stevens WC, Kingston HGG: Inhalation anesthetics. In Barash PG, Cullen BF, Stoelting RK, editors: Clinical anesthesia, ed 2, Philadelphia, 1992, JB Lippincott, pp. 439-65.

69. Korttila K, Ghoneim MM, Jacobs L et al: Time course of mental and psychomotor effects of 30% nitrous oxide during inhalation and recovery. Anesthesiology 1981; 54:220-6.

70. Cook TL, Smith M, Winter PM et al: Effect of subanesthetic concentrations of enflurance and halothane on human behavior. Anesth Analg 1978; 57:434-40.

71. Rodrigo MRC, Rosenquist JB: Isoflurane for conscious sedation. Anaesthesia 1988; 43:369-75.

72. Allan MWB, Laurence AS, Gunawardena WJ: A comparison of two sedation techniques for neuroradiology. Eur J Anesthesiol 1989; 6:379-84.

73. Boldy DAR, English JSC, Lang GS et al: Sedation for endoscopy: a comparison between diazepam and diazepam plus pethidine with naloxone reversal. Br J Anaesth 1984; 56:1109-12.

74. Milligan KR, Howe JP, McLoughlin J et al: Midazolam sedation for outpatient fiberoptic endoscopy: evaluation of alfentanil supplementation. Ann R Coll Surg Engl 1988; 70:303-6.

75. Ochs MW, Tucker MR, White RP: A comparison of amnesia in outpatients sedated with midazolam or diazepam alone or in combination with fentanyl during oral surgery. J Am Dent Assoc 1986; 113:894-7.

76. Geller E, Halpern P: Benzodiazepines and their antagonists in anesthesia. In International Anesthesia Research Society: Review course lectures, Baltimore, 1993, Williams & Wilkins, pp. 136-40.

77. Jensens S, Knudsen L, Kirkegaard: Flumazenil used for antagonizing the central effects of midazolam and diazepam in outpatients. Acta Anaesthesiol Scand 1989; 33:26-8.

78. Kestin IG, Harvey PB, Nixon C: Psychomotor recovery after three methods of sedation during spinal anaesthesia. Br J Anaesth 1991; 64: 675-81.

79. Philip BK, Simpson TH, Hauch MA et al: Flumazenil reverses sedation after midazolam-induced general anesthesia in ambulatory surgery patients. Anesth Analg 1990; 71:371-6.

80. Reves JG, Jacobs JR, Glass P: Intravenous anesthetic drug delivery in anesthesia. In International Anesthesia Research Society: Review course lectures, Baltimore, 1992, Williams & Wilkins, pp. 29-34.

81. White PF: Clinical uses of intravenous anesthetic and analgesic infusions. Anesth Analg 1989; 68:161-71.

82. Pace NA, Victory RA, White PF: Anesthetic infusion techniques—how to do it. J Clin Anesth 1992; 4(Supp 1): 45S-52S.

83. Jacobs JR, Reves JG, Glass PSA: Rationale and technique for continuous infusions in anesthesia. Int Anesthesiol Clin 1991; 29(4): 23-38.

84. Jacobs JR, Glass PSA, Reves JG: Opioid administration by continuous infusion. In Estafanous FG, editor: Opioids in anesthesia, Boston, 1991, Butterworth-Heinemann, pp. 241-55.

85. Shafer SL, Stanski DR: New intravenous anesthetics. In American Society of Anesthesiologists: Refresher courses in anesthesiology, Philadelphia, 1991, JB Lippincott, pp. 153-63.

86. Jacobs JR, Williams EA: Pharmacokinetics and pharmacodynamics of continuous intravenous infusion. Int Anesthesiol Clin 1991; 29(4):1-22.

87. Reves JG: Automated drug infusion systems in anesthesia. In American Society of Anesthesiologists: Annual refresher course lectures, Philadelphia, 1990, JB Lippincott.

88. Jacobs JR, Glass PSA, Reves JG: Technology for continuous infusion in anesthesia. Int Anesthesiol Clin 1991; 29(4):30-52.

89. Glass PSA, Jacobs JR, Quill TJ: Intravenous drug delivery systems. In Fragen RJ, editor: Drug infusions in anesthesiology, New York, 1991, Raven Press, pp. 23-61.

90. White PF, Vasconez LO, Mathes SA et al: Comparison of midazolam and diazepam for sedation during plastic surgery. Plastic Reconstr Surg 1988; 81:703-10.

91. Urguhart ML, White PF: Comparison of sedative infusions during regional anesthesia—methohexital, etomidate, and midazolam. Anesth Analg 1989; 68:249-54.

92. Sherry E: Admixture of propofol and alfentanil. Anaesthesia 1992; 477-9.

93. Lee W, Worthington J, Zahl K: An evaluation of alfentanil vs propofol for sedation in monitored anesthesia care during arthroscopy (abstract). Eighth SAMBA Annual Meeting, 1993.

94. Monk TG, Boure B, White PF et al: Comparison of intravenous sedative-analgesic techniques for outpatient immersion lithotripsy. Anesth Analg 1991; 72:616-21.

95. Fisher DM: Sedation of pediatric patients: an anesthesiologist's perspective. Radiology 1990; 175:613-5.

96. Splinter WM, Schaefer JD, Zunder IH: Clear fluids three hours before surgery do not affect the gastric fluid contents of children. Can J Anesth 1990; 35(5):498-501.

97. Lichenstein R, King JL, Bice D: Evaluation of chloral hydrate for pediatric sedation. Clinical Pediatrics 1993; 32(10): 632-3.

98. American Academy of Pediatrics Committee on Drugs and Committee on Environmental Health: Use of chloral hydrate for sedation in children. Pediatrics 1993; 92(3):471-3.

99. Tobias J, Phipps S, Smith B, Mulhern R: Oral ketamine premedication to alleviate the distress of invasive procedures in pediatric oncology patients. Pediatrics 1992; 90:573-41.

100. Feld LH, Negus JB: Oral midazolam preanesthetic medication in pediatric outpatients. Anesthesiology 1990; 73:831-4.

101. Yealy D, Ellis J, Hobbs G, Moscali R: Intranasal midazolam as a sedative for children during laceration repair. Am J Emerg Med 1992; 10:584-7.

102. Twersky RS, Berger BJ, McClain J, Beaton C: Midazolam enhances anterograde but not retrograde amnesia in pediatric patients. Anesthesiology 1993; 78(1):51-5.

103. Frieseu RH, Lockhart CH: Oral transmucosal fentanyl citrate for preanesthetic medication of pediatric day surgery patients with and without droperidol as a prophylactic antiemetic. Anesthesiology 1992; 76:46-51.

104. Green SM, Johnson NE: Ketamine sedation for pediatric procedures: review and implications. Ann Emerg Med 1990; 19(9):1033-46.

105. Hawk W, Crockett RK, Ochsenschlager DW, Klein BL: Conscious sedation of the pediatric patient for suturing: a survey. Ped Emerg Care 1990; 6(2):84-8.
106. Temme JB, Anderson JC, Matecko S: Sedation of children for CT and MRI scanning. Radiologic Technology 1990; 61(4):283-5.
107. O'Brien JF, Falk SL, Carey BE, Malone LC: Rectal thiopental compared with intramuscular meperidine, promethazine, and chlorpromazine for pediatric sedation. Ann Emerg Med 1991; 20(6):644-7.
108. Terndrup TE, Dine DJ, Madden CM et al: Comparison of intramuscular meperidine and promethazine with and without chlorpromazine: a randomized, prospective double-blind trial. Ann Emerg Med 1993; 22(2):206-11.
109. Bloomfield EL, Masaryk TJ, Caplin A et al: Intravenous sedation for MR imaging of the brain and spine in children: pentobarbital versus propofol. Radiology 1993; 186:93-7.
110. Schwanda AE, Freyer DR, Sanfilippo DJ et al: Brief unconscious sedation for painful pediatric oncology procedures. Am J Ped Hemat/Oncol 1993; 15(4):370-6.
111. Sievers T, Yee J, Foley M et al: Midazolam for conscious sedation during pediatric oncology procedures: safety and recovery parameters. Pediatrics 1991; 88:1172-9.
112. Vangerven M, Van Hemelryck J, Wouters P et al: Light anaesthesia with propofol for paediatric MRI. Anaesthesia 1992; 47:706-7.
113. Billmire D, Neale HW, Gregory RO: Use of IV fentanyl in outpatient treatment of pediatric facial trauma. J Trauma 1985; 25:1079-80.
114. Yaster M, Nichols DG, Deshpande JK, Wetzel RC: Midazolam-fentanyl intravenous sedation in children: case report of respiratory arrest. Pediatrics 1990; 86(3):463-7.
115. Henry RJ, Jerrell RG: Ambient nitrous oxide levels during pediatric sedation. Pediatric Dentistry 1990; 12(2):87-91.

Ambulatory Anesthesia Outside the Operating Room

Steven Hall

361

Sedation, monitored anesthetic care, and
anesthesia for minor procedures
Applicable techniques
Universal guidelines for sedation
Summary

The provision of anesthetic services outside the traditional operating room environment is a challenge to both the adaptability and
sensibility of the anesthesiologist. In an effort to increase the
comfort and safety of patients, and to assist other physicians, we
are increasingly asked to provide either anesthetic or monitored
anesthesia care (MAC) services for a variety of diagnostic and
therapeutic procedures. This enhanced role of the anesthesiologist
in patient care throughout the facility offers an opportunity to
improve patient care, increase the awareness of the services that
anesthesiologists can provide, and serve as an additional source of
revenue.

General Principles

Site Evaluation

The anesthetizing site must be surveyed before the clinician agrees
to provide anesthetic services. Generally, space requirements, electrical service, communications system, lighting, traffic control, personnel, and potential hazards should be evaluated (Box 10-1). If it
is not possible to deliver safe and effective care at the site, the
clinician should reevaluate the decision to make a commitment to
provide service. The survey of the site should be undertaken in the
presence of the personnel who will be providing the diagnostic or
therapeutic activity, so that they can ask questions about space, time
constraints, personnel, and traffic. The anesthesia department
should also enlist the help of the facility's biomedical engineers or
other technical personnel to determine whether the electrical outlet
supply, ventilation, and scavenging capability are adequate for the
additional demands of anesthetic equipment.

There might be local or state governmental building codes or
safety codes that must be considered in evaluating a potential site.
Storage of oxygen and nitrous oxide cylinders, use of enriched

---

Box 10-1 Principles of Site Evaluation

Space
Electrical service
Communications
Lighting
Traffic control
Personnel
Hazards

Box 10-2 Traffic Control

Patient reception area
Patient induction area
Patient transport
Recovery

---

oxygen, area ventilation, hazardous waste storage, corridor width, fire exits, lighting, and several other matters might be subject to local codes. The safety director or similar administrative officer of the facility should assist in these determinations.

Patient traffic flow should be considered (Box 10-2). The manner in which the patient (and accompanying responsible adult) is admitted and registered for the procedure, the area where the patient can change clothes and be examined by the anesthesiologist, the place where the accompanying adult can wait, and the recovery and discharge area should be evaluated. A routine for efficient admission and preparation of the patient should be developed before the first anesthetic is given. There will often be adjustments to this routine as experience is gained, but a reasonable approach should be in place before embarking on the coverage of care.

Space and Equipment Considerations (Box 10-3)

Each area will have its own unique requirements and restrictions. However, there are certain basics that should be present for every anesthetizing location. This is necessary not only for provision of

Box 10-3 *Principles of Site Evaluation*

Space

Room for anesthesia equipment
Room for anesthesia personnel
Access to patient
Storage
Interference from imaging or other equipment

Electrical Service

Adequacy of number of outlets
Line fault protection
Emergency, uninterrupted outlets

Communications

Dedicated, two-way system

Lighting

Room light
Procedure light
Emergency light

basic anesthesia care, but also for response to a reasonable range of potential emergencies. Remember, not all emergencies that may be encountered are medical in nature. There can also be problems such as loss of electricity, loss of lighting, absence of assisting personnel, or fire. The traditional operating room is designed and engineered with multiple safety systems in place,[1] and personnel in the operating room have been educated in safety procedures. In distant locations, however, this may not be the case. Therefore, one of the first items to identify is a reliable method of communication used to summon help. This can be a telephone, intercom, or other system, but it must be present before delivering anesthetic care. Additionally, personnel to be participating in the procedure and the sedation must be identified. The qualifications and responsibility of the nonanesthesia personnel should be delineated, and appropriate in-service training should be provided.

The area should be sufficiently spacious to allow the anesthesiologist immediate access to anesthetic machinery and other equipment that may be needed (Box 10-4). There should be adequate room to prepare and administer the anesthetic, and there

---

Box 10-4 Hazards to the Patient and Personnel

Poor patient access
Crowded conditions
Multiple extension cords
Radiation
High-energy magnetic fields

---

should be unimpeded patient access. A well-lit area is crucial, but the room should also have the capability of bright illumination of the patient for tasks such as obtaining vascular access. The anesthesia equipment and monitors should be easily seen at all times during the procedure. If equipment (such as a C-arm fluoroscopy unit) must be moved during the procedure, the access to the patient should be maintained. In some situations (e.g., radiation oncology), all personnel must leave the area during part of the procedure. If this is the case, the anesthesiologist must clearly understand when these periods will occur and what options exist for quick access to the patient.

There should be enough electrical outlets to accommodate all of the anesthetic and monitoring equipment without unduly over-taxing the circuits. Clearly labeled outlets to an uninterrupted emergency power supply should be designated for the sole use by the anesthesiologist. All outlets should be properly grounded and within easy reach. It is desirable to position equipment such that the electrical cords are not a potential source of tripping.

Equipment needs vary with location; however, certain require-ments must be met (Box 10-5). A reliable supply of oxygen adequate not only for the length of the intended procedure, but also for emergencies, is essential in all sites. Although a piped source of oxygen (and other gases like nitrous oxide) is ideal, it may be impractical. If piped gases are used, the anesthesiologist must be familiar with the source of the gas, its capabilities, and the procedure for enlisting backup sources. Likewise, if tanks of oxygen are the local source, there must be at least one full backup tank immediately available. It is prudent to have a freestanding tank-based backup system available, even if a piped source of oxygen is used.

Whenever anesthesia or MAC is administered, suction must be available. This suction must be adequate to deal with

---

Box 10-5 Equipment Evaluation

Anesthesia Equipment
Anesthesia machine and ventilator
Monitors
Backup nitrous oxide tanks
Airway equipment, drugs, intravenous fluid storage
Anesthesia work surface
Lighting

Oxygen Source
Presence of piped oxygen
Backup oxygen system and alarms
Additional tank backup

Suction

Scavenging
Validation of scavenging effectiveness

Emergency Cart and Defibrillator

---

any reasonable expected needs during anesthesia. Piped suction systems have the advantage of reliable power that is usually superior to small, independently powered machines that may be used in remote locations. The anesthesiologist must confirm that the available suction apparatus will be suitable for patient needs.

If administration of anesthetic gases or vapors is a possibility at the site, provisions must be made for adequate scavenging of waste gases. If a suction apparatus is used, the gases must not only be removed from the area, but also be directed out of contact with all personnel in the facility. If a passive system is used, the anesthesiologist must ensure that all waste gases are contained within the passive system. It is useful to test the area's atmosphere for appropriate trace anesthetic gases during an actual case to confirm that the system works and that the trace gas concentrations are within accepted standards.

Emergency equipment should be present whenever sedation or anesthesia is given. The minimum equipment should include a self-inflating, positive pressure ventilating resuscitation bag that is capable of delivering at least 90% oxygen;[2] airway supplies, such as a full range of sizes of airways, endotracheal tubes, and stylets; standard resuscitation drugs; a battery-powered source of lighting; a defibrillator; and any other usual equipment for resuscitation. There should be a clear policy about whose responsibility it is to check and maintain this emergency equipment.

Lastly, the functioning and safety of the anesthesia machine, monitors, and other equipment used in a remote location should be equivalent to those of equipment used in the traditional operating room. The American Society of Anesthesiologists (ASA) Standards for Basic Anesthetic Monitoring apply no matter where in the facility the anesthetic is given.[3] Distant sites should not be a "dumping ground" for outdated equipment. This equipment should be checked and maintained in the same manner as the operating room equipment. If this equipment is to be brought from the operating room area each time it will be used, excess equipment should be minimized and less bulky machines should be used. If some or all of the anesthesia equipment is stored on site, both maintenance and security of the equipment and supplies should be guaranteed.

Scheduling

If anesthesia services are to be supplied to remote locations, each area will have multiple unique problems that should be addressed. These relate, in general, to three specific questions: (1) Which patients and procedures are suitable candidates? (2) When will anesthetic services be provided? (3) Who is responsible for admission, preparation, and discharge of the patient?

There must be a clear understanding of which patients are suitable for this care (Box 10-6). In general, if the patient would normally be an appropriate candidate for an outpatient surgical procedure, he or she would also be a suitable candidate for a therapeutic or diagnostic procedure of similar length and intensity outside the operating room. This will vary by institution, and the anesthesiologist must feel comfortable with both the patient status and the procedure before agreeing to provide service.

If only a few patients are to be covered, it is often possible to provide service on short notice at the convenience of those outside the operating room. However, if requests are frequent, a more formal arrangement is necessary. Because of the potential for having to provide multiple coverages with only limited anesthesia

---

Box 10-6 *Patient Suitability Policies*

Age limitations
ASA physical status limitations
Duration and intensity of procedure
Necessity of preanesthetic visit
    Specific medical conditions
    Specific procedures

---

personnel, there should be specific guidelines concerning the times at which service will be provided. When giving anesthesia far from the operating room, it is usually necessary to devote experienced personnel who are usually covering only that case. If attending staff are usually assigned to more than one case simultaneously, this will alter the normal pattern of coverage. For this reason, it is more efficient to assign specific times when coverage will be provided and then ensure that adequate anesthesia personnel are available. Emergency coverage outside the operating room should be handled in the same fashion as emergency coverage in the operating room environment. There may be need for third-party payor insurance approval.

The routines and policies for patient admission, evaluation, and preparation are established and clearly understood before accepting coverage of the procedure. If there are facility, departmental, or state requirements for fasting, history, physical examination, laboratory, or consultation, these must be organized and obtained from assigned personnel (Box 10-7). For instance, if informed consent is necessary, it should be clear who is to obtain the consent. Likewise, after recovery from the anesthetic, it should be clear who has the responsibility to check the patient and approve discharge from the facility. Finally, if quality management activities, such as a postanesthetic phone check, are used for patients who have undergone surgery in the operating room, they should be used for patients having surgery outside the operating room (Box 10-8).

Radiology Suite

Radiation Safety

Whenever anesthesia personnel work in the radiology suite, computerized tomography (CT) scanner, nuclear medicine laboratory,

---

Box 10-7 Patient Preparation Policies

Preanesthetic instructions
  Fasting requirements
  Responsible accompanying adult
  Chronic medications
Method of obtaining medical consultation and clearance
Informed consent
History and physical examination
Laboratory studies

Box 10-8 Recovery and Discharge Policies

Dedicated recovery staff or operating room facility
Responsibility for discharge from recovery area
Responsibility for discharge from institution
Postanesthetic follow-up
Continuing quality management activities

---

or radiation therapy facility, they must be cognizant of the basics of radiation safety. Ionizing radiation can cause direct tissue damage, chromosomal damage, and an increased risk of malignancy.[4,5] Although it is the responsibility of the radiology personnel to help anesthesia staff understand what measures are needed to minimize exposure, it is the responsibility of the anesthesia staff to strictly adhere to safety guidelines.

The most basic concept in understanding radiation safety is that the closer the anesthesiologist is to the source of radiation, the higher the level of exposure. Because it is unusual for the anesthesiologist to be placed directly in the radiation beam, scatter radiation is the biggest danger. Because scatter radiation increases significantly when the power output of the beam increases or when the size of the imaged field increases, exposure is much higher when larger areas are imaged or techniques such as fluoroscopy are used. Techniques with a high intensity, focused beam (e.g., CT scanning) have lower scatter. Scatter radiation falls off with the inverse square of the distance from the field. For instance, the exposure 1 meter away is usually less than 1/1000 the exposure at the field. Radiation exposure limits, as established by the National Council on Radiation Protection and Measurements, have been based primarily on studies of civilians exposed to atomic bomb blasts during World War II.[6] This risk of genetic damage appears to be less than previously thought, though the risk of cancer is higher. Indeed, the risk of cancer is of greatest concern to those who have been repeatedly exposed to radiation. The primary cancer risks after excessive exposure include leukemia and thyroid cancer. However, this kind of excessive exposure rarely occurs.[7]

For anesthesiologists who are more likely to have multiple, smaller exposures, there are two important factors: the total amount of radiation exposure and the rate of exposure. A large total dose received over a long period of time is less likely to produce significant change than is the same dose received in a single exposure. There is special concern not only about total body exposure, but also localized skin or extremity exposure, and optic lens exposure because of the susceptibility of the lens to form cataracts.

Safety precautions observed by radiology staff should also be observed by anesthesiologists. They should wear a lead apron that covers the front, back, and sides. A thyroid collar should also be worn if prolonged exposure is expected. Leaded glass screens or treated glasses and goggles should be used for eye protection if there is repeated exposure to high scatter levels. If personnel have repeated exposures, it may be useful to use the same radiation monitoring devices that the radiology department uses. However, the most important safety precaution is to avoid exposure. This includes not only planning and using protective gear, but also having the radiologist inform anesthesia personnel when exposure is possible. Distance is important, because being 6 feet away from the beam decreases scatter exposure to the same level as having 2.5 mm of lead (the equivalent of 5 lead aprons) or 9 inches of concrete between the beam and the anesthesiologist.

Angiography, Myelography, and Embolization Procedures

The angiography/myelography suite is often a difficult place to administer an anesthetic because of limited space and access to the patient. Patients often have prolonged procedures on a hard table; proper attention to positioning, padding, access to the airway, lack of stretch on the brachial plexus or pressure on peripheral nerves, and adequate lighting of the patient and equipment are important. The patient may be repositioned or tilted during the procedure, and, after repositioning, the patient must be reevaluated for all of these factors.

Angiography is usually performed to identify the extent of peripheral or central vascular disease or malignancy. Central nervous system angiography is indicated for a variety of tumors, aneurysms, and arteriovenous malformations, while peripheral vascular angiography is used to identify both arterial and venous lesions, usually those associated with atherosclerosis. While patients with central nervous system lesions may otherwise be healthy, those with peripheral atherosclerotic lesions often have other vascular problems. Anesthesiologists may be asked to provide either MAC or general anesthesia during these procedures because of the discomfort of the procedure, problems with patient cooperation, or significant medical conditions that require monitoring and treatment. This last category is exceptionally challenging because the patient may be acutely decompensated and require aggressive resuscitation at the same time that the procedure is done. Because of this, the anesthesiologist must both understand the procedure and know the status of the patient before committing to providing coverage so that proper preparations of equipment and personnel can be made.

Monitoring for the patient undergoing angiography is based on the patient's medical condition and the anticipated procedure. For short procedures, sedation and monitoring may be the best choice. For longer procedures, it may be prudent to provide the ventilatory and hemodynamic control that general anesthesia gives. If there are special problems (e.g., increased intracranial pressure), both monitoring and anesthetic approaches will need to be tailored to address them specifically. Some of the medical problems that are common in the angiography or myelography suite include increased intracranial pressure (vascular and malignant lesions),[8] seizure disorder, coronary artery insufficiency, renal and peripheral vascular insufficiency, and cardiac failure (low output, coronary artery disease; high output, arteriovenous malformation). Proper preanesthetic evaluation, determination of whether the patient is an outpatient candidate, and preprocedure preparation should be the same for these patients as for a similar patient coming to the operating room.

Contrast media used in angiography can cause significant cardiovascular, central nervous system, and renal complications. The older high-osmolality agents (1400 to 1500 mOsm/L) have a higher incidence of reactions compared to newer low-osmolality agents (660 to 700 mOsm/L).[9] There are direct myocardial depressant, arrhythmic, and vasodilating actions that can cause transient hypertension followed by hypotension, as well as diuresis followed by hypovolemia. The agents can also cause seizures, cerebral edema, and renal damage. The total amount of dye used is recorded and monitored, and the amount is usually limited to 4 to 6 ml/kg. There can also be systemic responses, such as histamine release and complement activation. Reactions range from mild histamine release to life-threatening bronchospasm, angioneurotic edema, and anaphylaxis. These reactions must be treated promptly with diphenhydramine, steroids, oxygen, fluids, and, if necessary, epinephrine.[10] Pretreatment with prophylactic steroids and antihistamines has been used in patients having previous reactions to dye.

Embolization is occasionally utilized for lesions such as arteriovenous malformation.[11] Although these patients are usually admitted after the procedure, some adults with a stable medical status and no evidence of postprocedure instability may be sent home the same day after an extended observation period. This is especially appropriate if the embolization was in a superficial location; if the site was an extremity, distal perfusion should be checked and clearly be unimpaired before the patient is discharged. If materials such as pledgets or coils are used for the embolization, there is always the chance of bleeding or of migration of the object to a distal location that could require surgical intervention to remove. If toxic chemicals are used for sclerosing the area, there may be either local or systemic reactions.

When myelography is performed, it is common to tilt the patient to enhance the spread of the dye. The patient's position, padding, and adequacy of ventilation is checked after each move. Of particular concern is the risk of seizures; if the dye is allowed to flow to the supratentorial subarachnoid space, seizures may result. Another special concern with myelography is the decision to perform a CT scan after the myelogram. The anesthesiologist must decide whether to continue the sedation or anesthesia during the CT scan and how to safely transport the patient from the myelography suite to the CT suite.

Radiation Therapy

Radiation therapy treatment with high-energy beams is useful for treatment of specific tumors (e.g., retinoblastoma) and for total body irradiation before bone marrow transplantation. Although the exposure time is only a few minutes long, usually multiple exposures are administered over the course of a few weeks.[12] Anesthesiologists usually become involved only when the patient is a child because, even though the exposures are short, the patient must stay very still.

The radiation levels are so high that the anesthesiologist cannot be in the room during exposure. The heavily shielded door is sealed during the exposure, and usually it takes a couple of minutes to reopen the door and gain access to the room and the patient. The patient is appropriately sedated or anesthetized and then monitored with the usual monitors and two cameras, one focused on the patient and the other on the monitors. The patient is immobilized with padding and sandbags or a specially-designed frame. The sedation or anesthetic is individually tailored to each patient, but the goal is immobility, maintenance of the airway and ventilation, and rapid emergence so that the patient can return home. Several regimens have been used, including intravenous benzodiazepines or propofol, rectal methohexital, and halothane by mask.[12-16] It is desirable to develop a routine of sedation or anesthesia in which there is significant interaction with the patient and family. If the anesthesiologist develops a positive rapport with them, the provision of daily care is easier, and the negative effects of multiple hospital visits can be minimized. If an intravenous technique is chosen, it may be prudent to have a permanently implanted central line available to eliminate the discomfort of punctures with each procedure.

CT *and* MRI Scanner

Both CT and MRI (magnetic resonance imaging) scanners have become important diagnostic tools. They differ in the images they provide and the challenges they raise for the anesthesiologist. In general, it is much easier to provide care in the CT scanner suite.

Although the patient's remaining still while the examination bed is moved in and out of the imager may be a challenge, the equipment and mechanical problems are straightforward. All the usual-monitoring and anesthetic equipment used in the operating room is suitable for use in the CT suite; the only problem is the relatively small size of the room.

MRI Equipment Considerations

Unlike the situation with CT scanners, with MRI scanners there are several important equipment considerations that influence anesthetic management (Figs. 10-1 and 10-2). For an MRI, the patient is inserted into a tube that is surrounded by a powerful electromagnet. The generated field, which is 10,000 to 30,000 times as powerful as the earth's magnetic field, orients hydrogen molecules in the body so that they face one direction. The addition of radiofrequency signals alters the orientation of these molecules for a short time before they return to the baseline, during which they release a signal that is used to build the MRI picture.[17] Both components of this process have significance for anesthetic equipment.[18]

The magnetic field is so strong that it can draw ferromagnetic objects into the core of the magnet's bore, injuring the patient or anyone else that is between the object and the center of the magnetic field.[19] The magnetic force markedly decreases in strength, measured in gauss units (G), the farther from the magnet the object is, with the 5 G and 50 G limits most commonly used.[17] Items with high ferromagnetic content are drawn into a 50 G easily, pacemakers may not function properly in fields as low as 5 G, and cathode ray screens may be altered by fields as low as 1 to 2 G.[18] The functional ferromagnetic capability of an object can be assessed by placing a pacemaker magnet on the object and watching for noticeable attraction. Known ferromagnetic items should be kept at least 15 feet away from the magnet and, if at all possible, outside the scanning room.[17,19,20] Objects that can be drawn into the magnet include hemostats, keys, pens, ferromagnetic gas tanks, clipboards, and scissors; the magnetic field also can demagnetize watches and destroy the magnetic data strips on credit cards and magnetic tapes.[21]

The magnetic field can displace ferromagnetic vascular clips inside a patient, especially in the CNS where scar tissue does not form.[19,22] Cardiac pacemakers can be converted to the asynchronous mode or inactivated by the magnetic field.[23] Bioimplants

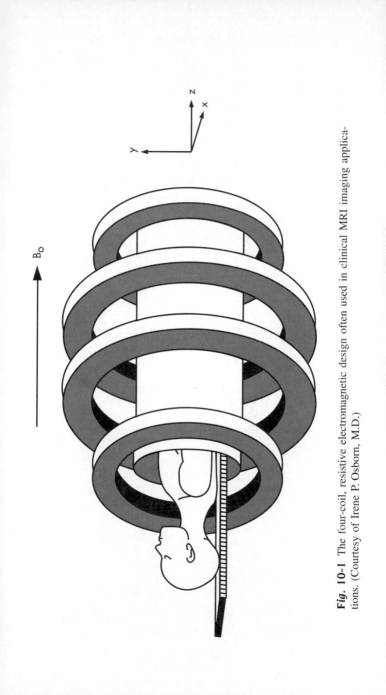

Fig. 10-1 The four-coil, resistive electromagnetic design often used in clinical MRI imaging applications. (Courtesy of Irene P. Osborn, M.D.)

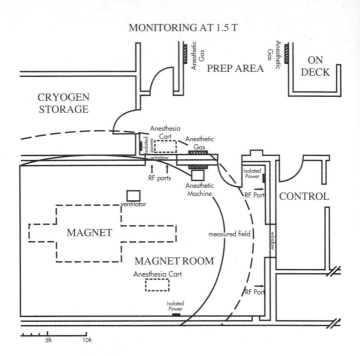

Fig. 10-2 Floor plan for MRI suite. (From Patient anesthesia and monitoring at a 1.5 Tesla installation. Magnetic Resonance Med 1988; 7:210-2.)

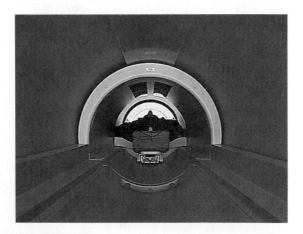

Fig. 10-3 Patient positioning inside MRI scanner. (Courtesy of Irene P. Osborn, M.D.)

Table 10-1   Anesthesia Equipment for MRI

Problematic	Usually compatible
ECG	Blood pressure measuring equipment
Anesthesia machines	Pulse oximetry
Automated IV infusion devices	Capnography
Laryngoscopes	Laryngeal mask airway
	Plastic stethoscopes
	Other miscellaneous plastic devices

made of stainless steel (high grades only), tantalum, aluminum, nickel, and most alloys are not attracted by the magnet and are safe.[24,25] If there is concern about possible internal metal, such as surgical implants or metal fragments, an initial x-ray or CT scan will identify the presence of a radiolucent object. The decision to proceed should be made with the radiologist and managing service.

The magnetic field can also draw anesthetic equipment into the magnet, and it can interfere with its function. Therefore, all anesthetic equipment in the scanning room should have a low ferromagnetic content. Also, any anesthetic equipment that can induce a radiofrequency signal can disrupt the patient's signal, producing an inadequate MRI picture. Monitors, in particular, can emit a radiofrequency signal that degrades the image. Because of this, many monitors have been evaluated for function in the MRI suite (Table 10-1).[20,25]

Some models of commonly available monitors have been found to work well in the MRI, but some models are not suitable. In addition, specially built monitors are available that contain low ferromagnetic content, extensive shielding, and in-line filters to prevent both degradation of the MRI picture and interference with the monitor's function. There are now a wide variety of pulse oximeter, capnograph, and noninvasive blood pressure monitors available that have been shown to work well in the MRI suite.[26,27] Plastic stethoscopes and mercury plastic film thermometers are also safe in the MRI suite.

Of all the standard monitors, the electrocardiograph (ECG) has been the source of most difficulty.[28] This monitor has been a source of patient burns and MRI signal degradation, as well as

Box 10-9 ECG Monitoring in the MRI Suite

Safety Precautions

Use 4-lead, 2-ground system.
Place all four electrodes close to center of trunk.
Check lead wires for fraying.
Place towel or sheet under lead wires.
Braid lead wires together to prevent loop formation.
Recheck lead wires periodically.

inadequate monitoring signal. Most of the attention has focused on the electrodes and lead wires. Because the lead wires are ferromagnetic, the strong magnetic field can distort the ECG signal. Also, there is a risk of burns at the site of the lead or over the course of the lead wires (Box 10-9). If the wire loops on itself, the loop acts as an antenna, and current is induced in this loop that leads to heat build-up and subsequent burn.[28] In our institution, we have used the following advice from engineers to decrease the risk of current generation:

- A 4-lead, 2-ground system is used instead of a 3-lead system. All electrodes are placed close to the center of the patient's trunk. The incidence of ECG artifacts has been lower with a 3-lead system than with any other system. Lead wires are checked before each use for evidence of fraying of the insulation.
- A towel or sheet is placed under the lead wires. The lead wires do not come in contact with the skin, which prevents burning even if the lead wires become heated.
- Lead wires are braided together as soon as possible. This prevents loop formation and subsequent induction of current.
- The position of the lead wires is rechecked each time the patient is moved, ensuring that a loop has not formed.

The positioning of anesthetic equipment, as well as monitors, is an important issue. It is possible to have the monitors either inside the MRI scanning room or, if so designed, have the sensors in the scanning room and the monitor display in the control room.[18,29,30] Likewise, if an anesthesia machine or other anesthetic equipment is used, it can be placed in the scanning room or in the control room. If equipment is used inside the scanning room, the anesthesiologist must ensure that it has low ferromagnetic content and works efficiently in the environment. There currently is a commercially available anesthesia machine that has had the ferromagnetic content markedly reduced to allow it to function in the scanning room. There also are a variety of ventilators that have been shown to work effectively in the scanning room. Remember that there is other anesthetic equipment besides an anesthesia machine, ventilator, and monitors that may be ferromagnetic. Fittings on the anesthetic circuit, the laryngoscope and its batteries, stylets, and other small equipment may be ferromagnetic and may need to be replaced.[20,25]

There are two alternatives to having anesthesia equipment in the scanning room.[31] The first alternative is to use standard anesthesia equipment and leave it in the control room. The anesthesia circuit must enter the room through a shielded conduit through the wall or door and be at least 20 to 25 feet long to reach the patient in the scanner. Two advantages of this approach include the ability to use an unmodified anesthesia machine and the lack of need for equipment or personnel to be in the scanner at all times. The disadvantage of this approach is the need to place the conduit at the time of initial construction or have it retrofitted. An alternative is to administer sedation or anesthesia without the use of an anesthesia machine. A vaporizer can be mounted on the piped oxygen source in the room and be used as an anesthetic source. Another technique involves intravenous or rectal medications. If an infusion pump is used, both its ferromagnetic content and ability to work in proximity to the magnet must be checked. Specific intravenous sedation techniques are discussed in Chapter 9.

Anesthetic Technique (Box 10-10)

An MRI scan often takes considerably longer to obtain than a CT scan, up to an hour. If the patient is cooperative, it may be possible to use sedation alone to provide adequate conditions. However, prolonged scanning is disturbing to many patients because of the loud noise produced by the scanning process and a sense of claustrophobia that may develop, especially in adults. As a practical matter, the anesthesiologist is usually summoned only when standard sedation regimens do not result in the desired immobility or if a child is medically unstable.[18]

A general anesthetic technique using any of a wide variety of agents is suitable in this setting. It is important to decide on the method used to provide a clear airway during the scan. Many

> ## Box 10-10 Anesthetic Care in the MRI Suite
>
> ### General Anesthesia versus Monitored Anesthesia Care
> Nonpainful procedure
> Varying degrees of patient cooperation (children are particularly difficult)
> Prolonged scan time compared with that of CT
> Availability of anesthesia or other trained personnel
> Inhalation, intravenous, or rectal-based techniques possible
>
> ### Control of the Airway
> Spontaneous ventilation
>   Unsecured airway
>   Laryngeal mask airway
>   Endotracheal intubation
> Controlled ventilation
>
> ### Anesthesia Equipment
> In-room nonferromagnetic equipment
>   Modified anesthesia machine
>   Specifically designed or tested equipment
>   Monitors
>   Intravenous pumps
>   Ventilators
> Out-of-room equipment
>   Shielded conduit through wall or door
> Scavenging

institutions prefer to place an endotracheal tube or laryngeal mask airway to maintain a secure airway, especially when the patient is out of sight in the scanner.[31] The anesthetic regimen is planned to provide an adequate level of anesthesia but rapid awakening when the scan is finished. The scan does not produce pain, and deep levels of anesthesia are not needed.

Alternative methods include total intravenous anesthesia, such as a propofol infusion, or bolus intravenous or rectal drugs to maintain sedation or anesthesia.[31-33] Box 10-11 provides recommendations for the use of propofol. If the airway is unprotected, the patient must be closely observed; this is difficult when a small patient disappears from ready site inside the bore of the magnet. It is possible to use an unsecured airway as long as the

---

Box 10-11 *Suggested Propofol Infusion Rates for MRI*[32,33]

Induction: 2 mg/kg of propofol *or* inhalation induction
Maintenance: Pediatrics 100 mcg/kg/min
          Adults 50 mcg/kg/min

Suggested Dilution and Infusion Rates for Nonautomated Infusions

1. 200 mg propofol (20 ml) is diluted to total volume of 66 ml (final concentration 3 mg/ml). Use only those solutions deemed compatible (i.e., dextrose, Lactated Ringer's)
2. Using calibrated drip chamber so that
   60 drops = 1 ml
   1 drop/kg/min = 50 μg/kg/min
   Titrate accordingly
   Example: For a 20 kg patient, count 20 drops/min = 50 μg/kg/min

For smaller children and infants:

1. 100 mg propofol (10 ml) is diluted to total volume of 66 ml (final concentration 2 mg/ml).
2. Using calibrated drip chamber so that
   60 drops = 1 ml
   2 drops/kg/min = 50 μg/kg/min

---

anesthesiologist is meticulous in monitoring and stops the scan if there is concern that the patient is not breathing adequately or has inadequate airway.

The need for the constant presence of an observer in the scanning room is controversial. The anesthesiologist must be certain that observation by monitors is adequate to assess the patient if there is no observer present in the scanning room. Concern has been raised about the potential danger of exposure to intense electromagnetic fields, but there is not definitive scientific evidence of an adverse effect from exposure to MRI fields.[34]

Recovery from anesthesia should be done in the same manner as it is for other anesthetized patients. The MRI scanner may be located far from the postanesthesia care unit. The anesthesiologist must decide whether it is better to transport the patient to this area for recovery or to develop the capability to recover these patients in the vicinity of the scanner. If recovery is done locally, the same personnel training, equipment, and discharge criteria should be used as that which is used after other anesthetics. Responsibility for discharge from the institution must be delineated.

Cardiac Catheterization

There is an increasing presence of anesthesiologists during cardiac catheterizations, especially for pediatric patients, because cardiologists understand the advantages of a cooperative subject who is cared for by a practitioner other than themselves. This allows the cardiologist to perform longer and more aggressive procedures on sick patients and to concentrate solely on the procedure, knowing that the anesthesiologist is providing sophisticated monitoring and evaluation of the patient.

As with most areas outside the operating room, the catheterization laboratory provides challenges to the anesthesiologist to ensure that there is adequate space, access to the patient, lighting, temperature control, electrical outlets, and radiation protection. However, the two biggest challenges are caring for patients with significant medical disease and interacting and anticipating the special needs of the cardiologist.

Patient Considerations

Providing anesthesia in the cardiac catheterization laboratory is a good example of the challenges we meet outside the operating room that are primarily related to the medical condition of the patient. These patients have heart disease that requires further evaluation, meaning that the anesthesiologist has some uncertainty about the exact anatomic and physiologic status of the patient.[35] Most of these patients have congenital heart disease that may be uncorrected, partially corrected, or repaired at the time of catheterization. These three anatomic conditions can be associated with a wide variety of functional states. Even a patient who has undergone surgical repair can have significant myocardial dysfunction, arrhythmias, pulmonary hypertension, or failure to thrive. The anesthesiologist should be familiar with anesthetic management of patients with these lesions and be comfortable caring for the patient in an environment that is not as well designed for anesthetic care as the operating room. There is sometimes a tendency to send the junior-most staff to give anesthesia in remote locations. When dealing with patients with significant medical disease, it is crucial that the staff be confident and experienced in the care of patients with these conditions. Additionally, only patients with stable cardiac disease should be catheterized as outpatients.

Anesthetic management can significantly alter the hemodynamics of a patient with congenital heart disease.[35,36] The anesthesiologist must have a clear understanding of the patient's current clinical status and probable anatomic lesion, as well as the likely consequences of anesthetic agents. Although a provisional evaluation based on clinical examination and echocardiography is made before the catheterization, the practitioner must be aware that the working diagnosis may not fully define the patient's pathophysiologic state. The preanesthetic evaluation is performed primarily to determine the functional status of the patient.[35] This includes identifying the probable anatomic lesion, the presence and magnitude of shunting, arrhythmias, dynamic or fixed obstruction or valvular insufficiency, adequacy of current cardiac output, and recent changes in the patient's exercise tolerance. Obtaining information about medications, allergies, previous anesthetic experiences, and other medical problems is also an important part of the evaluation. The anesthetic evaluation and preparation are the same as that done when preparing a patient for surgery in the operating room. Consultation with the cardiologist is useful in determining the patient's current status.

After assessing and preparing the patient, the anesthesiologist administers an anesthetic tailored to the patient's probable anatomic lesion and functional status. Experience has clearly demonstrated that it is possible to provide general anesthesia for virtually all patients safely. A wide variety of anesthetics, such as ketamine, propofol, the narcotics, and the volatile agents, have been used successfully.[35,37] The patient monitoring, evaluation, and management that is done by experienced practitioners is more important than the specific agents chosen. However, some anesthetic agents may be better suited to an individual patient, depending on his or her anatomic lesion, degree of shunting, and reserve. Careful titration of agents, coupled with meticulous monitoring and evaluation, are the basis of successful management. Although the anesthetic technique used for the eventual

---

Box 10-12 Cardiac Catheterization Considerations

Nonanesthesia personnel
Blood loss
Dysrhythmias
Effect of anesthesia on measured hemodynamic parameters

---

cardiac repair may be used for the catheterization, it is desirable to have the patient awake and extubated at the end of the procedure.

Catheterization Considerations

During the cardiac catheterization, there are certain matters that the anesthesiologist should understand (Box 10-12). The cardiologist, who often works without other physicians present, may not be familiar with direct communication with other physicians. There should be a continual exchange between the anesthesiologist and the cardiologist so that both understand the other's concerns. For instance, the cardiologist may cause considerable blood loss from cannulation of femoral vessels and withdrawal of samples. The anesthesiologist needs to keep close track of this loss and anticipate the need for transfusion. The cardiologist may not understand the hemodynamic consequences of dysrhythmias during anesthesia, since these do not have the same significance in the nonanesthetized patient. Finally, the measurement of pressures and saturations in the heart can be altered by the anesthetic. Enriched oxygen can invalidate shunting and pulmonary artery pressure studies, while volatile agents, hyperventilation, and muscle relaxants can change baseline values for heart rate, rhythm, and myocardial contractility. These matters should be discussed with the cardiologist as the case proceeds.

There are several exciting new developments in cardiac catheterization. These procedures are more likely to be done on an inpatient or 23-hour observation basis. Radiofrequency ablation of accessory pathways is a new technique that requires a prolonged catheterization and rhythm evaluation.[38] Conduction pathways can be altered by anesthetic agents, making induction of dysrhythmias difficult. The anesthesiologist may have to change the technique to provide optimal conditions for the study and ablation.

There is also interest in balloon dilation of stenotic pulmonary and aortic valves, as well as aortic coarctations.[39,40] These procedures produce a short, sudden cessation of blood flow during the expansion of the balloon and may result in significant disruptions in forward flow and subsequent hypotension. This brief period of absent cardiac output is usually well tolerated, but malignant arrhythmias or cardiac decompensation may occur in some patients, such as the infant with aortic stenosis and a small left ventricle. Although rupture is a rare complication, it can occur. Because of the potential for difficulty, the anesthesiologist must be prepared to deal with the range of complications quickly and efficiently; cardiostimulatory medications must be immediately available at the time of dilation.

Another potentially useful procedure is transcatheter closures of septal defects, patent ductus arteriosus, and the fenestrated Fontan using a clamshell-like umbrella device.[41] Two joined plastic umbrellas are introduced through the femoral sheath and positioned on either side of the septal defect. After ensuring proper placement by transesophageal echocardiography or fluoroscopy, the umbrellas are locked together, obliterating the defect. Complications have included dysrhythmias, significant cardiac decompensation, and embolism of the umbrellas. This procedure may become an important method of closing defects without the use of cardiopulmonary bypass.

As with anesthesia in other areas, it is useful to design the anesthetic technique to allow rapid awakening. Although most children stay in the facility after catheterization, some may be discharged. As with other remote surgical locations, it must be decided whether to transport the patient to the postanesthesia care unit or to establish a recovery facility closer to the catheterization lab.

Electroconvulsive Therapy

Electroconvulsive therapy (ECT) is used in the treatment of patients with affective disorders (e.g., depression) and schizophrenia. A grand mal seizure is induced by electrical current, and this seizure is accompanied by a wide range of cardiac and respiratory side effects. The duration of the seizure has been thought to be a determinant of effectiveness, with 30 seconds considered a minimum. However, this has been challenged.[42] There are several anesthetic considerations for patients having this procedure.[43]

The grand mal seizure starts with a short tonic phase, followed by a clonic phase. Initially there is vagally mediated bradycardia and hypotension, followed by several minutes of sympathetically mediated tachycardia and hypertension. This may be accompanied by significant dysrhythmias, myocardial ischemia, and, rarely, myocardial failure. There may also be apnea, hypoventilation, and increased cerebral blood flow and pressure in this period. Because clinical depression is more common in the elderly, these patients have reduced functional reserve to withstand the dramatic changes in hemodynamics during ECT. Their medical status, with an emphasis on the cardiac system, should be clear before administering anesthesia.

Before undergoing ECT, the patient should be questioned about the use of psychotropic medications. Tricyclic antidepressants and monoamine oxidase (MAO) inhibitors have significant anesthetic significance. They affect not only adrenergic tone, but also the response to sympathomimetic drugs. Because of the cardiac effects of lithium therapy, it has been suggested that patients should be off lithium therapy before receiving ECT. Because of the increase in cerebral blood flow, ECT should not be done on patients with intracranial masses.[44]

The goal of anesthetic management is to prevent injury, such as fractures, during the seizure; to provide amnesia but rapid emergence; to control the airway and ventilation; and to treat significant cardiovascular disturbances. After preoxygenation, a short-acting anesthetic (a barbiturate) and succinylcholine is usually administered to provide anesthesia and prevent injury from muscle spasms. Methohexital (0.5 to 1.0 mg/kg) is often preferred because of its short length of action. The associated hypertension commonly requires treatment, especially in patients with cardiovascular disease. A short-acting beta blocker or direct vasodilator is usually sufficient for this purpose. The use of propofol has been met with favor, despite concerns about shorter seizure duration.[45-51] It may be particularly useful for ambulatory ECT. However, recovery may be more influenced by the postictal state than by the anesthetic agent. Postanesthetic care should be given in the same manner as it is to other patients receiving general anesthesia.

Lithotripsy

The technique of lithotripsy as a noninvasive surgical approach for the disintegration of both urinary tract and biliary tract stones has gained wide acceptance. Over the past decade, the approach to the management of urinary tract stones has changed from their open removal from the kidney and the ureter, to the application of ultrasound for their disintegration, as well as laser removal of the stones from the ureter.[52,53] Placement of stents to maintain ureteral patency following removal of calculi or dilation of strictures has proven to be another great advancement in ureterolithotomy. The majority of renal calculi can now be managed by extracorporeal shock wave lithotripsy (ESWL), which may be considered the treatment of choice for renal stones smaller than 2 cm and for the majority of ureteral calculi, with success rates approaching 80% to 90%. The majority of these procedures are done on an ambulatory basis.

The principal underlying ESWL is the application of generated high pressure shock waves to the flank focused on the target stone. The shock wave is repeated several thousand times causing the stone to disintegrate. All lithotriptors share four main features (Box 10-13): an energy source, a focusing device, a coupling medium, and a stone localization system. The earlier form of ESWL provided by the original Dornier HM3 utilized a spark plug energy generator and required patients to be submerged in a hydraulically operated chair-like support. The water bath acted as the coupling medium to transmit the shock waves to the patient, with stone localization provided by biplanar fluoroscopy. Although the basic principles of shock wave lithotripsy remain unchanged, modifications of the four basic components of the first-generation lithotriptor have provided a class of second-generation lithotriptors, of which there are currently over 10 commercially available machines undergoing trials. Although ESWL is considered a noninvasive procedure, the impact of the shock waves at the entry site may cause a sharp stinging pain or visceral pain. While single low-impulse shock waves are easily tolerated, administration of multiple shocks requires anesthetic

---

Box 10-13 *Components of Lithotriptors*

Energy source
Focusing device
Coupling medium
Stone localization system

drugs. Because of the modification to shock waves generation, focusing devices, coupling medium, and stone localization system, some form of analgesia, sedation, or local anesthesia is usually required with the majority of second-generation electrohydraulic lithotriptors.[54] As the shock wave pressure (power) and focal region of the second-generation machines have been reduced, so has the requirement for anesthesia or analgesia. However, the price paid for anesthesia-free lithotripsy is a reduction in stone fragmentation efficiency. Thirty percent of patients treated with the second-generation lithotriptors may require a second treatment. To achieve an anesthesia-free status, one must expect the number of secondary treatments to increase and the efficiency of that lithotriptor to be diminished.[52]

Complications

Effectiveness of treatment is determined by eradication of calculus with minimal number and severity of complications. Complications of ESWL have been reported to occur in less than 3% of all cases and include medical problems (e.g., myocardial infarction, pulmonary embolism, congestive failure); nausea, pain, or fever; ureteral obstruction with colic and infection; perirenal hematoma, and urosepsis.[55] In addition, hemorrhagic blisters of the skin and the area where the shock waves enter and leave the body can occur, as well as edema of the kidney and bleeding into the renal pelvis or calices. There is an 8% incidence of new-onset hypertension reported; the etiology is unknown. Cardiac complications include arrhythmias (e.g., benign supraventricular and ventricular premature beats). The possibility of ventricular tachycardia or fibrillation by shock waves placed in the vulnerable period of the ECG led to the development of technology by which the shock wave is linked to the R wave of the ECG: The shock waves are delayed to avoid the vulnerable period of the cardiac cycle. The newer second-generation lithotriptors have further reduced these complications.[55]

Anesthetic Techniques

Newer lithotriptors require little or no anesthesia as shock-wave pain is reduced by lower voltage and a broader shock entry site pattern.[56] However, some patients still experience deep visceral pain and require intravenous sedation or analgesia. In addition, patients presenting for repeat ESWL may already have experienced the procedure under a certain anesthetic technique and be highly anxious. Patients requiring multiple anesthetics for repeated treatments and stent procedures related to ESWL may benefit from the use of continuous infusion techniques involving a combination of a short-acting analgesics (alfentanil or fentanyl), a sedative-hypnotic (propofol), and anxiolytics/amnestics (midazolam).[57] Monk et al. compared two intravenous sedation-analgesic outpatient lithotripsy techniques (midazolam/alfentanil and fentanyl/propofol) with continuous epidural anesthesia.[58] Both intravenous sedation techniques produced satisfactory analgesia, with mean anesthesia and recovery times significantly shorter than epidural anesthesia. In another study by the same researchers, sedative infusions of alfentanil and ketamine to supplement midazolam were both found to be acceptable techniques, with the alfentanil group having a shorter discharge time, more successful fragmentation, and fewer periods of confusion and disruptive movements than the ketamine group.[59] However, alfentanil infusion was associated with more periods of oxygen desaturation, itching, and intraoperative recall. The incidence of nausea was similar. Spinal and epidural anesthesia,[60] and intercostal blocks[61] have been used in this setting. EMLA (eutectic mixture of local anesthesia) has also been evaluated. Variability in the success of EMLA cream compared to a placebo[62,63] or lidocaine infiltration[64] have been reported; however, this may be due to differences in the models of lithotriptors used. EMLA must be applied at least 45 to 60 minutes before the procedure for adequate onset of dermal analgesia.

The lithotriptor and fluoroscopy do not interfere with the anesthesia machine or equipment; however, they force the patient to become positioned a distance from the anesthesiologist. Therefore, infusion pumps, supplemental nasal oxygen, precordial stethoscopes, blood pressure cuffs, ECG leads, capnography, and other equipment will require that sufficient extension tubing be used to reach the patient. Immersion-type lithotriptors, which are used less frequently, are associated with potential access problems because only the patient's head and arms are above the water level. Immersion itself is associated with compression of peripheral blood vessels, and subsequent increase in cardiac preload may be poorly tolerated in patients with cardiovascular disease. If a continuous epidural technique is used, fixation and sterility of the catheter site is of concern. More importantly, if vasodilation occurs secondary to the regional block, there can be a sudden decrease in preload and blood pressure during immersion because of the removal of compression of peripheral vessels.[54] During the procedure, the patient is repositioned constantly as fluoroscopy or ultrasonography is utilized to check the success of the stone disintegration. If fluoroscopy is used, exposure of the patient and staff to ionizing radiation becomes a hazard. Easy access to the patient, intravenous fluids and the applied monitors, and adequate ventilation and circulation should be ensured.

Miscellaneous Procedures

Other medical and surgical procedures, such as bronchoscopy, gastrointestinal endoscopy, and emergency room procedures may require anesthesia services. General principles of monitored care or general anesthesia as discussed below may be applied to any setting, provided that policies are in place and that the roles of the various providers are understood. In addition, open communication between the physicians, nurses, and ancillary personnel is vital for the provision of safe, high-quality services.

Sedation, Monitored Anesthetic Care, and Anesthesia for Minor Procedures

Applicable Techniques

There is increasing recognition of the benefits of analgesia and sedation for diagnostic and therapeutic procedures. In the past, both the analgesic and sedative needs of patients, especially children, have been underappreciated. In an effort to provide humane but safe patient care, a wide variety of drugs and techniques have been used. For instance, local anesthetic field blocks, local infiltration, and regional blocks are easy to administer, have a short duration, and are relatively safe. However, many patients require additional sedation to comfortably withstand the procedure. Although there is increased appreciation of the benefits of sedation of patients for minor procedures and studies, there is also recognition of the potential dangers of sedation. Practitioners have asked their anesthesia colleagues for help with both choice of drugs and recommendations on how to provide analgesia and sedation safely. Anesthesiologists can have a positive impact on the care of both adults and children in their facility by helping to institute reasonable practices. Guidelines and techniques for sedation are discussed in more detail in Chapter 9.

Universal Guidelines for Sedation

Anesthesiologists approach monitored anesthesia care with the same rational approach that they use with patients scheduled for general or regional anesthesia. It is second nature for anesthesiologists to evaluate and prepare patients, institute proper monitoring, titrate medication to effect, and ensure proper recovery before discharge. However, these basics of the anesthesiologist's approach are not necessarily appreciated by other clinicians who may provide sedation.[65] The anesthesia staff can have an important role in making sedation safer by participating in the development of institutional guidelines for sedation administration.[66] Guidelines that promote proper patient evaluation, monitoring, and documentation are powerful tools for improving care of these patients. The anesthesia staff may participate in setting medication dosage regimens, but the focus should be on patient evaluation and monitoring, which can have a significant impact on recovery.

There are several organizations that have developed standards and guidelines for sedating patients. The anesthesia staff can use these as a basis when assisting its institution to develop its own. An example of a published program that can be used as a resource is the 1992 version of sedation guidelines published by the American Academy of Pediatrics (AAP) (Box 10-14).[2] These guidelines are specifically tailored to the pediatric patient but have many elements that will be part of any guidelines, whether pediatric or adult.

In these guidelines, a distinction is made between conscious sedation and deep sedation, with conscious sedation considered a state of depressed consciousness in which the patient retains a patent airway and protective reflexes, and is arousable by verbal command or physical stimulation. Deep sedation is considered a state from which the patient is not easily aroused or does not maintain an adequate airway. Although the distinction is made in the guidelines, sedation can vary over the course of a procedure to encompass either state.

Some of the elements of the AAP guidelines should be considered for all patients. Equipment that *must* be available

Box 10-14 *Guidelines for Monitoring and Management*

Resuscitation cart
Oxygen source
Positive-pressure oxygen-delivery system that can deliver
    at least 90% oxygen for at least 60 minutes
Suction
Monitors:
    Continuous measurement of O_2 saturation, heart rate
    Intermittent respiratory rate
    Blood pressure
Person other than the one performing the procedure to
    monitor the patient
Documentation of vital signs and medication
Preanesthesia evaluation
Informed consent
Recovery parameters
Discharge instructions

Based on American Academy Pediatrics Guidelines Committee on Drugs:
American Academy of Pediatrics. Pediatrics 1992; 89:1110-15.

on-site includes a resuscitation cart, a source of oxygen, a
positive-pressure oxygen delivery system that can administer at
least 90% oxygen for at least 60 minutes, suction, and monitors.
Continuous measurement of oxygen saturation and heart rate by
pulse oximetry, and intermittent respiratory rate and blood pressure monitoring are required. An additional person should monitor
the patient, and, for patients receiving deep sedation, the monitoring personnel should have that monitoring as their only responsibility. There should be documentation not only of vital signs and
medication given, but also of a presedation health evaluation,
informed consent, recovery parameters, and instructions at discharge to the person responsible for the patient.

These and other guidelines are provided as suggestions for
care, not absolute standards.[67,68] They can be used as a framework
to guide sedation by nonanesthesiologists. When the anesthesia
staff participates in developing its own institution's parameters,
the individual needs of that institution should be incorporated.

It is useful for the anesthesia department to also consider
the circumstances under which it would be best to have an

anesthesiologist involved in sedative care. Often, help is requested after efforts at sedation by another service have failed to provide adequate conditions. It may or may not be reasonable to give additional sedation after multiple doses of drug(s) have already been administered. The anesthesiologist must evaluate the current status of the patient and then decide whether to give additional sedation or to recommend that the procedure be rescheduled. Although some departments may have the flexibility to offer assistance in sedation on short notice, this is often not the case with a busy service. In the latter situation, it is usually possible to help with sedation only when it has been scheduled in advance. By developing close communication between services, it is generally possible to find a mutually acceptable time when an anesthesiologist will be available to assist. Different arrangements that have been adopted by some include regularly scheduled time for services that often request help, involvement of the anesthesia department's acute pain service or intensive care service personnel, provision of a treatment room coverage at a fixed time of the day, or dedication of an otherwise underutilized operating room to patients needing sedation for procedures. Each anesthesia department's involvement in sedative care will be decided on a variety of factors, including frequency of use, complexity of patients' medical status, need for specialized equipment, and flexibility of staff schedules.

Summary

Anesthesiologists are increasingly asked to provide services outside the traditional operating room environment. This is an opportunity to deliver efficient, safe, and humane care for a wide variety of procedures, as well as to increase the recognition of our specialty in areas that previously have had little contact with anesthesiologists.

References

1. Ehrenwerth J, Eisenkraft JB: Anesthesia equipment; principles and applications, St Louis, 1993, Mosby, pp. 521-33.
2. Committee on Drugs, American Academy of Pediatrics: Guidelines for monitoring and management of pediatric patients during and after

sedation for diagnostic and therapeutic procedures. Pediatrics 1992; 89:1110-5.

3. American Society of Anesthesiologists: Standards for basic intra-operative monitoring. In ASA directory of members, Park Ridge, Ill, 1990, ASA, p. 735.

4. Report of the Advisory Committee on the Biological Effects of Ionizing Radiations: The effects on populations of exposure to low levels of ionizing radiation. Division of Medical Sciences, National Academy of Sciences, National Research Council, BEIR III 1980, Washington, D.C., 1980, National Academy Press.

5. Gordon I: Diagnostic imaging in paediatrics, London, 1987, Chapman and Hall, pp. 11-5.

6. National Council on Radiation Protection and Measurements: Limitation of exposure to ionizing radiation. NCRP Report No. 116, Bethesda, Md, 1993, National Council on Radiation Protection and Measurements.

7. Sprengler RF, Cook DH, Clarke EA et al: Cancer mortality following cardiac catheterization. A preliminary follow-up study on 4891 irradiated children. Pediatrics 1983; 71:235-9.

8. Brown TCK, Fisk GC: Anaesthesia for children, ed 2, London, 1992, Blackwell Scientific Publications, pp. 291-300.

9. King BF, Hartman GW, Williamson B et al: Low-osmolality contrast media: a current perspective. Mayo Clinic Proc 1989; 64:976-85.

10. Cohan RH, Dunnick NR, Bashore TM: Treatment of reactions to radiographic contrast material. AJR 1988; 151:263-70.

11. O'Mahoney BJ, Bolsin SNC: Anaesthesia for closed embolisation of cerebral arteriovenous malformations. Anaesth Intensive Care 1988; 16:318-23.

12. Griswold JD, Vacanti FX, Goudsouzian NG: Twenty-three sequential out-of-hospital halothane anesthetics in an infant. Anesth Analg 1988; 67:779-81.

13. Foesel TEH, Schrimer U, Wick C: Repeated rectal methohexitone as the sole anaesthetic agent for radiotherapy. Paediatric Anaesthesia 1992; 2:329-31.

14. Aldridge LM, Gordon NH: Propofol infusions for radiotherapy. Paediatric Anaesthesia 1992; 2:133-7.

15. Martin LD, Pasternak LR, Pudimat MA: Total intravenous anesthesia with propofol in pediatric patients outside the operating room. Anesth Analg 1992; 74:609-12.

16. Fisher DM, Robinson S, Brett CM: Comparison of enflurane, halothane, and isoflurane for diagnostic and therapeutic procedures in children with malignancies. Anesthesiology 1985; 63:647-50.

17. Menon DK, Peden CJ, Hall AS et al: Magnetic resonance for the anaesthetist. Part 1: Physical principles, application, safety aspects. Anaesthesia 1992; 47:240-55.

18. Tobin JR, Spurrier EA, Wetzel RC: Anaesthesia for critically ill children during magnetic resonance imaging. Br J Anaesth 1992; 69:482-6.

19. Gangarosa RE, Minnis JE, Nobbe J et al: Operational safety issues in MRI. Magnetic Resonance Imaging 1987; 5:287-92.

20. Peden CJ, Menon DK, Hall AS et al: Magnetic resonance for the anaesthetist. Part II: Anaesthesia and monitoring in MR units. Anaesthesia 1992; 47:508-17.

21. Kanal E, Shellock FG, Talagala L: Safety considerations in MR imaging. Radiology 1990; 176:593-606.

22. Gold JP, Pulsinelli W, Winchester P et al: Safety of metallic surgical clips in patients undergoing high-field-strength magnetic resonance imaging. Ann Thorac Surg 1989; 48:643-5.

23. Erlebacher JA, Cahill PT, Pannizzo F et al: Effect of magnetic resonance imaging on DDD pacemakers. Am J Cardiol 1986; 57:437-40.

24. Shellock FG, Curtis JS: MR imaging and biomedical implants, materials, and devices: an updated review. Radiology 1991; 180:541-50.

25. Patteson SK, Chesney JT: Anesthetic management for magnetic resonance imaging: problems and solutions. Anesth Analg 1992; 74:121-8.

26. Nixon C, Hirsch NP, Ormerod IEC, Johnson G: Nuclear magnetic resonance: its implications for the anaesthetist. Anaesthesia 1986; 41:131-7.

27. Shellock FG: Monitoring during MRI: an evaluation of the effect of high-field MRI on various patient monitors. Medical Electronics 1986; 17:93-7.

28. Dimick RN, Hedlund LW, Herfkens RJ et al: Optimizing electrocardiographic electrode placement for cardiac-rated magnetic resonance imaging. Invest Radiol 1987; 22:17-22.

29. Barnett GH, Ropper AH, Johnson KA: Physiological support and monitoring of critically ill patients during magnetic resonance imaging. J Neurosurg 1988; 68:246-50.

30. Shellock FG: Monitoring sedated pediatric patients during MR imaging. Radiology 1990; 177:586-7.

31. Cote CJ: Anesthesia outside the operating room. In Coté CJ, Ryan JF, Todres ID, Goudsouzian NG, editors: A practice of anesthesia for infants and children, ed 2, Philadelphia, 1993, WB Saunders, pp. 401-16.

32. Lefever EB, Potter PS, Seeley NR: Propofol sedation for pediatric MRI. Anesth Analg 1993; 76:919-20.

33. Frankville DD, Spear RM, Dyck JB: The dose of propofol required to prevent children from moving during magnetic resonance imaging. Anesthesiology 1993; 79:953-8.

34. Shellock FG: Biological effects of MRI: a clean safety record so far. Diagnostic Imaging 1987; 9:96-101.

35. Salem MR, Hall SC, Motoyama EK: Anesthesia for thoracic and cardiovascular surgery. In Motoyama EK, Davis PJ, editors: Smith's anesthesia for infants and children, ed 5, St Louis, 1990, Mosby, pp. 518-45.

36. Greeley WJ, Bushman GA, Davis DP, Reves JG: Comparative effects of halothane and ketamine on systemic arterial oxygen saturation in children with cyanotic heart disease. Anesthesiology 1986; 65:666-8.

37. Lebovic S, Reich DL, Steinberg LG et al: Comparison of propofol versus ketamine for anesthesia in pediatric patients undergoing cardiac catheterization. Anesth Analg 1992; 74:490-4.

38. Renwick J, Kerr C, McTaggart R, Yeung J: Cardiac electrophysiology and conduction pathway ablation. Can J Anaesth 1993; 40:1053-64.

39. Rao PS: Balloon pulmonary valvuloplasty: a review. Clinical Cardiology 1989; 12:55-74.

40. Choy M, Beekman RH, Rocchini AP et al: Percutaneous balloon valvuloplasty for valvar aortic stenosis in infants and children. Am J Cardiol 1987; 59:1010-3.

41. Hickey PR, Wessel DL, Streitz SL et al: Transcatheter closure of atrial septal defects: hemodynamic complications and anesthetic management. Anesth Analg 1992; 74:44-50.

42. Maletsky BM: Seizure duration and clinical effect in electroconvulsive therapy. Compr Psychiatry 1978; 19:541-50.

43. Baines GY, Rees DI: Electroconvulsive therapy and anesthetic considerations. Anesth Analg 1986; 65:1345-56.

44. Barash PG, Cullen BF, Stoelting RK: Clinical anesthesia, ed 2, Philadelphia, 1992, JB Lippincott, pp. 1165-6.

45. Rampton AJ, Griffin RM, Stuart CS et al: Comparison of methohexital and propofol for electroconvulsive therapy: effects of hemodynamic responses and seizure duration. Anesthesiology 1989; 70:412-7.

46. Mitchell P, Torda T, Hickie I, Burke C: Propofol as an anaesthetic agent for ECT: effect on outcome and length of course. Aust NZ J Psych 1991; 25(2):255-61.

47. Simpson KH, Snaith RP: The use of propofol for anaesthesia during ECT. Br J Psychiatry 1989; 154:721-2.

48. Boey WK, Lai FO: Comparison of propofol and thiopentone as anesthetic agents for electroconvulsive therapy. Anaesthesia 1990; 45:623-8.

49. Dwyer R, McCaughey W, Lavery J et al: Comparison of propofol and methohexitone as anaesthetic agents for electroconvulsive therapy. Anaesthesia 1988; 43:459-62.

50. McCall WV, Shelp FE, Weiner RD: Effects of labetalol on hemodynamics and seizure duration during ECT. Convulsive Ther 1991; 7:5-14.

51. Howie MB, Black HA, Zvara D et al: Esmolol reduces autonomic hypersensitivity and length of seizures induced by electroconvulsive therapy. Anesth Analg 1990; 71:384-8.

52. Koch M: Therasonics lithotripsy system. Sem Urol 1991; 9(4):275-8.

53. Wilson WT, Preminger GM: Update on urinary stone disintegration. Urol Clin North Am 1990; 17:231-42.

54. Mazze RI: Anesthesia and the renal and genitourinary systems. In Miller RD, editor: Anesthesia, ed 3, New York, 1990, Churchill Livingstone, pp. 1804-5.

55. Roth RA, Beckmann F: Complications of extracorporeal shock-wave lithotripsy and percutaneous nephrolithotomy. Urol Clin North Am 1988; 15:155-66.

56. Pettersson B, Tiselius HG, Andersson A, Eriksson I: Evaluation of extracorporeal shock wave lithotripsy without anesthesia using a Dornier HM3 lithotriptor without technical modifications. J Urol 1989; 142:1189-92.

57. Freilich JD, Brull SJ, Schiff S: Anesthesia for lithotripsy: efficacy of monitored anesthesia care with alfentanil. Anesth Analg 1990; 70:S115.

58. Monk G, Boure B, White PF et al: Comparison of intravenous sedative analgesic techniques for outpatient immersion lithotripsy. Anesth Analg 1991; 72:616-21.

59. Monk TG, Rater JM, White PF: Comparison of alfentanil and ketamine infusions in combination with midazolam for outpatient lithotripsy. Anesthesiology 1991; 74:1023-8.

60. Zeitlin GL, Roth R: Effects of three anesthetic techniques on the success of extracorporeal shock wave lithotripsy in nephrolithiasis. Anesthesiology 1988; 68:272-6.

61. Malhotra V, Long CW, Meister MJ: Intercostal blocks with local infiltration anesthesia for extracorporeal shock wave lithotripsy. Anesth Analg 1987; 66:85-8.

62. Bierkens AF, Maes RM, Hendrikx AJM et al: The use of local anesthesia in second generation extracorporeal shock wave lithotripsy: a study comparing eutectic mixture of local anesthetics cream and lidocaine infiltration. J Urol 1991; 146:287-9.

63. Monk TG, Ding Y, White PF et al: Effect of topical EMLA on pain response and analgesic requirements during lithotripsy procedures. Anesth Analg 1994; 79:506-11.

64. McDonald PF, Berry AM: Topical anaesthesia for extracorporeal shock wave lithotripsy. Br J Anaesth 1992; 69:399-400.

65. Fisher DM: Sedation of pediatric patients: an anesthesiologist's perspective. Radiology 1990; 175:613-5.

66. Coté CJ: Sedation for the pediatric patient: a review. Ped Clin North Am 1994; 41:31-58.

67. Fleischer D: Monitoring the patient receiving conscious sedation for gastrointestinal endoscopy: issues and guidelines. Gastrointestinal Endoscopy 1989; 35:262-6.
68. Feldscot AF: The new regulations on conscious sedation. NY State Dent J 1989; 55:8-10.

Postanesthesia Care Recovery and Management

Patricia A. Kapur

Anesthesia for same-day surgical patients is conducted in a variety of clinical situations. Ambulatory patients may be fully integrated with inpatients in the main operating rooms of a full-service hospital, handled in segregated operating rooms within a hospital, or cared for in a separate hospital-affiliated or freestanding building. Just as these arrangements affect patient selection and the types of surgery offered, they also affect recovery management. The following discussion will focus on generic aspects of postanesthesia care for the ambulatory patient that must be adapted for individual institutional circumstances.

Ambulatory Recovery Area Design and Function

Physically, a recovery unit for ambulatory anesthesia usually consists of an acute care recovery area (the postanesthesia care unit [PACU]) and a secondary recovery area (stepdown recovery area [SRA], short-stay recovery unit, and predischarge area). Ideally, the PACU and SRA are adjacent to each other and to the operating rooms so that anesthesiology staff are available for consultation and supervision during the recovery and discharge processes. This is not always possible when architectural modifications have been made to accommodate ambulatory patients within a full-service hospital. The patient intake area or the SRA may be distant from the operating rooms and PACU, perhaps even on another floor. Several inefficiencies result from this physical separation. First, there is a tendency for over-utilization of the PACU when patients are not moved as quickly to the SRA area (which has a lower staffing ratio) because the patient's physiological stability must be certain before he or she is moved to a remote area. Second, staff cannot be shifted between the PACU and SRA to compensate for changes in patient demand that occur throughout the course of the day. Finally, duplication of supplies and equipment may be necessary so that a remote SRA is independently equipped for rare postoperative complications.

Postanesthesia Care Unit

An ambulatory anesthesia PACU looks similar to any other PACU. If the ambulatory PACU is not integrated with that of a full-service hospital, options for treating the full range of postoperative complications must be provided and include cost-effective treatments for support of an occasional unstable patient until transfer to an acute care facility can take place. The PACU must be equipped to provide postoperative physiological monitoring for all patients, and backup supplies for invasive hemodynamic monitoring must be available if needed. Because the latter are rare-use items in the ambulatory setting, components can be stored together and in-service should be conducted at regular intervals so that staff maintain their familiarity and skills. Cardiac pacemaking capability is another rare need that must be considered. External pacing devices, including combined defibrillator/external pacing units or transesophageal pacing catheters,[1,2] are alternatives to transvenous pacemakers or pacing pulmonary artery catheters. A cardiac arrest cart is mandatory. However, to minimize duplicate stocking of rarely used cardiac medications (e.g., secondary antiarrhythmic drugs), the cart can be considered the principle source for these medications when needed, even in the absence of a cardiac arrest.

The ambulatory PACU also must address the respiratory care of the postoperative patient. Supplies and equipment are available for reintubation, oxygen delivery and humidification, and inhaled and nebulized medication delivery. A plan should be in place in case a patient needs prolonged postoperative mechanical ventilation. An intensive care unit ventilator is not mandatory. The plan could be manual ventilation until transfer to a better-equipped facility, or utilization of a back-up anesthesia machine with its ventilator.

Secondary Recovery Area

The SRA may share a space with the preoperative preparation area for ambulatory surgical patients, or it may be a separate area. By and large, patients are physiologically stable, awake, and oriented in the SRA. When the patient arrives in the SRA, a postoperative pain control plan should have already been initiated, and the intravenous catheter should still be in place. Nurse-to-patient ratios are lower in the SRA than in the PACU. It is frequently common to allow the family to participate in the secondary recovery process, during which time the patient is usually semirecumbent or sitting in a lounge-type chair. Activities such as nutrition, voiding, ambulation, dressing, and predischarge instruction are all carried out in the SRA. Staff must be prepared to treat the nausea and emesis that may occur in the setting of the SRA, and to continue to evaluate patients for late development of postoperative complications.

Extended Observation Unit

Physical design of ambulatory surgery facilities may now also incorporate space adjacent to the recovery areas for an extended observation unit (EOU). The EOU extends the recovery process in order to offer the benefits of ambulatory anesthesia and surgery techniques to a broader range of patients. Extended observation, per se, is not intended to substitute for a full-service hospital admission, but rather to offer skilled nursing observation for medically stable patients who may not be able to return home immediately because of postsurgical requirements such as continued parenteral analgesic therapy, unresolved nausea, or additional time for restricted movement to prevent hematoma formation. Extended observation may extend up to 24 hours after surgery, and it consists of limited services, most often at the level of surgical ward care. Patients who require care for medical instability (e.g., angina pectoris or bronchospasm) and patients with postsurgical conditions that require higher levels of care (e.g., potential airway obstruction or continued postsurgical bleed-ing) should be admitted to a full-service hospital.

Third-party insurance reimbursement for EOU care is variable and may depend on the surgical procedure or other justifiable indication. For specific procedures, EOU care may be favored over a full-service hospital admission (e.g., anterior cruciate ligament repair or superficial parotidectomy). At some facilities, postsurgical recovery care is available for up to 3 days following an operative procedure. This is most easily accomplished in a subdivided area of a full-service hospital. Freestanding recovery care centers have to evaluate individual state licensing regulations carefully if extension of patient care beyond 24 hours is contem-plated.

Transport Capability

All ambulatory surgery facilities must have complete plans in place to transport patients to a location where they may receive an increased level of care. This may involve stabilizing the patient's condition at the ambulatory center before transport, or transport-ing the patient emergently to a higher-level facility. The patient may need urgent additional surgery that may be better performed at a full-service facility. Alternatively, the patient may need transport for continued care of a postsurgical sequela or newly developed medical instability. All staff should be current in their knowledge of transport protocols.

Criteria-Based Recovery

The concept of criteria-based recovery triaging is an evolutionary development that has emerged along with the availability of short-acting anesthetic agents. As compared with arbitrary time-based recovery (where patients stay in each phase of the recovery process for a minimum amount of time), criteria-based recovery allows patients to move through the recovery process at their own speed, determined by their meeting specified criteria for each transition. Patients who have received short-acting anesthetics, who are awake, alert, and responsive, with stable vital signs, who are able to move with minimal assistance, and who have manage-able pain and nausea may pass directly from the operating room to the SRA, or alternatively to the SRA after a brief stay in the PACU. Some centers have eliminated the requirement for a PACU stay for stable patients following monitored anesthesia care, as well as for patients with satisfactory upper-extremity regional blocks or distal lower-extremity blocks, if such patients already meet the PACU discharge criteria before leaving the operating room.

The advantages of criteria-based recovery are obvious in terms of patient throughput in an ambulatory setting. However, reduced utilization of the PACU will only translate into cost savings if utilization of staff and supplies is actually reduced. Furthermore, such a plan will not succeed if long distances between the PACU and the SRA lead to staff reluctance to implement the program fully because of concerns that a patient might need increased attention at a remote SRA soon after arrival from the operating room.

Management of Ambulatory Recovery Issues

Postoperative Pain

The plan for postoperative pain management should be developed and initiated before the patient leaves the operating room. Because the anesthesia practitioner must go on to care for other patients, the recovery staff must have a clear understanding of analgesic protocols and be prepared to treat pain early to optimize recovery time. Narcotics, despite concerns for potential respiratory effects and/or nausea, help to minimize autonomic responses during surgery and to provide postoperative pain relief. Neither propofol nor inhalation anesthetics alone provide patients with good postoperative analgesia. Alfentanil, which has a short half life that provides beneficial altering levels of narcosis during surgery, is too short acting for reasonable postoperative pain control in the absence of a patient-controlled analgesia (PCA) device. The new ultrashort acting opioid, remifentanil, undergoes ester hydrolysis such that continuous delivery by infusion pump may be necessary during transport to the recovery area until the postoperative pain management plan is implemented.[3,4] Following the administration of anesthetics with little or no postoperative analgesic properties, intermediate narcotics such as fentanyl (1 to 2 µg/kg) can be used for immediate pain control in the PACU. Although likely to produce prolonged drowsiness and emetic symptoms, longer-acting narcotics (e.g., dihydromorphine, morphine), may be added if needed. Then a

Table 11-1   Oral Preparations of Opioid and Nonopioid
Analgesic Combinations*

Drug	Duration of action
Acetaminophen/propoxyphene napsylate (Darvocet)	4-6 hours
Acetaminophen/oxycodone (Percocet)	6 hours
Acetaminophen/codeine (Tylenol with codeine)	4 hours
Acetaminophen/hydrocodone (Vicodin)	4-6 hours

*Aspirin and salicylate compounds are not recommended postoperatively.

smooth transition to oral medications (e.g., codeine, oxycodone, hydrocodone, or propoxyphene with or without acetaminophen) should follow by the time the patient is in the SRA (Table 11-1).

Adjuncts to decrease narcotic requirements (see Box 11-1) include local anesthetic infiltration of the surgical site, nonsteroidal antiinflammatory drugs (NSAIDs), regional anesthetics planned to yield residual analgesia,[5] and intraarticular opioids.[6,7] Local anesthetic infiltration at the surgical site can interfere with neuronal wind-up, which amplifies painful signals to the central nervous system, resulting in diminished pain perception beyond the duration of action of the local anesthetic at the peripheral site.[8,9] NSAIDs can be administered orally (e.g., ibuprofen, diclofenac, naproxen) or parenterally (ketorolac 30 to 60 mg) for mild to moderate pain, provided sufficient time is allowed for effects to accrue, subsequent to interference with prostaglandin synthesis.[10] Older, less expensive NSAID preparations are showing promise similar to the newer NSAIDs to reduce narcotic requirements in appropriate patients after ambulatory surgery.[11]

Box 11-1 *Alternatives to Narcotic Analgesics*

Wound infiltration with local anesthetics
Regional anesthetics planned for residual analgesia
Nonsteroidal antiinflammatory drugs
Intraarticular opioids

However, decreased nausea or analgesic requirements, or short-ened discharge times, have not been proven.[12-14] The newer NSAIDs can also trigger so-called "aspirin-induced asthma" in susceptible patients, which may manifest itself during the recovery period (Table 11-2).[15,16]

Regional anesthesia techniques can contribute to a successful plan for the management of postoperative pain (Box 11-2). These may include blocks of the upper extremity or hand, ankle blocks for foot surgery, and intercostal blocks. It is usually not appropriate to instill intrathecal or epidural narcotics for the ambulatory surgical patient who will be returning home, because of the possibility of delayed respiratory sequelae after discharge.

Intraarticular opioids are currently being studied as possible adjuncts for postoperative pain management of patients who have undergone arthroscopic procedures (e.g., 1 to 5 mg of morphine in the knee joint has been evaluated). Intraarticular bupivacaine 0.25% administered before tourniquet release has reportedly provided good postoperative analgesia during the intermediate recovery period. The role of peripheral opioid receptors, interactions with intraarticular local anesthetics, dosages, etc., are all subjects of study.[6,7,17]

New delivery systems for narcotics are also the subject of study and controversy (see Box 11-3). Transdermal, transmucosal, and PCA may all have applications in ambulatory postoperative pain management.[18-20] PCA may be particularly helpful for the management of certain patients with challenging postoperative

---

Box 11-2 *Perioperative Pain Control*: *Common Nerve Blocks*

Wound infiltration
Ilioinguinal-iliohypogastric
Penile and dorsal nerve block
Extremity blocks: Bier, axillary, interscalene, ankle
Spinal
Epidural
Caudal

***Table* 11-2**   Selected Preparations of Nonopioid Analgesics for Adult Outpatient Postoperative Pain Management*

Drug	Dose range	Time to onset (minutes)	Duration of action (hours)
NSAIDs			
Ibuprofen (Advil, Motrin, Nuprin)	400-800 mg PO	30	2-4
Naproxen Sodium (Anaprox)	550 mg PO	60	6-8
Naproxen (Naprosyn)	500 mg PO	60	6-8
Ketorolac (Toradol)	10-20 mg PO 30-60 mg IM/?IV	30-60 15-45	4-6
Ketoprofen (Orudis)	25-50 mg	30	4-6
Diclofenac (Voltaren)	75 mg IM (not available in the United States)	30	4-6
Indomethacin (Indocin)	100 mg rectal suppos. 25-50 mg PO	30	4-6
p-Amino-phenols			
Acetaminophen	500 mg	30	2-4

*This list is not intended to be exhaustive because new compounds become available.

pain problems. Examples include those patients who have had orthopedic procedures such as cruciate ligament repairs or open fixation of fractured bones of the distal extremities who may benefit from the availability of PCA in an extended observation mode.

Box 11-3 Modes of Opioid Delivery

Intravenous with or without PCA
Intramuscular
Oral
Epidural/intrathecal with or without PCA
Transdermal
Transmucosal

Nonpharmacologic methods of treating acute pain postoperatively, including thermal or ice packs, massage, relaxation techniques, and reassurance and transcutaneous electrical nerve stimulation (TENS), have been used with mixed success.

Cardiovascular Alterations

Hypertension

Elevated blood pressure is frequently encountered during the recovery from anesthesia and surgery in patients with good myocardial function.[21] A search should be made for obvious etiologies (see Box 11-4), such as pain, bladder distention, hypoxemia, hypercarbia, agitation, or abrupt preoperative cessation of chronic antihypertensive medications. In patients with prior good health, in the absence of an identified cause, treatment should be approached cautiously because of wide interpatient variability in the response to antihypertensive medications. Patients with a history of chronic hypertension, with or without discernable end-organ damage, need to be treated promptly, taking into account possible pharmacologic interactions of acutely administered drugs with chronic medications. The concern is that, for the at-risk cardiac patient, increased blood pressure may reflect an increased afterload that may cause an imbalance in myocardial oxygen supply and demand. Unless remedied, a spiraling course of cardiac compromise may result.

Treatment of hypertension in the recovering surgical patient consists of either vasodilator or myocardial depressant drugs (see Table 11-3). The former category includes the vasodilating calcium channel blocking drugs in the nifedipine family, as well as the short-acting agents that can be given by intravenous bolus or infusion, such as nitroglycerin or nitroprusside for prolonged or severe hypertension. Beta-adrenergic antagonists may be

---

Box 11-4 Etiology of Postoperative Hypertension

Pain
Bladder distention
Hypoxemia
Hypercarbia
Agitation
Cessation of chronic antihypertensive medications

Box 11-5 Etiology of Hypotension

Reduced myocardial preload
Decreased systemic vascular resistance
Decreased cardiac output

---

employed to lower blood pressure by reducing cardiac output. Esmolol, propranolol, and metoprolol are all available for intravenous administration, though with differences in pharmacokinetic properties and relative cardiac selectivity. Labetalol, a mixed alpha- and beta-adrenergic antagonist with predominant nonselective beta-adrenergic antagonist properties, can be used to treat postoperative hypertension,[22] but also causes a lowered cardiac output. All of the beta-adrenergic antagonists have the potential to exacerbate bronchoconstriction in a dose-dependent manner in individual patients. All beta-adrenergic antagonists should be used with extreme caution in patients with poor ventricular function.

Hypotension

Systemic hypotension is another cause for concern during the recovery period (see Box 11-5). For the appropriate intervention to be undertaken, the etiology of hypotension must be sought among the broad general categories of reduced myocardial preload, decreased systemic vascular resistance, or decreased cardiac output secondary to reduced myocardial performance or dysrhythmias.

Decreased cardiac filling results from insufficient perioperative fluid administration to replace maintenance fluid requirements and surgical losses. Ongoing postoperative blood loss must be one of

Table 11-3 Treatment Modalities for Postoperative Hypertension

Drug	Dose range	$t_{1/2}\beta^*$
β Blockers		
Propranolol (Inderal)	0.5-1.0 mg IV	2-4 hours
Labetalol (mixed α&β) (Trandate, Normodyne)	5-10 mg bolus IV	4-6 hours
Esmolol (β₁ selective) (Brevibloc)	0.25-0.5 mg/kg bolus IV; may be followed by an infusion of 50-200 ug/kg/ min	9 minutes
Metoprolol (β₁ selective) (Lopressor)	5-25 mg IV increments	2.5-4.5 hours
Smooth-muscle Vasodilators		
Hydralazine (Apresoline)	2.5-5.0 mg IV increments	4-6 hours
Nitroglycerin	50-100 μg IV bolus; 0.1 ug/kg/min	
Calcium Channel Blockers		
Nifedipine (Procardia)	10-20 mg PO, SL	4-6 hours
Nicardipine (Cardene)	2.5 mg IV	6 hours
ACE Inhibitors		
Enalapril/ Enalaprilat (Vasotec)	2.5 mg IV	4-6 hours

$^*t_{1/2}\beta$ half-life may not predict clinical duration of action.
Adjust dosing recommendations in presence of impaired renal/liver function.

the considerations when assessing the recovering patient. Residual venodilating effects of anesthetic drugs and adjuvants may exacerbate effects of hypovolemia. Specific treatment includes using the head down position, administering volume resuscitation with appropriate fluids, and making a diligent search for and consideration of possible reoperation to remedy sources of continuing blood loss.

Decreased afterload may result from vasodilating medications or sympathectomy (e.g., residual effects of spinal or epidural anesthesia), or large arteriovenous shunts, hyperthermia, or sepsis (less likely in the ambulatory setting). Vasoconstricting medications may be needed to counter the effects of vasodilators or until the effects of a spinal or epidural anesthetic wane. In the case of severe hypotension in the absence of ongoing myocardial ischemia, myocardial stimulating medications, such as direct- and indirect-acting sympathomimetics, may serve to temporize until the proximate cause of the hypotension can be diagnosed and treated.

Hypotension associated with poor myocardial performance results from inadequate pump function or from arrhythmias that result in impaired chamber filling and/or ejection. Inadequate pump function of the heart may, in turn, be on a chronic or acute basis. Chronically depressed myocardial function would presumably be detected during the prescreening process before anesthesia at an ambulatory center. It would be a factor in determining appropriate patient selection before the procedure is undertaken, because one of the presumptions of ambulatory anesthesia is that patients will be chosen whose chronic medical disease processes will not be significantly worsened by ambulatory anesthesia techniques and, therefore, will not require prolonged postoperative observation for sequelae or for adjustments in medical management.

Acute myocardial pump decompensation during the recovery period typically indicates ongoing myocardial ischemia with decreased perfusion of the affected segment of myocardium. In this situation, reversal of hypotension will result from improving myocardial oxygen supply and demand imbalance, whether by administering a coronary vasodilator such as nitroglycerin or a vasodilating calcium channel blocker; by reducing myocardial-oxygen demand by reducing afterload with a vasodilator or heart rate with a beta-adrenergic antagonist, if the episode was preceded by a high catecholamine state; and/or by improving perfusion pressure per se across coronary arteries if reduced myocardial perfusion precipitated the incident.

Myocardial ischemia may also develop in the absence of measurable hemodynamic alterations, as a result of intrinsic changes in coronary artery vascular tone. Coronary vasoconstriction may occur with or without concomitant obstructive coronary artery disease. The occurrence of unexpected chest pain or unexpected symptoms of congestive heart failure in the postoperative period must be thoroughly evaluated, the former to rule out chest wall or gastrointestinal/esophageal etiologies of parasternal pain and the latter to rule out noncardiogenic causes of pulmonary edema. If a cardiac diagnosis is made, treatment is similar to that for myocardial ischemia. A caveat exists for the specific diagnosis of coronary vasospasm for which beta-adrenergic antagonists are contraindicated (alpha-mediated coronary constriction thus unopposed). Vasodilating calcium channel blockers are the treatment of choice.

The issue inevitably arises whether or not to admit a patient who has experienced a postoperative episode of either hypertension or hypotension to a full-service hospital. There is not one answer that can be applied to all patients. If a discernable cause for the cardiovascular alteration has been identified, and if the patient has responded predictably and promptly to the treatment and has experienced no recurrence or sequelae, discharge to home may be the most appropriate measure. However, patients who have experienced unanticipated cardiovascular instability, who have responded unpredictably to treatment or have required continuous infusion therapy, or who experience repeated episodes or develop secondary symptoms such as a dysrhythmia or chest pain, may well deserve hospital admission for observation and further treatment.

Rhythm disturbances

Rhythm disturbances in the postoperative period may be the cause or result of impaired cardiac performance (see Box 11-6). In all cases of rhythm disturbances, adequacy of respiration must be assessed to rule out and/or treat hypoxia or hypercarbia as an inciting cause of the dysrhythmia. Dysrhythmias associated with myocardial ischemia are treated primarily by improving myocardial oxygen supply or reducing myocardial oxygen demand, as

Box 11-6 Etiology of Dysrhythmias in the
          Postoperative Period

Hypoxia/hypercarbia
Myocardial ischemia
Electrolyte imbalance
Drug toxicity
Excessive catecholamine activity
Breakthrough chronic dysrhythmias upon cessation of
    chronic antiarrhythmic medications

indicated by clinical assessment, to prevent the development of
malignant ventricular arrhythmias. Definitive treatment of dysryth-
mias associated with electrolyte imbalance, drug toxicity, or
excessive catecholamine activity requires treatment of the underlying cause. Bradyarrhythmias, in the absence of hypoxia, hypercarbia, or other treatable causes, are treated to prevent potential
compromise of vital organ perfusion, with an anticholinergic drug,
such as atropine, a beta$_1$ agonist, or by cardiac pacing. Resurgence
of chronic arrhythmias when medication levels wane (e.g., chronic
atrial fibrillation) requires acute treatment and reestablishment of
therapeutic drug levels by resumption of the chronic medication
regimen.

Management of Chronic Cardiac Medications

The main types of cardiovascular disease encountered in the
ambulatory surgical population will be stable hypertensive cardiovascular disease, ischemic cardiovascular disease, or valvular
abnormalities, including mitral valve prolapse. In general the
surgical procedure will not be related to the patient's cardiovascular diagnosis. Patients should continue taking their cardiac
medications until the time of surgery and then reinstitute the
medications following surgery. Since many perioperative phar-
macy areas do not carry a wide array of oral medications, patients
should be instructed to bring their daily chronic medications with
them so that doses can be administered as closely on schedule as
possible after surgery. If nausea and/or vomiting is a problem

postoperatively, other plans must be made to afford the patient uninterrupted pharmacologic control of the cardiovascular problem. Topical preparations are available for some medications, such as nitrates and clonidine, though in the latter case time is required for effective plasma levels to be obtained. Nifedipine may be administered sublingually. Some drugs such as digoxin or nadolol are given at long intervals and can be administered before surgery for that day's dose. With other drugs, intravenous substitutions may be administered if oral intake is temporarily precluded postoperatively.

Oral antiarrhythmic drugs of particular note are tocainide, mexilitine, encainide, flecainide, and amiodarone, which are all indicated for the management of ventricular arrhythmias. Tocainide and mexilitine have pharmacodynamic and toxicity profiles similar to lidocaine. Encainide and flecainide may depress cardiac contractile function, and flecainide, in particular, may even potentiate certain dysrhythmias. Amiodarone has beta-blocking, calcium-blocking, and thyroid hormone–interfering properties. It can cause eye, skin, and pulmonary problems and has an extremely long half life (weeks to months). Because of the serious nature of the arrhythmias for which these medications are prescribed, they should be continued throughout the perioperative period. Serious consideration should be given to whether patients with indications for these medications need to be observed longer postoperatively than is afforded by the usual protocols.

Nausea and Emesis

Perioperative nausea and emesis is the most common overall postoperative complication in adults and children.[23,24] A preliminary report by Orkin[25] indicated that, given the choice, individuals would choose to have more pain, somnolence, etc., if only they were not nauseated postoperatively. Despite resolution of numerous other surgical and anesthesia sequelae, nausea and emesis can unduly postpone discharge and even result in unanticipated admission.[26] Clearly, the causes of perioperative nausea and emesis are multifactorial, including age, gender, time of the menstrual cycle, early pregnancy, history of motion sickness, obesity, increased gastric volume, administration of narcotics or inhaled anesthetics, specific procedures (e.g., laparoscopy, strabismus repair), pain, and so forth.[27]

Because no entirely satisfactory pharmaceutical agent exists as yet for the reliable prevention of nausea and emesis, most centers do not routinely administer prophylactic antiemetics to all ambulatory patients. Drowsiness, extrapyramidal effects, and a sense of dysphoria after dopamine antagonists, dry mouth and blurred vision after the scopolamine patch, and high cost for newer agents such as ondansetron, for example, have meant that nausea prophylaxis is usually reserved for patients perceived to be at a higher risk for its occurrence because of past history or a specific proposed procedure.[27] Various alterations in anesthetic technique may have been incorporated before the recovery period in attempts to minimize postoperative nausea and emesis (e.g., include propofol;[28-30] avoid nitrous oxide, potent inhalation agents, and/or narcotics; or provide adjunctive methods for postoperative pain management to minimize narcotic use). Adequate hydration of ambulatory surgical patients is important because nausea can also result from postural hypotension,[27] which frequently occurs when the patient stands to move to a chair, to dress, or to void.

If nausea or emesis ensues in the postoperative period, parenteral therapy may be given (Table 11-4). Examples of the range of drugs with antiemetic activity include the dopamine antagonist, droperidol; the benzamide, metoclopramide; the phenothiazine, prochlorperazine; the antihistamine, hydroxyzine; and the new serotonin antagonists exemplified by the first available agent in that class, ondansetron.[27,31-33] Antiemetics are also available in rectal suppository form, such as prochlorperazine. The scopolamine patch marketed for the treatment of motion sickness may be effective in some patients when applied sufficiently in advance of the procedure.[34] Unfortunately, none of these drugs are completely effective in every patient. Reports using propofol (10 to 15 mg IV)[35] and ephedrine (25 to 50 mg IM) have met with mixed results.

Airway and Pulmonary Complications

Pulmonary sequelae of anesthesia and surgery may include atelectasis, bronchospasm, croup, or aspiration. Fortunately, many ambulatory procedures are of reasonably short duration such that atelectasis is rarely tabulated as an ambulatory surgery complication. Reduced functional residual capacity may, however, compromise respiratory sufficiency during recovery in patients such as the supine obese patient, the advanced pregnant patient, and the patient nursed in the head down position.

Bronchospasm

Selected patients with a prior known history of stable, well-controlled bronchospastic disease can be safely cared for on an

Table 11-4 Postoperative Antiemetic Therapy

Drug	Dose	Side effects
Butyrophenones		
Droperidol (Inapsine)	0.625-1.25 mg IV, IM	Extrapyramidal effects, dysphoria, drowsiness, dizziness
Phenothiazines		
Prochlorperazine (Compazine)	5-10 mg IV, IM, PO; 25 mg rectal suppos.	Sedation, drowsiness, hypotension
Antihistamines (H$_1$ Antagonists)		
Promethazine (a phenothiazine) (Phenergan)	25-50 mg PO, IV 12.5-50 mg rectal suppos.	Sedation
Hydroxyzine (Vistaril)	25-50 mg IV, IM	
Diphenhydramine (Benadryl)	10-50 mg IV, IM, PO	
Benzamides		
Metoclopramide (Reglan)	0.15 mg/kg or 10 mg IV, IM	Extrapyramidal effects, dysphoria, drowsiness, anxiety, dizziness
Trimethobenzamide (Tigan)	100-200 mg IV, IM; 200 mg rectal suppos.	
Anticholinergics		
Scopolamine patch (Transderm Scop)	1.5 mg transdermal	Delayed onset, diplopia, hallucinations, dry mouth
5-HT$_3$ Serotonin Antagonist		
Ondansetron (Zofran)	4-8 mg IV	Headache, dizziness

ambulatory basis. Such patients should be carefully evaluated preoperatively regarding the severity, predictability, and degree of control of their symptoms. Those judged suitable for ambulatory anesthesia and surgery should continue taking their medications up until surgery and bring their inhalers with them to the ambulatory center. An additional dose of inhaled medications may be administered just before moving into the operating room, with inhalers available for additional perioperative doses if needed. Steroid-dependent patients can have a booster dose of intravenous hydrocortisone administered, if indicated. Airway instrumentation should only take place when the patient is thoroughly anesthetized.

In the recovery area, these patients should be carefully assessed for the degree of bronchospasm. Preoperative medication regimens should be reinstituted as soon as practicable. Center personnel should be able to deliver aerosolized bronchodilators by nebulizer, if required. Intravenous theophylline compounds and beta-adrenergic agonists should also be available, and the staff should be comfortable with their use. Persistent postoperative bronchospasm requiring repeated treatments or continuous intravenous therapy may indicate the need for hospital admission for additional observation and treatment.

Postintubation stridor

The prevention of postoperative stridor,[36] particularly in pediatric ambulatory anesthesia patients, requires careful screening for predisposing factors (e.g., prior intubation difficulties, prolonged neonatal intubation with subsequent narrowed airway, recent upper respiratory infection, etc). Care should be taken intraoperatively to ascertain that a slight air leak is present around an endotracheal tube in infants and young children. Recovery staff should be qualified to administer humidified oxygen, dexamethasone, and/or aerosolized racemic epinephrine treatments to pediatric patients, and to resecure an airway at risk of obstruction. Additional postanesthetic observation is indicated, and careful assessment should be made regarding discharge. See Chapter 4 for further discussion of postintubation stridor in pediatrics.

Pulmonary aspiration

With careful patient selection, preoperative preparation, and modern intraoperative precautions, the incidence of pulmonary aspiration is quite low. Aspiration in the presence of oropharyngeal gastric contents or blood may occur at any time during the perioperative period including at the time of tracheal extubation or in the recovery suite. In the latter environment, special attention should be paid to patients with compromised airway reflexes caused by residual anesthetics, sedatives, or narcotics, or in patients with neurologic compromise of the airway for any reason. Some patients at higher risk during the perioperative period include those with hiatal hernia, obesity, pregnancy, upper abdominal surgery, compromised gastroesophageal sphincter function, or recent ingestion of solid foods.[37] It is now recognized that clear liquids are emptied from the normal stomach quite quickly, resulting in shortened preoperative restrictions for clear liquids to as little as 2 hours at some centers.[38,39]

Symptoms and sequelae of pulmonary aspiration are related to the volume, type of fluid, and acid content of the aspirate. The airway should be cleared and oxygenation of the patient assured. Assessment includes chest x-ray, which may or may not show changes early on, and arterial blood gas measurement. If severe aspiration is indicated by a low PaO_2 value, possibly with pulmonary edema, vigorous therapy including mechanical ventilation may be required. If the patient is experiencing no respiratory distress and oxygenation is adequate, the aspiration may have been mild and careful observation to rule out development of a worsening clinical presentation may be all that is required.[40]

Surgical Complications

Surgical complications include postoperative bleeding, more extensive surgery than originally anticipated, or a surgical mishap that requires additional postoperative care (e.g., perforated viscus). These surgical complications are not usually within the capabilities of the anesthesiologist to prevent, although certainly prompt recognition and appropriate supportive measures can contribute to an optimized outcome. Many potential surgical complications have implications for recovery care, including initial identification during the recovery period for complications such as persistent postoperative bleeding.

Several procedures common to the ambulatory arena have their own unique complications. Abdominal insufflation associated with laparoscopy can cause either subcutaneous emphysema that may dissect into the mediastinum or pericardium, or cause pulmonary gas embolism. The main concern during the recovery period for either of these complications is the appropriate ongoing management of any severe cardiopulmonary sequelae, including continued ventilatory and/or inotropic support while awaiting transport to an acute care facility.

Hemodilution syndrome is another complication, which can result from visceral irrigation during transurethral prostate surgery or hysteroscopy. Intravascular absorption of irrigation fluid occurs via prostatic sinuses or from severed uterine venous channels or possibly from peritoneal absorption of irrigation fluid that has passed out the fallopian tubes into the abdominal cavity during hysteroscopy.[41] If dilutional hyponatremia is symptomatic, treatment to restore normal serum sodium levels is based on the patient's central nervous system status and/or current serum sodium level and may require diuresis or intravenous administration of hypertonic saline solutions. Air embolus has also been reported as a complication of hysteroscopy.[42]

Temperature Abnormalities

Hypothermia

Wide changes in patient core temperature are less common with brief ambulatory surgeries. Hypothermia can occur, however, in some longer procedures for which the usual intraoperative supportive measures, including warmed intravenous fluids, humidification of inspired gases, warming blankets of various types, wrapping of extremities, etc., may be helpful to prevent postoperative sequelae,[43] which include excessive metabolic oxygen consumption with the potential to cause increased cardiac output, prolonged time in PACU, and patient discomfort from thermoregulatory shivering. Patients undergoing surgery under monitored anesthesia care with sedation, or regional anesthesia techniques, are very appreciative of efforts to keep them warm in the cold operating room environment.

If lowered core temperature is detected postoperatively, particularly in the presence of shivering, warming lights and blankets are utilized. Small doses of intravenous meperidine, or if it should become available in the United States, intravenous clonidine, may be helpful to reduce shivering.[44,45]

Malignant hyperthermia

As in any center in which anesthetics are administered, ambulatory centers must be able to differentiate causes of elevated

---

Box 11-7 *Minor Complications After Ambulatory Surgery*

Postdischarge nausea
Headache/myalgias
Sore throat/hoarseness
Dizziness/light-headedness
General malaise

---

core temperature, including malignant hyperthermia. Patients at risk for malignant hyperthermia have been safely anesthetized in ambulatory centers, taking the precautions in anesthetic technique recommended for such patients, with an adequate postoperative observation period.[46] Prompt access to dantrolene sodium should be available. Consideration can be given to accessibility of blood gas and/or serum electrolyte determinations for the treatment of this condition if it arises unexpectedly.[47] Diagnosis and management is discussed on pages 465-467.

Minor Complications

In general, ambulatory anesthesia patients and their families expect very little morbidity from their perioperative experience (see Box 11-7). Nevertheless, ambulatory patients may experience one or more of a host of minor complications, including postdischarge nausea, sore throat, hoarseness, myalgias, dizziness/light headedness, general malaise, etc., related to the physiologic trespass of the surgery and related maneuvers. Laparoscopy patients may not recover their general sense of well being for 3 to 5 days postoperatively. Care must be taken throughout the entire perioperative period to prevent other minor complications such as corneal abrasion, dental damage, tape irritation, multiple needle puncture marks, and residual iodinated antiseptic stains after procedure preps.

Resumption of Normal Activities

Influence of Anesthetics and Anesthesia Techniques on Recovery

Anesthetic techniques currently being used for ambulatory anesthesia include monitored anesthesia care or regional anesthesia with or without intravenous sedation and general anesthesia. In ambulatory surgical care, anesthetic cost-saving strategies center on choosing techniques that result in reduced drug acquisition costs versus achieving savings from improved patient flow through the facility. Ambulatory anesthesia settings are certainly one of the areas where justification for the use of newer, albeit more expensive, shorter acting sedative/hypnotic, anesthetic, and muscle-relaxant drugs can reasonably be supported if, indeed, offsetting savings can be achieved. Cost savings from better patient flow can occur from improved efficiency of operating room utilization, from reduced consumption of recovery room supplies and staff when patients have shortened times to return of baseline faculties, and from reduced need for observation and treatment of anesthetic sequelae such as persistent sedation or nausea. Adaptation of full-service hospital recovery facilities to accommodate quick-to-wake up, stable, ambulatory surgery patients may require that systems, procedures, and staffing patterns all be reexamined to truly achieve any fiscal benefits. If, for example, staffing patterns, postoperative monitoring requirements, and mandatory observation times are unchanged from those necessary for the care of critically ill patients, regardless of the more favorable patient recovery profiles of ambulatory patients, savings from the use of more costly short-acting anesthetic drugs will never be realized.

In considering anesthetic drugs, recent studies have compared the newer alternatives for ambulatory anesthesia, specifically desflurane and propofol.[48] While minor differences may be apparent in measures of immediate recovery on the operating table between desflurane and propofol (i.e., eye opening), very little difference—if any—can be shown in overall recovery times, which have been quite prompt in most centers using modern agents for sedation and general anesthesia.[49,50] Desflurane has recently been demonstrated to cause sympathetic nervous system activation when inspired concentrations are increased.[51] This presumably could have implications for the recovery period in higher-risk patients in whom myocardial instability has resulted from precipitous increases in blood pressure and heart rate.

For longer surgeries necessitating general anesthesia, drugs with lower acquisition costs, such as the older, less expensive, longer acting inhalation anesthetics, muscle relaxants, and anticholinest-erase drugs, can be incorporated into combined techniques.

An example could be inducing anesthesia with propofol to avoid prolonged barbiturate effects, maintaining anesthesia with isoflurane, then discontinuing the isoflurane 20 to 30 minutes before the end of the procedure and finishing the anesthetic with propofol so the patient can have the benefits of a quick propofol emergence, as well as the benefit of any residual antiemetic effect from propofol administration.[28-30]

As mentioned previously, various attempts to replace or reduce narcotic utilization (e.g., with NSAIDs) may or may not be associated with reduced nausea and/or emesis and have not necessarily shortened the mean time to patient discharge. As anesthetic techniques improve, small differences in the recovery profiles of the heterogeneous patient populations encountered every day in busy ambulatory surgical centers are difficult to recognize.

In patients who are not at risk for pulmonary aspiration of gastric contents, quality of recovery may be improved by the intraoperative use of the laryngeal mask airway (LMA) (see Box 11-8), particularly when inconvenience or difficult application of a traditional face mask may have been the only indication for endotracheal intubation.[52] The LMA is suitable for the many ambulatory surgical procedures requiring general anesthesia that do not require intraoperative muscle relaxation, for which spontaneous respiration is suitable, and that can be performed in the supine position with potential access to the head and neck throughout the anesthetic. The LMA frees up the anesthesiologist's hands during long cases, avoids endotracheal intubation for procedures in which the practitioner's hand and the face mask would be in the way, is not associated with elevations in intraocular pressure,[53] and eliminates the need to administer muscle relaxants and reversal agents. Sequelae of the latter drugs as well as postoperative morbidity from laryngoscopy (e.g., oropharyngeal injury, dental damage, etc.) are avoided. Progress from the

---

Box 11-8 Benefits of Laryngeal Mask Airway for Recovery

Avoids sequelae of laryngoscopy and tracheal manipulation
May allow lower doses of anesthetic agents
Avoids sequelae of muscle relaxants and reversal agents

intraoperative to the postoperative period proceeds smoothly without a disruptive respiratory transition associated with tracheal extubation. In addition, evidence indicates that an LMA is tolerated by patients at lighter levels of anesthesia than an endotracheal tube,[54] which may contribute to quicker recovery times.

The appropriate use of regional anesthesia techniques has been associated with shorter recovery stays. This is the case particularly when the regional anesthetic incorporates residual pain relief, when the regional block does not interfere with ambulation or bladder function, or when the avoidance of general anesthetics is associated with reduced recovery sequelae such as nausea and emesis. Alternatively, recovery can be prolonged in the case of spinal or epidural anesthesia if the duration of the local anesthetic applied has been poorly matched to the length of the procedure and the patient must be kept until motor, sensory, and sympathetic blockade has abated to allow ambulation and voiding before discharge.

Oral Nutrition

In the absence of disabling nausea, most patients are able to resume oral nutrition on the day of surgery. This is an advantage for the continuity of administration schedules for chronic medications, and also simplifies the management of patients with diabetes mellitus undergoing anesthesia and surgery. It is highly likely that ambulatory patients will have some caloric intake postoperatively on the day of surgery.

If the patient is awake and alert, not nauseated, and desires oral intake, ice chips, water, or clear juice can be offered. Parents of bottle fed infants can bring their favorite bottle to the center for use postoperatively, being advised that clear liquids will be the first thing offered. If the clear liquids are ingested without difficulty, crackers, fruit-flavored gelatin, or even sandwiches may be available in the SRA for patients to consume before discharge. There are relatively no postanesthetic contraindications to the awake, stable patient whose airway reflexes are intact to resume oral nutrition. However, postsurgical requirements may limit the patient to liquids or soft foods initially (e.g., following procedures in the oropharyngeal area).

If patients are nauseated or simply do not desire anything by mouth, recent experience has indicated that insisting on oral intake in order to meet arbitrary discharge criteria is not necessary and possibly can serve to worsen or bring on nausea.[55] Some centers will allow such patients to return home with clear instructions to caregivers of where to seek assistance if the patient has not taken anything by mouth after a reasonable period of time. Even resistant pediatric patients will usually resume oral intake voluntarily upon return to the familiar environs of home.

Bladder Function

Short surgeries with short recovery stays have also led to a re-evaluation of a mandatory postoperative requirement to void in order to meet discharge criteria. Frequently, patients have not eaten or taken liquids since the prior evening, have emptied their bladder upon arrival at the preoperative area, and have received less than 1 liter of intravenous fluid during their brief surgical procedures. In many instances, insistence that all such patients must then void predischarge, particularly those with little likelihood of having experienced any urinary compromise as a result of their procedure or anesthetic, just consumes recovery time and may even necessitate intravenous volume loading to precipitate voiding. Centers can consider discharging such low-risk patients to reliable caregivers without having voided predischarge if clear instructions are given for where to obtain assistance if voiding does not resume within a reasonable length of time. However, patients who have received spinal or epidural anesthesia or who have undergone urological or gynecological procedures, inguinal herniorrhaphy, or other procedures that may interfere with urinary function should be held in the recovery suite until they can void satisfactorily. Caudal analgesia in the pediatric age group has been noted not to prolong the time to first micturition even if the patients returned home.[56]

Appropriate postsurgical and postanesthetic discharge instructions should be given in both verbal and written form to patients and their caregivers and be appropriately documented in the medical record. A responsible adult should accompany the patient home. Discharge criteria and instructions are discussed in depth in Chapter 12.

Special Considerations for Recovery of Pediatric Patients

Appropriate Facilities

Other than pediatric hospitals, most ambulatory surgical facilities do not have a completely separate pediatric recovery area. A variety from simple to elaborate attempts are made to address the needs of the pediatric age group. The principle recovery needs for children are to reunite parent and child as soon as safety and the facility design allows, as well as to provide some noise barrier between the recovering adults and children, at least in the SRA, to improve patient satisfaction overall. Additional amenities in distinct pediatric areas include bright wall coverings, age-appropriate playthings, and staff who by nature enjoy being with children.

Other considerations for the recovery of children include having equipment and supplies in pediatric sizes in the recovery areas. Examples are blood pressure cuffs and oximeter probes; pediatric laryngoscope blades, face masks, and airway equipment for emergencies; pediatric-sized defibrillator paddles; medications needed for children, such as elixirs of codeine, oxycodone, acetaminophen, and/or ibuprofen, pediatric naloxone, and bronchodilator preparations; and equipment and supplies for supplemental oxygen delivery to children. Adjunctive equipment such as cribs, rocking chairs, and infant feeding bottles are also needed for ambulatory pediatric patients who are expected to be up and about before leaving the recovery area.

Role of Parents

Not every center is designed, equipped, or staffed to allow parents in the PACU, but most allow parents in the SRA. Favorite objects, such as a special blanket or toy, are helpful during parental separation in the preoperative period and can be available as the child awakens. Since ambulatory pediatric patients are expected to become quite alert during the recovery process, postsurgical pain, thirst, and separation from the parents are physical and emotional needs that may become difficult to distinguish, particularly in the preverbal recovering child. An early parental reunion in the SRA can often help. Parents who are calm and attuned to their child's signals and needs can assist the SRA staff in assessing postoperative pain, giving the child oral liquids, dressing the child, etc., essentially freeing up the staff to assist more than one patient.

Pediatric Postoperative Pain Management

General principles of modern pediatric postoperative pain management are similar in concept to those for adults. These include modalities to reduce total narcotic use, such as intraoperative wound infiltration with local anesthetics; use of regional blocks where appropriate; and the use of NSAIDs, including

***Table** 11-5*   Commonly Used Pediatric Analgesic Drugs and Dosages

Drug	Route	Dose	Duration of action (hours)
Acetaminophen	Rectally/PO	10-15 mg/kg*	4-6
Ketorolac	IM/?IV	1 mg/kg (Max 30 mg)	6-8
	PO	1 mg/kg (Max 10 mg)	4-6
Ibuprofen	PO	5 mg/kg	6-8
Codeine	PO	0.5-1 mg/kg	4-6
Naproxen	PO	10 mg/kg	6-8
Fentanyl	IV	1-2 mcg/kg	0.5-1
Meperidine	IV/IM	0.5-1 mg/kg	2-4
Morphine	IV/IM	0.05-0.1 mg/kg	2-4

*Acetaminophen suppositories are available in 120, 325, and 650 mg sizes. Usually the calculated dose is rounded up or down to the nearest whole or half size suppository.

acetaminophen suppositories and syrup, ibuprofen syrup, etc. When narcotics are required, centers may wish to avoid intramuscular injections in awake children. Intravenous opioids can be utilized in appropriate doses. Then, similar to adults, pediatric patients must be able to be managed on oral analgesics by the time of discharge. Codeine and oxycodone are two opioids that are available in elixir form (Table 11-5).

Single injection of dilute concentrations of bupivacaine in the caudal epidural space can be useful to aid the management of postoperative pain following lower abdominal procedures, urological surgery, and lower extremity procedures in young children.[56,57] In pediatric patients, a caudal block is quick and simple to perform and provides excellent postoperative analgesia for approximately 6 hours. The caudal block can be placed after the child is asleep with a general anesthetic. If the block is placed before the skin incision, it will be functional to provide pain relief immediately at the conclusion of surgery. If the block is placed at the end of the surgical procedure, the child may still require other means of pain relief in the early postoperative period until the block is effective. Parents are advised not to allow the child to ambulate unsupervised for at least 6 to 8 hours postoperatively.

Older children are not suitable for discharge with functional caudal blocks if there is a possibility of orthostatic changes or an inability on the part of the family to restrict ambulation in the early postoperative period.

Summary

The design, staffing, and medical treatment rendered in the recovery areas of an ambulatory surgery center are integrally related to achieving the goal of safe, high quality, efficient, cost-effective, patient-oriented perioperative care that incorporates the most up-to-date concepts in ambulatory surgery and anesthesia. In contrast to the fact that patients and their families may remember or know little of the operating room events, the generally alert recovering ambulatory anesthesia patient is able to fully appreciate the care and concern shown during the recovery process. A center that is prepared to prospectively and proactively address the range of potential postoperative events, from prevention of discomfort and possible complications, to preparation for post-recovery discharge, is appreciated by patients, their surgeons and referring physicians, and ultimately by third-party payors, who ever more frequently determine to which ambulatory facilities patients will be directed.

References

1. Kelly JS, Royster RL: Noninvasive transcutaneous cardiac pacing. Anesth Analg 1989;69:229-38.
2. Pattison CZ, Atlee JL, Krebs LH et al: Transesophageal indirect atrial pacing for drug-resistant sinus bradycardia. Anesthesiology 1991; 74:1141-4.
3. Westmoreland CL, Hoke JF, Sebel PS et al: Pharmacokinetics of remifentanil (GI87084B) and its major metabolite (GI90291) in patients undergoing elective inpatient surgery. Anesthesiology 1993; 79:893-903.
4. Rosow C: Remifentanil: a unique opioid analgesic. Anesthesiology 1993; 79:875-6.
5. Bridenbaugh LD: Regional anaesthesia for outpatient surgery—a summary of 12 years' experience. Can Anaesth Soc J 1983; 30:548-52.
6. Allen GC, St Amand MA, Lui ACP et al: Postarthroscopy analgesia with intraarticular bupivacaine/morphine. Anesthesiology 1993; 79:475-80.

7. Joshi GP, McCarroll SM, O'Brien TM, Lenane P: Intraarticular analgesia following knee arthroscopy. Anesth Analg 1993; 76:333-6.

8. Woolf CJ, Chong MS: Preemptive analgesia—treating postoperative pain by preventing the establishment of central sensitization. Anesth Analg 1993; 77:362-79.

9. Ejlersen E, Bryde Anderson H, Eliasen K, Mogenson T: A comparison between preincisional and postincisional lidocaine infiltration and postoperative pain. Anesth Analg 1992; 74:495-8.

10. Wong HY, Carpenter RL, Kopacz DJ et al: A randomized double-blind evaluation of ketorolac tromethamine for post-operative analgesia in ambulatory surgery patients. Anesthesiology 1993; 78:6-14.

11. Rosenblum M, Weller RS, Conard PL et al: Ibuprofen provides longer lasting analgesia than fentanyl after laparoscopic surgery. Anesth Analg 1991; 73:255-9.

12. Ding Y, White PF: Comparative effects of ketorolac, dezocine and fentanyl as adjuvants during outpatient anesthesia. Anesth Analg 1992; 75:566-71.

13. Smith I, Shively RA, White PF: Effects of ketorolac and bupivacaine on recovery after outpatient arthroscopy. Anesth Analg 1992; 75:208-12.

14. Ding Y, Fredman B, White PF: Use of ketorolac and fentanyl during outpatient gynecologic surgery. Anesth Analg 1993; 77:205-10.

15. Haddow GR, Riley E, Isaacs R, McSharry R: Ketorolac, nasal polyposis, and bronchial asthma: a cause for concern. Anesth Analg 1993; 76:420-2.

16. Zikowski D, Hord AH, Haddox JD, Glascock J: Ketorolac-induced bronchospasm. Anesth Analg 1993; 76:417-9.

17. Khoury GF, Chen ACN, Garland DC, Stein C: Intraarticular morphine, bupivacaine, and morphine/bupivacaine for pain control after knee videoarthroscopy. Anesthesiology 1992; 77:263-6.

18. Sevarino FB, Naulty JS, Sinatra R et al: Transdermal fentanyl for postoperative pain management in patients recovering from abdominal gynecologic surgery. Anesthesiology 1992; 77:463-6.

19. Striebel HW, Koenigs D, Kramer J: Postoperative pain management by intranasal demand-adapted fentanyl titration. Anesthesiology 1992; 77:281-5.

20. Ashburn MA, Lind GH, Gillie MH et al: Oral transmucosal fentanyl citrate (OTFC) for the treatment of postoperative pain. Anesth Analg 1993; 76:377-81.

21. Gal TJ, Cooperman LH: Hypertension in the immediate postoperative period. Br J Anaesth 1975; 40:70-74.

22. Leslie JB, Kalayjian RW, Sirgo MA et al: Intravenous labetalol for treatment of postoperative hypertension. Anesthesiology 1987; 67:413-6.

23. Hines R, Barash PG, Watrous G, O'Connor T: Complications occurring in the postanesthesia care unit: a survey. Anesth Analg 1992; 74:503-9.

24. Patel RI, Hannallah RS: Anesthetic complications following pediatric ambulatory surgery: a 3-year study. Anesthesiology 1988; 69:1009-12.

25. Orkin F: What do patients want? Preferences for immediate postoperative recovery. Anesth Analg 1992; 74:S225.

26. Gold BS, Kitz DS, Lecky JH, Neuhaus JM: Unanticipated admission to the hospital following ambulatory surgery. JAMA 1989; 262:3008-10.

27. Watcha MF, White PF: Postoperative nausea and vomiting: its etiology, treatment and prevention. Anesthesiology 1992; 77:162-84.

28. Weir PM, Munro HM, Reynolds PI et al: Propofol infusion and the incidence of emesis in pediatric outpatient strabismus surgery. Anesth Analg 1993; 76:760-4.

29. Borgeat A, Wilder-Smith OHG, Saiah M, Rifat K: Subhypnotic doses of propofol possess direct antiemetic properties. Anesth Analg 1992; 74:539-41.

30. Martin TM, Nicolson SC, Bargas MS: Propofol anesthesia reduces emesis and airway obstruction in pediatric outpatients. Anesth Analg 1993; 76:144-8.

31. Leeser J, Lip H: Prevention of postoperative nausea and vomiting using ondansetron, a new, selective, 5-HT$_3$ receptor antagonist. Anesth Analg 1991; 72:751-5.

32. Scuderi P, Wetchler B, Sung Y-F et al: Treatment of postoperative nausea and vomiting after outpatient surgery with the 5-HT$_3$ antagonist ondansetron. Anesthesiology 1993; 78:15-20.

33. Alon E, Himmelseher S: Ondansetron in the treatment of postoperative vomiting: a randomized double-blind comparison with droperidol and metoclopramide. Anesth Analg 1992; 75:561-5.

34. Bailey PL, Streisand JB, Pace NL et al: Transdermal scopolamine reduces nausea and vomiting after outpatient laparoscopy. Anesthesiology 1990; 72:977-80.

35. Borgeat A, Wilder-Smith OHG, Suter PM: The nonhypnotic therapeutic applications of propofol. Anesthesiology 1994; 80:642-56.

36. Koka BV, Jeon IS, Andre JM et al: Postintubation croup in children. Anesth Analg 1977; 56:501-5.

37. Kallar SK, Jones GW: Postoperative complications. In White PF, editor: Outpatient anesthesia, New York, 1990, Churchill Livingstone, pp. 397-415.

38. Maltby JR, Lewis P, Martin A, Sutherland LR: Gastric fluid volume and pH in elective patients following unrestricted oral fluid until three hours before surgery. Can J Anaesth 1991; 38:425-9.

39. Nicolson SC, Dorsey HT, Schreiner MS: Shortened preanesthetic fasting interval in pediatric cardiac surgical patients. Anesth Analg 1992; 74: 694-7.

40. Warner MA, Warner ME, Weber JG: Clinical significance of pulmonary aspiration during the perioperative period. Anesthesiology 1993; 78:56-62.

41. Fleisher IK, Boudreaux AM: Hyponatremia and possible uterine perforation during endometrial rollerball ablation. Anesth Analg 1993; 77:860-1.

42. Perry PM, Baughman VL: A complication of hysteroscopy: air embolism. Anesthesiology 1990; 73:546-7.

43. Slotman GJ, Jed EH, Burchard KW: Adverse effects of hypothermia in postoperative patients. Am J Surg 1985; 149:495-501.

44. Macintyre PE, Pavlin EG, Dwersteg JF: Effect of meperidine on oxygen consumption, carbon dioxide production, and respiratory gas exchange in postanesthesia shivering. Anesth Analg 1987; 66:751-5.

45. Delaunay L, Bonnet F, Liu N et al: Clonidine comparably decreases the thermoregulatory thresholds for vasoconstriction and shivering in humans. Anesthesiology 1993; 79:470-4.

46. Yentis SM, Levine MF, Hartley EJ: Should all children with suspected or confirmed malignant hyperthermia susceptibility be admitted after surgery? A 10-year review. Anesth Analg 1992; 75:345-50.

47. Strazis KP, Fox AW: Malignant hyperthermia: a review of published cases. Anesth Analg 1993; 77:297-304.

48. Rapp SE, Conahan TJ, Pavlin DJ et al: Comparison of desflurane with propofol in outpatients undergoing peripheral orthopedic surgery. Anesth Analg 1992; 75:572-9.

49. Spear RM, Yaster M, Berkowitz IP et al: Preinduction of anesthesia in young children with rectally administered midazolam. Anesthesiology 1991; 74:670-4.

50. Weldon BC, Watcha MF, White PF: Oral midazolam in children: Effect of time and adjunctive therapy. Anesth Analg 1992; 75:51-5.

51. Ebert TJ, Muzi M: Sympathetic hyperactivity during desflurane anesthesia in healthy volunteers: a comparison with isoflurane. Anesthesiology 1993; 79:444-53.

52. Brain AI: Laryngeal mask airway. Anesthesiology 1992; 76:1061.

53. Watcha MF, White PF, Tychsen L, Stevens JL: Comparative effects of laryngeal mask airway and endotracheal tube insertion on intraocular pressure in children. Anesth Analg 1992; 75:355-60.

54. Wilkins CJ, Cramp PGW, Staples J, Stevens WC: Comparison of the anesthetic requirement for tolerance of laryngeal mask airway and endotracheal tube. Anesth Analg 1992; 75:794-7.

55. Schreiner MS, Nicolson SC, Martin T, Whitney L: Should children drink before discharge from day surgery? Anesthesiology 1992; 76:528-33.

56. Fisher QA, McComiskey CM, Hill TL et al: Postoperative voiding interval and duration of analgesia following peripheral or caudal nerve blocks in children. Anesth Analg 1993; 75:173-7.

57. Warner MA, Kunkel SE, Offord KO et al: The effects of age epinephrine, and operative site on the duration of caudal analgesia in pediatric patients. Anesth Analg 1987; 66:995-8.

Discharge Process 12

Frances Chung

Ambulatory surgery has increased in popularity because of the rising costs of inpatient hospital care. The technological developments in medicine, surgery, pharmacology, and anesthesia management have also advanced ambulatory surgery. Today there are more patients with health problems requiring extensive surgery and longer durations of anesthesia on an ambulatory basis. It is predicted that 60% to 70% of future surgeries will be performed on an ambulatory basis. The shortage of nurses, limitation of bed

431

space, and the popularity of ambulatory surgery with patients all encourage the growth of ambulatory surgery with the emphasis on efficiency.

The question of how long patients should remain in ambulatory surgical facilities following ambulatory surgery and anesthesia is crucial to future developments in this area. It is important to anesthetize patients to provide a fast recovery, with as little postanesthetic cognitive and psychomotor impairment as possible, and to judge when patients can be safely sent home after outpatient anesthesia. A major concern in the quality of patient care is the safe timing of patient discharge, in relation to recovery from general anesthesia or conscious sedation. At the time of discharge from the ambulatory surgery unit, the patients should be home ready; i.e., they should be clinically stable and able to rest at home under the care of a responsible adult.

Definition of Recovery Period

The time course of recovery includes early, intermediate, and late recovery (Table 12-1).[1] **Early recovery** is defined as the time during which patients emerge from anesthesia and recover their protective reflexes and motor activity. **Intermediate recovery** is defined as the period where coordination and physiological function normalize, and the patient may be considered in a state of "home readiness" and able to return home in the company of a responsible adult. **Late recovery,** which can last for hours to days, is the time after which the patient has fully recovered and is capable of full psychomotor functioning, including returning to work and driving.

Table 12-1   Stages of Recovery

Stage of recovery	Clinical definitions
Early recovery	Awakening and recovery of vital reflexes
Intermediate recovery	Immediate clinical recovery
	Home readiness
Late recovery	Full recovery
	Psychologic recovery

Ordinarily, patients undergo early recovery in the postanes-thetic care unit (PACU), phase 1, which contains all the usual equipment found in any recovery area. Intermediate recovery to home readiness occurs in a phase 2 area, where patients are transferred to a reclining lounge chair for progressive movement to a sitting position and ambulation.

Discharge in Practice

The success of ambulatory surgery depends on appropriate and timely discharge of patients who have been anesthetized. Prema-ture release of patients who later experience postoperative com-plications requiring unanticipated admission to the hospital or emergency care should occur infrequently, or not at all.[2]

The major accreditation bodies in the United States (Joint Commission of Accreditation of Hospitals [JCAHO], Accredita-tion Association for Ambulatory Health Care [AAAHC]), and in Canada (the Canadian Anaesthetists' Society) require that certain policies and procedures be implemented to ensure safe recovery after anesthesia. This includes examining the patient and requiring that the patient have an escort home. Each patient must also receive written postoperative instructions, which include instruc-tions to contact an appropriate physician if problems develop. Each facility must develop its own policies and adhere to estab-lished criteria.

Legal Considerations

Legal considerations are important in ambulatory anesthesia, especially in regard to discharge. The anesthesiologist practicing ambulatory anesthesia must be aware that he or she faces risks of liability.

Ogg studied 100 patients undergoing outpatient anesthesia during its early development in the 1970s.[3] Thirty-one percent went home unaccompanied by a responsible adult. There were 41 car owners: 9% drove themselves home, 30% drove within 12 hours, and 73% drove within 24 hours. A patient who had a dental extraction under methohexitone anesthesia had no escort and, subsequently, sustained a knee fracture. He won a $40,000 settlement.[3] A more recent survey also found that 30% of patients drank alcohol or drove a car within 24 hours of surgery.[4]

Thus, it is important that all safety measures are implemented and that they are documented in the patient's medical record. To protect against a possible challenge of inappropriate discharge, a physician must have evidence that the patient's home readiness was carefully assessed. Even when a physician may not be physically present at the time of discharge, institutionally approved discharge criteria and policies must be adhered to.[2]

Clinical Discharge Criteria

Scoring systems have been developed to guide the transfer from recovery room to ward. The most commonly used method, described by Aldrete and Kroulik in 1970, assigns a score of 0, 1, or 2 for activity, respiration, circulation, consciousness, and skin color. A score of 10 indicates that the patient is in the best possible condition for discharge from the recovery room (Table 12-2).[5] This scoring system is often used in phase 1 recovery of ambulatory surgery patients. The discharge of patients from phase 1 PACU should be criteria-based, not time-based. It is not necessary for intubated patients to stay for 60 minutes.

Criteria used for discharging patients from the PACU cannot be applied to ambulatory surgery patients. Inpatients may be responsive and in no acute distress, but they also may be heavily medicated and unable to walk. These patients are also transported to a hospital room with a bed and are monitored by nursing personnel after being discharged from the PACU. In comparison, ambulatory surgical patients must be able to walk before being discharged. The ability to ambulate, the level of hydration, and the ability to tolerate oral intake are unique to the ambulatory surgery patient. The patient's readiness to be discharged should be addressed in a simple, clear manner, and this should be documented.

Phase 2 postanesthetic care unit patients should be offered oral fluids. Once they have tolerated oral fluids, they should walk to the bathroom and attempt to void. If patients have successfully tolerated oral fluids and voided, have no excessive pain or vomiting, and are able to walk out by themselves, they may be discharged with an escort.[6]

Guidelines for safe discharge after ambulatory surgery have been developed and clinical discharge criteria are often used in phase 2 PACU to determine home readiness of ambulatory patients. Several clinical discharge criteria have been described,

Table 12-2   Aldrete Scoring System

Activity

Able to move voluntarily or on command	
4 extremities	2
2 extremities	1
0 extremities	0

Respiration

Able to deep breathe and cough freely	2
Dyspnea, shallow or limited breathing	1
Apneic	0

Circulation

Preoperative blood pressure _____ mm	
BP ± 20 mm of preanesthesia level	2
BP ± 20 to 50 mm of preanesthesia level	1
BP ± 50 mm of preanesthesia level	0

Consciousness

Fully awake	2
Arousable on calling	1
Not responding	0

Color

Normal	2
Pale, dusky, blotchy	1
Cyanotic	0

From Aldrete JA, Kroulik D: A postanesthetic recovery score. Anesth Analg 1970; 49:924-34.

and, although readily applicable, have been nonstandardized. The minimal clinical criteria for safe discharge as suggested by Korttila[6] is summarized in Box 12-1. Wetchler of the Methodist Medical Center of Illinois Ambulatory Surgicare used the policy shown in Box 12-2.[7]

Postanesthesia Discharge Scoring System (PADSS)

A simple cumulative index, the Postanesthesia Discharge Scoring System (PADSS), was designed by this author to measure home

Box 12-1 Guidelines for Safe Discharge After
         Ambulatory Surgery

1. Patient's vital signs must be stable for at least 1 hour.
2. Patient must have no evidence of respiratory depression.
3. Patient must be:
   a. Oriented to person, place, time.
   b. Able to maintain orally administered fluids.
   c. Able to void.
   d. Able to dress himself or herself.
   e. Able to walk without assistance.
4. Patient must not have:
   a. More than minimal nausea and vomiting.
   b. Excessive pain.
   c. Bleeding.
5. Patient must be discharged by both the person who administered anesthesia and the person who performed surgery, or by their designees. Written instructions for the postoperative period at home, including a contact place and person, need to be reinforced.
6. Patients must have responsible "vested" adult escort them home and stay with them at home.

Adapted from Korttila K: Recovery period and discharge. In White PF, editor: Outpatient anesthesia, New York, 1990, Churchill Livingstone, pp. 369-95.

readiness of ambulatory surgical patients.[8] A patient's readiness for discharge needs to be addressed in a simple, clear manner, to be documented, and to meet medical and anesthesia national standards. Nursing staff need to be able to evaluate the postoperative course of the patient in a systematic way and, when necessary, meet guidelines to seek physician consultations.

The PADSS is based on several main criteria: (1) vital signs—blood pressure, heart rate, respiratory rate, and temperature; (2) activity and mental status; (3) pain, nausea, and/or vomiting; (4) surgical bleeding; and (5) intake and output (Box 12-3). The perfect score is 10. When patients have a score ≥ 9, they are considered to be fit for home discharge.

Box 12-2 *Guidelines for Safe Discharge After Ambulatory Surgery*

1. Vital signs stable: These include temperature, pulse, respiration, and blood pressure when appropriate. Vital signs should remain stable for a period of not less than a half-hour and be consistent with the patient's age and preanesthesia levels.
2. Ability to swallow and cough: The patient must demonstrate the ability to swallow fluids and to cough.
3. Ability to walk: The patient demonstrates ability to perform movement consistent with age and developmental level (sit, stand, walk).
4. Minimal nausea, vomiting, dizziness:
   a. Minimal nausea: Absence of nausea, or if nausea is present, the patient can still swallow and retain some fluids.
   b. Minimal vomiting: Vomiting is either absent or, if present, does not require treatment. Following vomiting that requires treatment, the patient should be able to swallow and retain fluids.
   c. Minimal dizziness: Dizziness is either absent or present only upon sitting, and the patient is still able to perform movement consistent with age.
5. Absence of respiratory distress: The patient exhibits no signs of snoring, obstructed respiration, stridor, retractions, or croupy cough.
6. Alert and oriented: The patient is aware of surroundings and what has taken place and is interested in returning home.

From Wetchler BV: Problem solving in the postanesthesia care unit. In Wetchler BV, editor: Anesthesia for ambulatory surgery, Philadelphia, 1990, JB Lippincott, pp. 375-436.

For any scoring system to be useful, it must be practical, simple, easy to remember, and it should be applicable to all postanesthesia situations. Using only the commonly observed physical signs will avoid any added duties for the postanesthesia

> ## Box 12-3 *Postanesthesia Discharge Scoring System* (PADSS)*
>
> 1. Vital signs
>   2 = Within 20% of preoperative value
>   1 = 20-40% of preoperative value
>   0 = 40% of preoperative value
> 2. Ambulation and mental status
>   2 = Oriented × 3 AND has a steady gait
>   1 = Oriented × 3 OR has a steady gait
>   0 = Neither
> 3. Pain, or nausea/vomiting
>   2 = Minimal
>   1 = Moderate
>   0 = Severe
> 4. Surgical bleeding
>   2 = Minimal
>   1 = Moderate
>   0 = Severe
> 5. Intake and output
>   2 = Has had PO fluids AND voided
>   1 = Has had PO fluids OR voided
>   0 = Neither

*The total score is 10. Patients scoring ≥ 9 are considered fit for discharge.

care personnel. By assigning numerical values to parameters indicating patient recovery, progress or lack of it becomes more objective and more easily identified. This scoring system is a simple way of providing uniform assessment for all patients, and it may have added medicolegal value for assessment of home readiness. It can determine the patient's optimal length of stay in the ambulatory surgery unit, reducing nursing time per patient and increasing the efficiency of nursing staff.

In a comparison of the PADSS with conventionally established clinical discharge criteria, Chung et al. found that patients can be discharged earlier if PADSS is used.[8] Thirty thousand patients were discharged safely from the Toronto Western General

Hospital using PADSS. The majority of patients can be discharged within 1 to 2 hours after outpatient anesthesia. A minority of patients may have persistent symptoms such as pain, nausea and vomiting, hypotension, dizziness, or unsteady gait delaying their discharge.[9] Delay in discharge can also be attributed to the lack of an escort being immediately available.[10]

Modified Discharge Criteria

Drinking Before Discharge

The necessity to drink and to void before discharging ambulatory patients is not universally adopted in most institutions. Research shows that 20% of patients can be potentially discharged earlier by eliminating the drinking and voiding criteria.[11] A modified postanesthetic discharge scoring system has been suggested by this author (Box 12-4), which eliminates input and output.

The ability to tolerate oral fluids remains controversial as a clinical criterion for discharge. It is unacceptable to discharge a patient when he or she is actively vomiting. However, it is also undesirable to continue to administer oral fluids when he or she is vomiting. The decision to discharge the patient should be based on a number of factors such as age, medical condition, distance from home, availability of a responsible adult, state of hydration, and anticipation of whether or not the patient is likely to suffer any complication if fluids are not taken on the day of surgery.

Schreiner et al. found that requiring children to drink before hospital discharge appeared to increase the incidence of vomiting and prolong the duration of hospital stay.[12] The Children's Hospital of Philadelphia has discharged more than 6000 day-surgery patients without requiring them to drink before discharge. Within this group, only three patients required admission for vomiting, and one required readmission for intractable vomiting and dehydration.[12] Thus, drinking may not be a necessary criterion for discharge.

Voiding Before Discharge

The requirement to void before discharge is another controversial issue during recovery of the adult patient. Inability to void, urinary retention, and subsequent catheterization have been related

Box 12-4 A Modified Postanesthetic Discharge
Scoring System (MPADSS)*

1. Vital signs
   2 = Within 20% of preoperative value
   1 = 20% to 40% of preoperative value
   0 = 40% of preoperative value
2. Ambulation
   2 = Steady gait/no dizziness
   1 = With assistance
   0 = None/dizziness
3. Nausea/vomiting
   2 = Minimal
   1 = Moderate
   0 = Severe
4. Pain
   2 = Minimal
   1 = Moderate
   0 = Severe
5. Surgical bleeding
   2 = Minimal
   1 = Moderate
   0 = Severe

*The total score is 10. Patients scoring ≥ 9 are considered fit for
discharge.

to reflex urethral spasm, or reflex inhibition of normal bladder
detruser muscle activity by pain, distension of the anal canal, and
prolonged block of bladder autonomic inneration.

Kallar of The Medical College of Virginia found that 86% of
patients could be discharged more rapidly by using PADSS
assessment than with clinical discharge criteria. However, 14% of
patients had not reached the discharge criteria of PADSS when
clinical discharge criteria were already satisfied. This was due to
failure to void before discharge in the PADSS assessment,
whereas the ability to void was optional in the clinical discharge
criteria.[13] At Loyola University, patients were catheterized if they
failed to void within 4 hours of recovery room stay after spinal

anesthesia. None of these patients encountered delayed voiding problems following discharge. If voiding is not a criterion for discharge, the patient must be fully informed about his or her role, when to call a physician, or when to return to the facility. Certain urological or gynecological procedures, or spinal or epidural anesthesia, interfere with urinary function, and following those procedures, patients should be evaluated for voiding before discharge.

Discharge After Regional Anesthesia

Patients recovering from regional anesthesia must meet the same discharge criteria as patients who are discharged after general anesthesia. When is it safe to permit patients to ambulate following spinal or epidural anesthesia? Suitable criteria for ambulation after spinal anesthesia include normal perianal (S4-5) pinprick sensation, plantar flexion of the foot, and proprioception of the big toe.[7] No motor block should be present when a patient tries to stand or walk. To test the motor block, one can ask the patient to touch both the right and left heel to the opposite big toe and to run each heel up and down the opposite leg to the knee. A patient's ability to walk to the bathroom and urinate may be the best recovery test after epidural or spinal anesthesia because these abilities indicate recovery of motor and sympathetic functions. Patients should be able to void before discharge following spiral or epidural anesthesia, but need not following pediatric caudal analgesia. Patients receiving spinal anesthesia should be warned about the possibility of spinal headache.

The central nervous system effect of local anesthetics may prolong complete recovery after regional anesthesia. In one study, a patient's postural stability was impaired 40 minutes after perivascular axillary block with mepivacaine.[6] Because of the prolonged block and analgesic duration that may occur following regional anesthesia (i.e., upper or lower extremity nerve blocks), patients can be discharged postoperatively even before complete block resolution. Philip recommended discharging patients with axillary block with their arms in a sling, and providing them with written discharge instructions reminding them that they did not have 24-hour protective pain sensation in the arm and to contact their physician if a problem occurred.[14]

Malignant Hyperthermia

Isolated postoperative myoglobinuria has been reported as a presenting symptom in a malignant hyperthermia ambulatory patient.[15A] Should all children with suspected or confirmed malignant hyperthermia susceptibility (MHS) be admitted after surgery? A retrospective review of the history, management, and outcome of all suspected or proven MHS patients ($n=285$) who required surgery was examined to ascertain the incidence of complications. No malignant hyperthermia reactions occurred.[15B] It was suggested that same-day discharge of malignant hyperthermia–susceptible patients after uncomplicated ambulatory surgery would be unlikely to be associated with a malignant hyperthermia event after discharge. An information sheet outlining signs of a malignant hyperthermia reaction can be explained to the parents of malignant hyperthermia–susceptible children. Following trigger-free anesthesia, the children can be monitored for 4 to 6 hours in the postanesthesia care unit, after which they may be discharged if there is no evidence of a malignant hyperthermia reaction.[15B] Provisions for transfer to an inpatient facility or to an extended observation unit should be in place before anesthetizing an MHS patient.

Discharge Instructions and Street Fitness

Discharge instructions should be given to the patient and the escort responsible for the care of the patient at home. General postoperative instructions for any surgical procedure are shown in Box 12-5. In addition, procedure-specific instructions should be given to the patient. Examples are given in Boxes 12-6 to 12-8.

Recovery from the patient's standpoint signifies the return to normal function, such as driving a car or returning to work. Carefully selected batteries of psychomotor tests or driving simulation can be employed to assess the patient's psychomotor recovery. These tests are complex and cannot be used clinically. Herbert et al. monitored ambulatory surgery patients for 2 days following hernia surgery with a choice reaction time test. Reaction times were impaired for as long as 1 to 2 days.[16]

Baskett indicated that patients who had had a good night's sleep after an anesthetic should be able to drive the following day.[17] Kortilla studied the effects of different analgesics, sedatives,

Box 12-5 General Postoperative Instructions for Patients Following Ambulatory Surgery

1. Postsurgery activities
   a. Rest today.
   b. You may experience some dizziness or drowsiness following the surgery or procedure.
   c. Do NOT consume alcohol, drive, or make important personal or business decisions for 24 hours.
   d. Activity level: See procedure-specific instructions.
2. Postsurgery diet
   a. Progress as tolerated without nausea and vomiting.
3. Postsurgery medications
   a. Medications taken before surgery should be resumed as ordered by your physician.
   b. Mild aches and pains are not unusual and may be relieved by acetaminophen (Tylenol) or similar non-aspirin pain medication after surgery.
   c. A prescription for other pain medication may be given by your physician after surgery. Take as instructed.
4. Emergency situation
   Call your physician immediately, if any of the following occurs:
   a. Bladder difficulties.
   b. Persistent nausea or vomiting.
   c. Bleeding that does not stop.
   d. Unusual pain.
   e. Fever.
   f. Redness/swelling or drainage of pus.
If unable to contact your physician, you may contact or go to the hospital emergency department.

Box 12-6 Discharge Instructions for Patients Following Laparoscopy

1. You may be up and about as much as you can tolerate, but avoid any strenuous exercise or activity for 1 to 2 days.
2. You may shower or bathe the day after surgery.
3. There may be slight bleeding for 1 to 2 days.
4. You may experience some abdominal discomfort, sore muscles, sore throat, and/or shoulder tip pain. This is due to the anesthetic or procedure and usually subsides in 1 to 2 days.
5. You may take your prescribed medication or acetaminophen (Tylenol) for pain.
6. If the pain becomes severe, or if you develop excessive bleeding, fever, or chills, rest and call your physician. If you are unable to contact your doctor, go to the nearest emergency department.
7. You may remove the Band-Aid in 1 to 2 days. There are no stitches to be removed. They will fall out themselves in 7 to 10 days.
8. If required, wear sanitary pads instead of tampons for the vaginal bleeding or discharge that may be present postprocedure for 1 to 2 days.
9. You may resume sexual intercourse in 1 to 2 weeks or when comfortable, unless otherwise instructed by your physician.
10. You may return to work in 2 days if able, unless otherwise instructed by your physician.
11. If you have concerns or problems, contact your physician or visit the nearest emergency department.
12. Phone your physician regarding your follow-up appointment.
13. Follow-up appointment: Doctor/clinic: _____
                              Date & time:

Box 12-7 Discharge Instructions for Patients
           Following Breast Biopsy

---

1. You may be up and about, but avoid any strenuous activity for 24 hours.
2. When you shower, avoid getting the dressing wet. You may take a sponge bath. You may remove the initial bulky dressing in 48 hours, after which you should wear a soft support bra without stays (underwires).
3. There may be some discomfort at the breast and axillary area. If so, you may take your prescribed medication, or you may take one or two acetaminophen tablets (Tylenol) every 3 to 4 hours, if required.
4. Move your fingers and arm on the operative site to prevent stiffness.
5. You may return to work in 48 hours, unless otherwise instructed by your physician.
6. Phone your physician for a follow-up appointment and the results of the biopsy.
7. If you have any concerns or problems and are unable to reach your physician, return to the nearest emergency department.
8. Follow-up appointment: Doctor/clinic: _____
                          Date & time: _____

---

and anesthetics on the psychomotor skills of volunteers[18] and recommended that patients refrain from driving for 24 hours if the duration of anesthesia was less than 30 minutes. If the duration of anesthesia was 2 hours or more, it was safer to advise them not to drive for 48 hours.[6]

Postoperative Follow-up

Since ambulatory patients are discharged shortly after the procedure, a traditional postoperative follow-up visit cannot be conducted. Alternative means for obtaining patient's assessment, such as postoperative telephone interview, postoperative questionnaire or

---

Box 12-8 Discharge Instructions for Patients Following Knee or Ankle Arthroscopy

---

1. You may be up and walking with full weight bearing as you can tolerate, unless you were given specific orders by your physician.
2. The tensor bandage is to be left on. Loosen the tensor bandage if it is too tight. After the first 24 hours, it should be loosely worn for 1 week.
3. You may shower after 48 hours and swim after your postoperative check-up, unless otherwise instructed by your physician.
4. The suture line may be covered with a Band-Aid. Do not remove Steri-Strips, they will fall off. Steri-Strips are used instead of stitches. The Band-Aid may be changed after each shower.
5. Take your pain pills as directed to minimize pain and discomfort. Do not drink any alcohol when taking the medication, and avoid taking the pain pills on an empty stomach.
6. If there is any swelling, rest and elevate the affected limb.
7. If there is any excessive swelling, excessive bleeding, or discoloration, call your physician. If you are unable to see your physician, return to the nearest emergency department.
8. Keep your clinic appointment or phone your physician the day after your discharge for a postoperative appointment, results, and/or further instructions (i.e., when stitches are to be removed [usually 7 to 10 days]).
9. Follow-up appointment: Doctor/clinic: _____
                            Date & time: _____

---

postcards, are used in the ambulatory surgery unit. Each facility must develop a method of postoperative follow-up suited to its needs.

There are very few studies that have examined return to normal activities after ambulatory anesthesia. One study included 777 patients 24 hours after surgery. There was a considerable number of adverse outcomes at 24 hours postoperatively,[19] the reduction of which may hasten the return of daily function of these patients. Patients with adverse outcomes have recovered only 61% of their daily function versus 78% in patients with no adverse outcomes. The return of daily function also depends on the type of surgery. On the first day after surgery, dilatation and curettage patients have recovered 81%, ophthalmic patients 70%, and orthopedic/general surgery patients 60% of their daily function. Philip found that 38% of patients were able to return to their usual activities the day after surgery, the remainder required 3.2 ± 2.0 additional days. The main reasons for delayed recovery included general malaise (57%) and surgical discomfort (38%). Assessing their overall satisfaction, 97% would choose day surgery again.[20]

Summary

The use of a practical discharge criteria or a postanesthesia discharge scoring system should be implemented in every ambulatory surgery center to ensure safe recovery and discharge after anesthesia. The postanesthesia recovery score (Aldrete score) is used to evaluate the initial recovery of the patient. Once the Aldrete score is satisfied, home readiness can be evaluated using clinical criteria that assess recovery of vital signs, level of activity, intake and output, degree of pain control, and degree of orientation. Modification of these criteria have been adapted in ambulatory surgery facilities. Described in this chapter is the author's postanesthesia discharge scoring system (PADSS), a simple, practical systematic scoring system. However, the application of any discharge criteria scoring system must be used with common sense and clinical judgment. Home readiness of an outpatient does not mean street fitness. Once the patient has satisfied the clinical criteria, the patient can be discharged in the presence of a responsible adult escort. Written instructions and provisions for follow-up are discussed. The safe and expeditious conduct of ambulatory surgical care can only succeed by careful selection of patients and surgical procedures, appropriate intraoperative and postoperative anesthetic care, and prudent and timely discharge of patients.

References

1. Steward DJ, Volgyesi G: Stabilometry: a new tool for the measurement of recovery following general anaesthesia. Can Anaesth Soc J 1978; 25:4-6.
2. Korttila K: Practical discharge criteria. Problems in Anesthesia 1988; 2:144-51.
3. Ogg TW: An assessment of postoperative outpatient cases. Br Med J 1972; 4:573-5.
4. Lichtor JL, Sah J, Apfelbaum J et al: Some patients may drink or drive after ambulatory surgery. Anesthesiology 1990; 73:A1083.
5. Aldrete JA, Kroulik D: A postanesthetic recovery score. Anesth Analg 1970; 49:924-34.
6. Korttila K: Recovery period and discharge. In White PE, editor: Outpatient anesthesia, New York, 1990, Churchill Livingstone, pp. 369-96.
7. Wetchler BV: Problem solving in the postanesthesia care unit. In Wetchler BV, editor: Anesthesia for ambulatory surgery, Philadelphia, 1990, JB Lippincott, pp. 375-436.
8. Chung F, Ong D, Seyone C et al: PADSS—A discriminative discharge index for ambulatory surgery. Anesthesiology 1991; 75:A1105.
9. Chung F, Baylon GJ, Michaloliakou C: Persistent symptoms after ambulatory anaesthesia. Can J Anaesth 1993; 40:A21.
10. Chung F, Baylon GJ, Michaloliakou C: Home readiness with postanesthetic discharge score: a report on 500 cases. Can J Anaesth 1993; 40:A21.
11. Michaloliakou C, Chung F: Does a modified postanesthetic discharge scoring system determine home readiness sooner? Can J Anaesth 1993; 40:A32.
12. Schreiner MS, Nicolson SC, Martin T, Whitney L: Should children drink before discharge from day surgery? Anesthesiology 1992; 76:528-33.
13. Kallar SK, Chung F: Practical application of postanesthetic discharge scoring system—PADSS. Anesthesiology 1992; 77:A12.
14. Philip BK: Ambulatory anesthesia. Semin Surg Oncol 1990; 6:177-83.
15A. Birmingham PK, Stevenson GW, Uejima T, Hall SC: Isolated postoperative myoglobinuria in a pediatric outpatient: a case report of malignant hyperthermia. Anesth Analg 1989; 69:846-9.
15B. Yentis SM, Levine MF, Hartley EJ: Should all children with suspected or confirmed malignant hyperthermia susceptibility be admitted after surgery? Anesth Analg 1992; 75:345-50.
16. Herbert M, Healy EGJ, Bourke JB et al: Profile of recovery after general anesthesia. Br Med J 1983; 286:1539-42.
17. Baskett P, Vickers M: Driving after anaesthetics. Br Med J 1979; 1:686-7.

18. Korttila K: Recovery and driving after brief anaesthesia. Anaesthesist 1982; 30:377-82.

19. Chung F: Return to daily living function after outpatient anesthesia. Anesth Analg 1994; 78:S62.

20. Philip BK: Patient's assessment of ambulatory anesthesia and surgery. J Clin Anesth 1992; 4:355-8.

Complications and Quality Assurance

13

Barbara S. Gold

A major evolutionary advance in surgical and anesthetic care during the past few decades has been the growth and development of outpatient surgery. During the 1970s only the healthiest of patients were considered appropriate candidates for outpatient surgery. Consequently, only 10% to 15% of all surgical procedures were performed on an outpatient basis. Currently, outpatient surgery accounts for 50% of all procedures and includes patients at the extremes of age and those with coexisting medical problems. Despite the increase in patient volume and case complexity, complication rates have remained fairly static. This is borne out by unanticipated admission rates following outpatient surgery, which have hovered around 1% to 2% over the past decade.[1] Low complication rates have contributed to the tremendous growth of ambulatory surgery and anesthesia. Complication rates have remained at a level that is sufficiently low to be acceptable to patients, physicians, and third-party payors. However, as outpatient anesthesia and surgery evolve with respect to procedures, patient population, and societal expectations, it is important to continuously evaluate the type, prevalence, and severity of complications that occur in the outpatient surgical setting.

Complications in the outpatient setting encompass a broad spectrum and include not only major adverse events such as cardiac arrest, but also seemingly minor events such as postoperative pain, nausea and vomiting, and difficulty with urination. These minor complications become major issues because they impede patient discharge and interfere with patients' resuming their usual level of function shortly after surgery. Therefore, when evaluating outpatient complications, one must consider minor yet distressing problems as well as life-threatening adverse events.

Complications: An Overview

Unanticipated Admission

One of the best indicators of complications in the ambulatory anesthesia setting is the rate of unanticipated admissions to the hospital following outpatient surgery. Unanticipated admissions are easily quantifiable endpoints that signify that the outpatient procedure did not go according to plan. Analysis of data from unanticipated admissions enables us to identify groups of patients or procedures that may not be well suited for ambulatory surgery and anesthesia. In this way ambulatory patient and procedure selection can be refined. Although retrospective, this type of analysis is important since, due to insurance reimbursement pressures, it is no longer possible to compare similar groups of inpatients with outpatients in randomized, prospective controlled trials.

Although unanticipated admissions reflect complications, it would be too simplistic to equate them, because admissions are influenced by multiple confounding medical and nonmedical variables. For example, a patient without a competent adult to escort and care for them at home may be admitted for "social reasons." Furthermore, each ambulatory surgery facility will have its own guidelines for admitting patients. For example, a free-standing facility may restrict its practice to healthier patients having limited procedures to avoid complications and hence admissions. Alternatively, a surgery unit based in a tertiary care center may have a larger proportion of patients at the extremes of age who have complex coexisting disease and poor social support that may lead to hospital admission. Thus, when comparing unanticipated admission rate, the facilities and patient population should be similar.

The reported rates of unanticipated admission range from 0.1% to 9.5% with most facilities averaging around 1% (Table 13-1). The reasons for this variability include type of patient population and scheduling practices of a given facility. For example, some facilities may routinely care for patients undergoing diagnostic procedures who subsequently require more extensive surgery necessitating admission. However, if the multiple confounding variables mentioned above are taken into account, then close examination of the reasons for admission often yields useful information about medical complications following outpatient surgery.

The reasons for unanticipated admissions in adult and pediatric patients are shown in Table 13-2. In study after study over the past decade vomiting, pain, bleeding, and extensive surgery have been the leading causes of unanticipated admission, with subtle differences between pediatric and adult patients.

Three surveys of unanticipated admissions at pediatric hospitals found the leading causes of admissions among children to be vomiting, extensive surgery, and respiratory complications such as croup and apnea.[2,3,4] In a survey of complications among 10,000 children undergoing ambulatory surgery at Children's National Medical Center between 1983 and 1986, the unanticipated admission rate was 0.9%, and the three leading causes of admission were protracted vomiting (33%), extensive surgery (17%), and croup (9%).[2] In a follow-up study at the same institution conducted between 1988 and 1991, the admission rate declined to 0.3%, even though the patient volume increased ($n = 15,245$). The leading causes of admission, however, remained unchanged.[5] In another survey, which spanned 30 years of pediatric ambulatory surgery among 39,654 children, the unanticipated admission rate remained relatively constant at 1%. The leading cause, by far, was

Table 13-1 Admission Rates

Year surveyed	Admission rate	Type of facility	Number of patients	% ASA 1 & 2	Comments
1983-86[2]	0.90%	Hospital based	10,000	Not reported	Pediatric, teaching, tertiary care
1955-85[3]	1.10%	Hospital based	39,654	Not reported	Pediatric, Canada, teaching hospital
1982-86[4]	1.60%	Hospital based	2160	Not reported	Pediatric, Canada
1988-91[5]	0.30%	Hospital based	15,245	97%	Pediatric, teaching, tertiary care
1977-87[6]	0.28%	Hospital based	90,234	Not reported	10-year survey, Canada
1984-86[7]	1.04%	Hospital based	9616	96%	Teaching, tertiary care, adult
1987[8]	9.50%	Hospital based	1971	Not reported	Community teaching hospital
1985-86[9]	1.30%	Hospital based	2268	Not reported	Ophthalmic surgery
Not reported[10]	2.10%	Hospital based	236	Not reported	Cataract surgery only, average age = 72 years, United Kingdom
1986-89[11]	3.64%	Hospital based	2470	Not reported	Teaching hospital, gynecologic surgery only
1989[12]	5%	Hospital based	2039	Not reported	United Kingdom
1984-90[13]	1.20%	Freestanding	18,321	Not reported	Australia
1983-87[14]	0.70%	Hospital based	10,348	Not reported	United Kingdom
1980-88[15]	0.50%	Freestanding	3340	Not reported	T and A only

Freestanding: ambulatory surgery facilities that are not associated with a hospital except for emergencies.

Hospital based: ambulatory surgery centers that are associated with a main hospital and may be located within that hospital's operating room complex or on hospital grounds.

Admission rate: rate of unanticipated admissions following ambulatory surgery for the years reported.

T and A: tonsillectomy and adnoidectomy.

Table 13-2 Reasons for Admission

Year surveyed	Admission rates	Number of patients	Reasons	Comments
1983-86[2]	0.90%	10,000	Protracted vomiting, extensive surgery, croup	Pediatric
1955-85[3]	1.10%	39,654	Vomiting, extensive surgery, respiratory	Pediatric
1982-86[4]	1.60%	2160	Extensive surgery, hemorrhage, apnea/bradycardia	Pediatric
1988-91[5]	0.30%	15,245	Protracted vomiting, extensive surgery, croup	Pediatric
1977-87[6]	0.28%	90,234	Bleeding, surgical complication, extensive surgery	Canada, hospital based
1984-86[7]	1.04%	9616	Pain, bleeding, vomiting	University based, adult
1987[8]	9.50%	1971	Extensive surgery, dizziness, pain	Hospital based
1985-86[9]	1.30%	2268	Vomiting, pain, drowsiness	Ophthalmic
Not reported[10]	2.10%	236	Extensive surgery, vitreous loss, slow awakening	Cataract surgery
1986-89[11]	3.64%	2470	Vomiting, extensive surgery, hemorrhage	Gynecological surgery only
1989[12]	5.00%	2039	Vomiting, hemorrhage, postoperative pain	United Kingdom
1984-90[13]	1.20%	18,321	Extensive surgery, hemorrhage, perforated viscus	Australia
1983-87[14]	0.70%	10,000	Extensive surgery, vomiting, drowsiness	England
1980-88[15]	0.50%	3340	Hemorrhage, dehydration, emesis	Freestanding T and A only

vomiting, accounting for approximately 20% of unexpected admissions.[3] Although postoperative vomiting is a common postoperative complication in pediatric outpatients, other less frequent but life-threatening complications can account for admission. This is illustrated by a review of complications such as apnea and bradycardia, aspiration, and cyanosis among 2160 children undergoing general ambulatory surgery.[4] In this series, 11 experienced anesthetic complications necessitating admission. The vast majority (9 of 11) occurred in children younger than 3 months of age, some of whom had preexisting anomalies such as prematurity, Pierre Robin syndrome, and tracheoesophageal fistula.

In spite of the numerous challenges encountered with pediatric anesthesia, these studies demonstrate that certain types of complications, such as vomiting and respiratory compromise, are commonly seen in many facilities. Nevertheless, despite an increase in the number of children having ambulatory surgical procedures, unexpected admissions, which reflect complications, have remained constant or decreased. The challenge we face is to identify improved means of treating and preventing postoperative vomiting and preoperatively identifying children who are at risk for postoperative respiratory insufficiency.

The spectrum of perioperative complications as represented by unanticipated admissions among adult outpatients is also documented in several studies (Table 13-2). Again, vomiting, bleeding, and extensive surgery are common reasons for admission. In contrast to children, adults are often admitted for control of postoperative pain. The reasons for this are unclear, but may include the more liberal use of regional anesthesia for postoperative pain management in children (e.g., caudal blocks) and the nature of the surgical procedures.

Infrequent, but life-threatening, complications that contribute to admissions do occur even with "minor" surgery among adult patients. These complications, although small in number, deserve emphasis because they represent the scope of adverse events that any ambulatory surgical facility is expected to manage. In a survey of over 90,000 patients who underwent ambulatory surgery over a 10-year period, the admission rate was 0.28%.[6] As with other centers, common causes of admission were bleeding and extensive surgery. Relatively rare reasons for admission over this 10-year period were syncope ($n = 14$), aspiration ($n = 6$), and cardiac arrest ($n = 2$). In another study of 9616 adult outpatients having surgery at a university-based facility, the admission rate was 1%. The common diagnoses such as pain, hemorrhage, and vomiting accounted for over half of all admissions. However, 20% of all admissions were from various rare adverse events such as aspiration pneumonia ($n = 3$), suspected myocardial infarction ($n = 3$), suspected airway obstruction ($n = 2$), and diabetic control ($n = 1$).[7]

Deaths have occurred in the ambulatory surgery setting; however, these are extremely rare events, chronicled in the form of case reports. Causes of death have included CO_2 embolus during laparoscopy and undiagnosed cardiomyopathy.[8,16]

These data demonstrate that the vast majority of complications that lead to admission are common problems such as pain, vomiting, and bleeding. Nevertheless, rare life-threatening events can and do occur in the outpatient surgery setting. Although these events happen rarely, their occurrence demonstrates the need for every ambulatory surgical facility to be equipped to handle such emergencies.

Perioperative Events

Analysis of unexpected admissions is only one of the tools available for measuring complications in the ambulatory surgery setting. Other tools include surveys of perioperative complications that do not necessarily result in admission.

A recent multicenter, prospective evaluation of perioperative complications among adult outpatients confirms clinical intuition: ambulatory surgery patients with preoperative coexisting medical conditions are at higher risk for adverse events in the perioperative period.[17] This study surveyed 6914 adult outpatients who received general or regional anesthesia. The attending anesthesiologist listed any adverse perioperative events that may have occurred. Such events were broadly defined and included cardiac arrest, bronchospasm, difficult intubation, and damage to dentition. The majority of patients (97%) were ASA 1 or 2, with only 3% more than 70 years old. The most common event was nausea and/or vomiting. With respect to preoperative medical conditions and complications, patients with asthma, chronic obstructive pulmonary disease (COPD), or other respiratory diseases were at least twice as likely to have an adverse event as compared with patients without such coexisting disease. Similarly, patients with preoperative hypertension or gastrointestinal disorders were also more likely to have an adverse event. Patients with neurological disease or diabetes were almost four times as likely to have cardiovascular adverse events.

While previous investigations have focused on the immediate postoperative period, Warner and colleagues prospectively evaluated 38,598 adult outpatients for mortality and major morbidity (such as myocardial infarction and respiratory failure) up to 30 days postoperatively.[18] This study took place in a tertiary care referral facility where 24% of patients were ASA 3 and ranged in age from 18 to 96 years. The incidence of major morbidity or mortality within the 30 days following ambulatory surgery was rare (1:1366). The leading cause of major morbidity was perioperative myocardial infarction (1:3220). Only 2 of 14 myocardial infarctions occurred within 8 hours of surgery. Central nervous system (CNS) deficit accounted for 23% of major morbid events (1:6441). Only 1 of 7 CNS events occurred before the patients were discharged and 4 of 7 occurred within 48 hours of surgery. Respiratory failure accounted for 16% of all morbidity ($n = 5$); this includes one patient who aspirated intraoperatively. The remaining patients developed aspiration or pneumonia after discharge. To put the risk of mortality following ambulatory procedures into perspective, in this large study a total of four patients died within 30 days of surgery—two of myocardial infarction and two as passengers in automobile accidents. Taking this analysis one step further, would these morbid events have occurred anyhow, or did the surgical procedures and anesthetics contribute? The authors predicted, based on extensive epidemiologic data from the region, that after adjusting for age and unusual perioperative events, the three major types of morbidities (myocardial infarction, CNS deficit, and pulmonary embolus) occurred less often in the outpatient surgery population than in a comparable population not having ambulatory anesthesia. The authors attribute this to preoperative patient screening and selection. From this relatively long-term study, it appears that in the population examined the risk of overall major morbidity following outpatient anesthesia and surgery is very low, especially when compared with everyday risks, such as riding in an automobile.

Although major perioperative morbidity in the ambulatory setting is rare, minor sequelae occur with surprising frequency. In a postoperative mail-in questionnaire survey of patients who mainly had gynecologic outpatient surgery, 86% of responders reported one or more minor morbidity that persisted after discharge.[19] These morbidities included nausea, vomiting, myalgias, and sore throat. However, 38% of patients were able to resume their usual activities the day after surgery, and the remaining patients required an additional 3 ± 2 days. The reasons cited for the additional recovery days were general malaise and surgical discomfort. As expected, the frequency and the type of minor sequelae depended on the surgical procedure performed, with laparoscopy being associated with the greatest number of minor adverse events. In this series, the frequency and type of minor sequelae following ambulatory surgery was similar to that reported in studies from the early 1970s.[20-24] This frequency of minor side effects has remained relatively constant despite an outpatient population that is medically more complex than 20 years ago, and the use of an array of drugs marketed specifically for the ambulatory setting. Furthermore, in this study, almost two thirds of patients were not able to resume their usual activity on the first postoperative day. Thus, while available data consistently demonstrate that serious adverse events following outpatient surgery are extremely rare, minor sequelae that interfere with daily function occur frequently. These findings need to be appreciated by health care providers, patients, and their families so that expectations of ambulatory surgery and anesthesia are realistic.

Specific Complications

Nausea and Vomiting

Postoperative nausea and vomiting are among the most common postoperative complaints and occur in approximately 20% to 30% of patients.[25-28] In the outpatient setting, nausea and vomiting delays discharge, may result in unanticipated admission, and interferes with patients' resuming their usual activities. One of the reasons that effective management of this problem has remained so elusive is due to many variables that affect emesis. The emetic center, located in the parvicellular reticular formation, receives afferent stimuli from the pharynx, gastrointestinal tract, and mediastinum, as well as higher cortical centers such as the chemoreceptor trigger zone and the vestibular portion of the eighth cranial nerve (Fig. 13-1).[25] The chemoreceptor trigger zone (CTZ) is located in the area postrema, which is a highly vascularized region lacking an effective blood brain barrier. Therefore, the CTZ may be stimulated by substances in the blood as well as

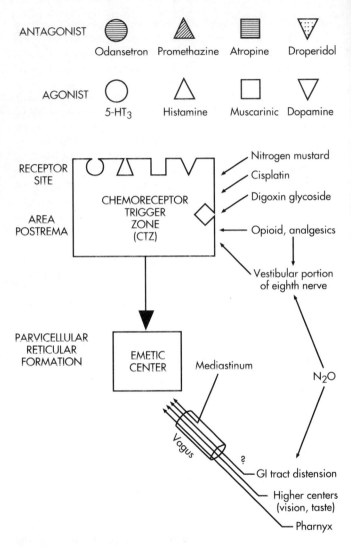

Fig. 13-1 Relation of emetic center with chemoreceptor trigger zone, various stimuli, and antagonists. (From Watcha MF, White PF: Post-operative nausea and vomiting. Anesthesiology 1992; 77:162-84.)

cerebrospinal fluid (CSF). The area postrema has receptors for dopamine, serotonin (also known as 5-hydroxytryptamine), muscarinic compounds, histamine, and opioids. Activation of these receptors is postulated to transmit impulses to the emetic center, which results in vomiting. Blockade of these receptors with drugs such as ondansetron and droperidol has been the rationale for antiemetic therapy to date.[25,28] However, the emetic center receives impulses from many sources, of which the CTZ is just one. The complex nature of afferent transmission to the emetic center helps explain why prevention and treatment of postoperative nausea and vomiting remains a challenge.

There are also several patient- and procedure-related factors that contribute to postoperative nausea and vomiting (Box 13-1). Younger patients (especially preadolescent), women, the obese, and anxious patients all have a preponderance for postoperative vomiting. In addition, patients with a history of motion sickness, postoperative vomiting, or gastroparesis are also at increased risk.[25,28] Recently, menses has also been implicated in contributing to postoperative vomiting. Specifically, the incidence of postoperative vomiting was found to be highest in women undergoing laparoscopy during their menstrual cycle (especially days 4 and 5). The authors speculate that this phenomena is secondary to increased levels of estrogen relative to follicle stimulating hormone that occurs on about day 5.[29] In a follow-up study, droperidol was not as effective in preventing postoperative vomiting in menstruating women as compared with nonmenstruating women following laparoscopic tubal ligation.[30]

The type of surgical procedure also influences postoperative nausea and vomiting. Specifically, strabismus repair, laparoscopy, middle ear surgery, and orchiopexy are all associated with a relatively high incidence of postoperative vomiting in several studies using a variety of anesthetic techniques (Box 13-1).[25,28]

Numerous anesthetics have also been implicated in contributing to postoperative emesis. Nitrous oxide has been frequently associated with causing vomiting.[31,32] However, more recent studies have found no causal relationship.[33,34] Opioids have also been linked with postoperative vomiting, but patients who develop vomiting with one opioid may not with another. Although the respiratory depressant effects of opioids have been associated with a specific opioid receptor, emetic effects have not. In fact, administration of naloxone, a pure opioid antagonist, can itself

Box 13-1 *Common Causes of Nausea and Vomiting in Outpatients*

Predisposing Factors

Female gender
Motion sickness
Morbid obesity
Early pregnancy

Increased Gastric Volume

Excessive anxiety
Noncompliance

Premedicants

Narcotic analgesics (e.g., fentanyl)

Anesthetic Agents

Inhaled gases
Intravenous drugs (e.g., etomidate)

Surgical Procedures

Laparoscopy
Strabismus correction
Insertion of PE tubes
Orchiopexy

Postoperative Factors

Hypotension
Pain

From White PF, Shafer A: Nausea and vomiting: causes and prophylaxis. Semin Anesthesia 1987; 6:300.

result in vomiting.[25] Consequently, development of a narcotic that is devoid of emetic side effects has been elusive. Propofol is promoted as an anesthetic that reduces the incidence of nausea and vomiting. Several studies have shown that propofol used for induction, or induction and maintenance, of anesthesia is associated with less postoperative nausea and vomiting than thiopental-isoflurane–nitrous oxide anesthesia.[35,36] For example, among outpatients receiving propofol the incidence of emesis was 5% versus 27% in patients receiving isoflurane.[35] In women undergoing in vitro fertilization, a comparison of total intravenous anesthesia with propofol and alfentanil versus enflurane–nitrous oxide found substantially lower rates of postoperative emesis in the propofol group (64% versus 39%).[37]

Similar results with propofol have been reported in children. Among pediatric outpatients having strabismus surgery, the use of propofol for induction and maintenance was associated with significantly shorter discharge times and less postoperative emesis than anesthetics containing halothane/N_2O/droperidol or propofol/ N_2O ± droperidol.[38] However, the incidence of oculocardiac reflex was significantly greater in the children receiving propofol exclusively. In another study of 143 children undergoing various outpatient procedures with either propofol or inhaled anesthetics, the propofol group experienced significantly less postoperative emesis in the PACU (0% versus 7%) and at home (18% versus 34%). Furthermore, there were more episodes of airway obstruction during induction of anesthesia in the inhalation group (34% versus 10%). In spite of these differences, however, the duration of postoperative stay was the same in both groups.[39]

With both pediatric and adult use, it is unclear whether propofol has an antiemetic effect or is just associated with less vomiting than other currently available anesthetics.[40] Nevertheless, this feature, coupled with relatively rapid emergence, has helped to make propofol an extremely popular outpatient anesthetic.

Not to be forgotten are postoperative factors that contribute to postoperative nausea and vomiting. These include postoperative pain, postural hypotension, ambulation, and oral intake.[25,28] Prompt treatment of pain, adequate intravenous hydration, and delaying oral intake until the patient is so inclined may all help to relieve postoperative causes of nausea and vomiting.

Given the complex physiology and multifactorial nature of postoperative emesis, as well as expectations of prompt ambulation and oral intake following surgery, it is not surprising that postoperative nausea and vomiting remains one of the most common complications in the outpatient surgery setting.

Aspiration

Pulmonary aspiration of gastric contents is a serious but rare complication. Since this adverse event is not common in modern anesthetic practice, large studies involving varying patient populations are necessary to determine the frequency of aspiration and associated risk factors. In one large study of over 185,000 anesthetics, the incidence of aspiration was 4.7 per 10,000 anesthetics.[41] A large prospective multicenter French study of 198,103 patients documented 27 cases of aspiration yielding an incidence of 1.4 per 10,000.[42] In a survey of more than 500,000 outpatient anesthetics during 1985, there were 1.7 episodes of aspiration per 10,000 anesthetics.[43] In the ASA Closed Claim Study, of the 522 adverse respiratory events, aspiration accounted for only 5% of cases.[44]

Among children the risk of aspiration is somewhat higher, perhaps due to difficulties encountered with airway management. In a prospective multicenter study of 40,240 inpatient and outpatient anesthetics in France, the incidence of aspiration was <1:10,000 in children more than 1 year old and 1:1000 in infants.[45] Manchikanti and colleagues compared gastric pH and volume in pediatric (6 months to 12 years old), adult, and geriatric (more than 65 years old) patients. Mean gastric pH was significantly lower in the pediatric group as compared with the adult and geriatric group pH (1.99, 2.40, and 3.32). Mean gastric volumes were also higher in pediatric patients when compared with adult and geriatric patients (0.49 ml/kg, 0.37 ml/kg, and 0.24 ml/kg).[46] Coté and colleagues found that, compared with historical controls, children had a lower gastric pH and higher gastric volume than adults, but that there was no significant difference in the gastric contents among inpatient or outpatient children who fasted.[47]

From these studies and others, several risk factors for aspiration have been identified. They include conditions that delay gastric emptying, such as obesity, diabetes, peptic ulcer disease, stress, pain, trauma, and opioid use. An incompetent lower esophageal sphincter and symptoms of gastric reflux are also risk factors. There are also other less predictable factors such as emergency surgery (especially at night) and difficult airway management.[48] Outpatients had been considered to be at increased risk of aspiration because of the stress associated with arriving at the hospital on the day of surgery. This belief was based on a study of comparing the gastric volume and pH of inpatients with outpatients.[49] Outpatients had greater gastric volume than inpatients (mean 69 ml versus 33 ml), while the gastric pH was essentially the same between groups. However, there was considerably more variability in the range of gastric volumes among outpatients (15 ml to 355 ml), even though all had reportedly fasted. These findings are in contrast to more recent studies that have found no difference in the gastric pH and volume of inpatients and outpatients.[47,50-54] In current practice, healthy outpatients are not generally assumed to be at increased risk for aspiration.

Using gastric pH and volume as a marker for aspiration risk, several studies over the past decade have examined the impact of clear fluids taken up to 2 hours before elective surgery in otherwise healthy adults and children. Based on numerous investigations conducted over the past decade, ingestion of clear liquids up to 2 to 3 hours preoperatively does not appear to affect gastric volume or pH.[48,51,53,55-60] It is important to emphasize that these results were obtained from healthy patients having elective surgery who were not taking medication that delayed gastric emptying. In these studies, there was not an increased incidence of aspiration if patients were allowed clear liquids preoperatively. However, given the rarity of aspiration, very large populations will have to be evaluated. Whether the practice of allowing clear liquids to healthy adults having elective outpatient surgery will afford benefits without increasing risks remains to be determined. Among children, however, clear liquids up to 2 hours preoperatively may not only make them more comfortable, but potentially minimize dehydration in small infants and hypoglycemia in neonates.

Malignant Hyperthermia

Malignant hyperthermia (MH) is a rare but potentially fatal complication. Even though MH is rare, it may develop unexpectedly. Furthermore, malignant hyperthermia is more common in children than adults, and children account for a sizable proportion of surgical outpatients. Therefore, it is imperative that each ambulatory surgical facility have the means and expertise to immediately and aggressively manage malignant hyperthermia.

The incidence of MH is estimated to be 1:50,000 to 1:100,000 in adults and 1:3000 to 1:15,000 in children.[61] However, the exact incidence in outpatients is unclear. Given the catastrophic nature of this complication, a major goal is to prevent an episode from occurring. Prevention includes a thorough preoperative evaluation including history of past anesthetics, family history of MH, or major anesthetic complications. Recognition of possible risk factors for MH is also important. These include history of strabismus, muscular dystrophy (especially Duchenne), and central core disease. Noninvasive screening tests (such as serum CPK) to rule out MH are not conclusive, thereby necessitating a muscle biopsy.[61,62] Even in the absence of a definitive diagnosis of MH, many patients with suggestive histories or risk factors are considered to be MH–susceptible and managed as if they had MH. Triggering agents, such as halogenated inhaled anesthetics and succinylcholine, must be avoided. Other precautions include using a clean anesthesia machine that does not have vaporizers but has a new CO_2 absorber and hoses, and has been flushed with oxygen at 10 liters/min for several minutes.[62,63] Pretreatment with dantrolene in MH–susceptible patients remains controversial.

Prompt recognition of MH is essential for effective treatment. Since MH involves an increase in the metabolic rate of skeletal muscles, one of the first systemic signs of MH will be a response to increased metabolic demand, namely tachycardia, tachypnea, and a rise in measured end-tidal CO_2. Other signs include ventricular ectopy that occurs without other obvious causes, acidosis, and eventually hyperthermia (Box 13-2). Treatment of MH depends on prompt, aggressive management as outlined in Box 13-3. Dantrolene is the cornerstone of therapy and, therefore, needs to be readily available in each ambulatory surgery unit.

Should patients who have confirmed MH or are MH–susceptible have outpatient surgery? This issue is controversial and was the subject of a recent 10-year retrospective review.[64] In this

---

Box 13-2 *Signs and Symptoms of Malignant Hyperthermia*

Tachycardia	Hyperkalemia
Arrhythmias	Cyanosis
Respiratory acidosis	Coagulopathy
Tachypnea	Muscle rigidity
Metabolic acidosis	Myoglobinuria
Fever	

From Ryan JF: Malignant hyperthermia. In Coté CJ, Ryan JF, Todres ID, Goudsouzian NG, editors: A practice of anesthesia for infants and children, ed 2, Philadelphia, 1993, WB Saunders, pp. 417-28.

Box 13-3 Malignant Hyperthermia Treatment Regimen

1. Stop anesthesia and surgery immediately.
2. Hyperventilate patient with 100% oxygen.
3. Administer dantrolene (Dantrium), 2.5 mg/kg IV, and procainamide (up to 15 mg/kg IV slowly if required for dysrhythmias) as soon as possible.
4. Initiate cooling.
5. Correct acidosis.
6. Secure monitoring lines: electrocardiogram, temperature, urinary catheter, arterial pressure, central venous pressure.
7. Maintain urine output.
8. Monitor patient until danger of subsequent episodes is past (48 to 72 hours).
9. Administer dantrolene PO or IV for 48 to 72 hours.

From Ryan JF: Malignant hyperthermia. In Coté CJ, Ryan JF, Todres ID, Goudsouzian NG, editors: A practice of anesthesia for infants and children, ed 2, Philadelphia, 1993, WB Saunders, pp. 417-28.

---

chart survey of 303 MH–susceptible children, triggering agents were avoided in all cases and prophylactic dantrolene was given before 1985. Over half of the patients were admitted because they were labeled as MH–susceptible. There were no cases of intraoperative pyrexia (temperature more than 38.5°C) and 10 cases of postoperative pyrexia. Of these 10 patients, there were alternative explanations for fever, such as otitis media and radiographic evidence of atelectasis or resolution of fever with acetaminophen. Four patients who developed postoperative pyrexia had received prophylactic dantrolene. Based on this retrospective analysis, the authors do not recommend admission to the hospital because a child is labeled as MH–susceptible.[64] This recommendation is not universally accepted, and other experts take a more conservative approach.[65,66] This issue may remain controversial until results of large prospective studies become available. However, guidelines for prevention and treatment of MH are well developed so that this catastrophic complication can either be avoided or promptly managed in any ambulatory surgery facility.

Advanced Age, Coexisting Disease, and Complications

During the past several years many procedures, including cataract removal, have shifted to the outpatient setting. Cataract surgery is one of the most common outpatient surgical procedures.[67] Usually, cataract excision requires local anesthesia with mild sedation. However, the vast majority of patients are elderly and many have chronic illness and/or poor social support systems. To help define the types of complications in elderly outpatients, it is useful to examine the population undergoing eye surgery.

In a study of 2268 patients with a mean age of 63 years who received either local or general anesthesia for eye surgery, the rate of unanticipated admissions was 1.3%.[9] Risk factors associated with unplanned admission were completion of surgery late in the afternoon and elevated white blood cell count. Remarkably, variables not associated with admission were age, underlying medical illness, and ASA physical status. In over a quarter of patients, the reason for admission was persistent nausea and vomiting. A British survey of outpatients having cataract surgery with either local or general anesthesia found an unanticipated admission rate of 2.1%. Admissions were not a function of the patient age or distance traveled.[10]

These geriatric patients having eye surgery may do well because they often receive local anesthesia with little or no sedation. One important question is whether complication rates are low in geriatric patients who receive general or regional anesthesia for other procedures. In a case-control study of 9616 adult outpatients not having ocular procedures, advanced age independently correlated with unanticipated admissions.[7] Older patients were more than twice as likely to be admitted as their younger counterparts (as measured in 30-year intervals). In this study, patients with coexisting disease were also twice as likely to be admitted. However, this association lost significance when the analysis was controlled for age. This suggests that age is a surrogate of other factors that influence admission, such as underlying medical illness, weak social support systems, and perhaps slower recovery from anesthesia and surgery.[7] Similar findings are reported in a multicenter Canadian study of ambulatory surgery complications. In almost 7000 patients, those with well-controlled preoperative medical disease were more likely to have an adverse perioperative event.[17] For example, patients with diabetes were more likely to have labile blood pressure, and those with asthma or COPD experienced more adverse events involving the lower respiratory tract.[17] The relationship between adverse events and unexpected admissions, however, was not evaluated in this study.

There is similar evidence from other studies that advanced age is associated with perioperative complications, at least as measured by unexpected admissions. In a survey of 1971 outpatients undergoing a variety of procedures, most of the patients were in the 20 to 40 year age range. However, the age distribution of patients who were unexpectedly admitted was bimodal. One peak occurred at 20 to 30 years and another at 70 to 80 years.[8] In another study of women having outpatient gynecologic surgery, the presence of coexisting medical disease was associated with unexpected admission, but age was not.[11]

These data suggest that there is an association between advanced age, coexisting medical conditions, and complications in the ambulatory surgery setting. The extent and significance of this association need to be examined in detail especially as the indications for outpatient anesthesia and surgery expand and the population becomes more complex.

The Child with an Upper Respiratory Tract Infection

The child with an upper respiratory tract infection (URI) who presents for elective outpatient surgery poses a difficult dilemma. On the one hand, URIs occur frequently and to varying degrees. The child (and his or her parents) may have had to travel great distances and taken time away from work and school. Of concern, however, is that administration of general anesthesia will exacerbate the URI. During an acute URI, airways will be hyperreactive, which may progress to bronchospasm. There may be mucous plugging and atelectasis, which can lead to hypoxia and pneumonia. What criteria should be used in deciding when and if to proceed with general anesthesia in a child with a URI?

This question raises several other questions such as: Are there adverse outcomes with asymptomatic viral infections? Which symptoms are important? What is the effect of age? Intubation? Procedure? Bacterial infection versus viral infection? How long should one wait after a URI before proceeding with elective surgery? There are no prospective studies that definitively answer all these questions, but recent data provide some useful guidelines.

In children with URIs having only myringotomies via mask general anesthesia, there was no increase in the incidence of laryngospasm, bronchospasm, dysrhythmias, or apnea; none of these patients were intubated and the mean duration of surgery was 12.6 minutes. Among patients classified with URIs, only 22% had the virus isolated, which questions whether "URI" patients had a respiratory infection or merely rhinitis.[68]

In a subsequent study of children undergoing a variety of otolaryngological procedures, children with URI symptoms were significantly more likely to experience desaturation in the PACU as compared with controls. This occurred even though oxygen saturation was more than 95% preinduction in both groups. At the time of this study, oxygen saturation was not measured routinely; therefore, the incidence of intraoperative desaturation was not assessed.[69]

Cohen et al.[70] prospectively evaluated 1283 children with a URI and 20,876 children without URI who underwent elective surgery. In this study children who had mucopurulent nasal secretions, an elevated white blood count, or positive chest findings did not present to the operating room and were not included. Therefore, children with a URI were those who had clear nasal secretions and a possible fever, but also had chest sounds that were clear to auscultation. The majority of procedures involved ears, eyes, nose and throat, and the extremities. Children with a URI were more likely (2:7) to have an adverse event related to the respiratory system. For example, children with a URI were almost five times more likely to suffer airway obstruction intraoperatively than children without a URI. This increased risk applied to all age groups. Children with a URI who were not intubated were almost nine times more likely to experience an adverse respiratory event as compared with children without a URI who were also not intubated. Given their results and the frequency of URIs, the authors concluded that (1) children less than 1 year old with asymptomatic or mild URI should have elective surgery postponed, and the decision to proceed in children more than 1 year old should be made on an individual basis; (2) children (regardless of age) with symptomatic URIs should have elective surgery rescheduled, because children with even mild URI symptoms are at risk for adverse perioperative respiratory events.

Complications Following Tonsillectomies and Adenoidectomies

Tonsillectomy and adenoidectomy are among the most common operations performed nationally, and frequently the patients are children.[71] Several factors have moved this procedure to the outpatient setting, including low complication rates, pediatric population, and cost effectiveness. Although complications following tonsillectomy and adenoidectomy may be rare, they usually involve the airway. These complications, which include hemorrhage and airway obstruction, may have a precipitous onset.

In light of these life-threatening, albeit rare, complications there have been several investigations of the safety of outpatient tonsillectomy and adenoidectomy. A retrospective review of 3340 outpatient adenoidectomy and/or tonsillectomy procedures at a freestanding surgical center reported a complication rate of 1.4%.[71] Primary tonsillar hemorrhage (postoperative bleeding within 24 hours of surgery) occurred in 0.35% of patients. A somewhat larger number of patients (0.9%) experienced secondary hemorrhage (bleeding occurring more than 24 hours after the surgery). Other complications included dehydration and persistent emesis, which brought the total unanticipated admission rate to 0.5%.[71]

Another study examined complications after inpatient tonsillectomy and adenoidectomy among children less than 36 months old to assess the appropriateness of performing this procedure in such a young population on an outpatient basis.[72] Airway complications occurred postoperatively in over half of the patients, and the majority of the patients required more than routine care after discharge from the PACU (supplemental oxygen, dexamethasone, droperidol, etc.). Based on these findings, the authors recommended that children less than 3 years old have tonsillectomies and adenoidectomies as inpatients.

Other earlier surveys of complication rates following tonsillectomy and adenoidectomies have shown similar results.[73-75] Postoperative hemorrhage occurred in up to 7% of patients, with primary hemorrhage being relatively rare (under 1%).[73-75] Children less than 3 years old with preexisting medical illness (such as cerebral palsy or congenital heart disease) were more likely to have major airway complications requiring reintubation.

These retrospective studies and others suggest that complications following tonsillectomies and adenoidectomies are rare and that these procedures may be safely performed in certain children only after rigorous patient selection criteria are met, families are educated regarding potential complications, and the threshold for admission is low. Larger, prospective studies would provide even more compelling evidence for the safety, efficacy, and limitations of outpatient tonsillectomies and adenoidectomies.

Quality Assessment and Quality Improvement

Given the nature of medical practice, some complications are bound to occur. The process by which we recognize and minimize complications while providing efficient, quality health care that is satisfying to both patient and health care provider is the foundation for quality assessment and improvement programs. This is a very complex process that involves local health care providers, hospital and government regulators, and third party payors. There are assumptions about what constitutes "quality," which outcomes should be measured, and how to measure them. Problems need to be identified and solved in a nonthreatening, objective, and systematic manner. This process is changing as we struggle with controlling health care costs and improving access to health care while maintaining high standards of care. Nevertheless, even with the given state of flux there exist basic principles that can guide "quality improvement."

Quality improvement programs evaluate and monitor the standard of care delivered by a given health care facility. For ambulatory surgery, these programs are governed by the major accreditation and licensing organization, namely the Joint Commission on Accreditation of Healthcare Organizations (JCAHO). The JCAHO operates peer-based assessment and accreditation programs, the criteria for which are detailed in its yearly manuals.[76,77] The JCAHO establishes broad criteria, which ambulatory surgery facilities must meet in order to be accredited. However, each facility needs to have its own specific policies, procedures, and means for assessing and implementing quality care that are also consistent with the standards established by the JCAHO.

Theoretically, there are several approaches to assessing quality. One approach, which is supported by the JCAHO, involves the assessment of "structure, process and outcome."[76,78] "Structure" refers to human and physical resources (e.g., qualifications of personnel, physical plant, equipment) and organizational structure (e.g., medical staff organization, reimbursement methods). "Process" is the actual giving and receiving of health care. For example, in the ambulatory surgery setting, part of this process is documented in the anesthesia and PACU records. "Outcome" refers to the effects of the care on the patients.[76,78] Several different outcomes need to be monitored to assess the quality of care. For example, the unanticipated admission rate should be evaluated in the context of the type of facility, patient volume, patient population, and PACU stay.

The rationale for this three-part approach to quality assessment is that each part affects the other. A strong structure contributes to a good process, which in turn leads to positive outcomes. Consequently, quality improvement programs need to evaluate each of these parts and the relationship between them. For example, if a piece of laser equipment is faulty (structure) and the patient cannot receive the planned treatment (process), then the procedure will have to be rescheduled resulting in a cancellation and possible delays (outcome).

While the JCAHO has provided very general guidelines, it is the responsibility of the individual facility to identify, monitor, and practice quality care. How does this process happen? Specifically, who should be involved, which clinical indicators should be examined, how should deficiencies be corrected, how should progress be monitored, and how should this information be documented and reported?

An example of a quality improvement program at a hospital-integrated ambulatory surgery unit is described by Twersky et al.[76] In this model, persons actively involved in the delivery of care at the ambulatory surgery facility form the basis for the quality improvement committee, which meets approximately monthly. This committee includes the medical director (anesthesiologist), nursing director, and representatives of each of the surgical specialties who use the unit. The medical director chairs the meetings and is responsible for documenting them as required by regulatory agencies. The medical director also communicates with the hospital quality improvement committees and the operating room committees. Clinical indicators that are assessed in this program include patient satisfaction questionnaires, incident

---

Box 13-4 *Sample of Clinical Indicators for Quality Improvement Programs*

Unanticipated admissions
Cancellations
Prolonged PACU stay
Delays
Inadequate medical record documentation
Adequacy of preoperative evaluation
Patient follow-up
Patient satisfaction questionnaires
Equipment performance
Adherence to infection control standards

---

reports (including delays), patient follow-up (including readmission within 30 days of surgery), prolonged PACU stay, unanticipated admissions, cancellations, and adequacy of medical record documentation. Other clinical indicators that may need to be examined include the adequacy of the preoperative evaluation, equipment performance, and proper adherence to infection control standards (Box 13-4). When problems are recognized, the persons involved are requested to submit a report, which is reviewed by the committee. At this point, a determination is made as to which factors contributed to the problem and how it could have been avoided, if possible. If necessary, corrective action is then taken.

As part of the transition from quality assurance to continuous quality improvement, the JCAHO— in its accreditation process— seeks to involve administrators and hospital leaders in the monitoring and evaluation of health care. The focus should be on collecting data that ". . . may be used by the organization to meet the demands of patients, payors, and others who want to make informed health care decisions."[79] Several indicators (or outcomes) will need to be assessed. These include documentation of patients who develop central or peripheral neurologic deficit, myocardial infarction, or cardiac arrest within 2 days postprocedure in procedures involving anesthesia administration. These events need to be categorized by the procedure, ASA physical status, and patient age. Indicators that the JCAHO now recommends for internal hospital use only include assessment of patients who develop either intraoperative or postoperative pulmonary edema, aspiration pneumonitis, postdural puncture headache, dental injury, ocular injury, and unplanned admission within 2 days of outpatient anesthesia.[79] This is only a partial list of outcomes that need to be monitored to comply with quality assessment guidelines.

Although outcomes analysis is an essential component of any quality assessment program, it is only one measure of "quality." As we have learned from colleagues in industry, it is not sufficient just to inspect products as they leave the factory. Rather, quality needs to be built into the production process.[80] In an ambulatory surgery center, this translates to assessing care from the preoperative evaluation to the postoperative follow-up telephone call with the ultimate goal of continuously improving the quality of care our patients receive.

Summary

While ambulatory anesthesia and surgery practice has rapidly expanded to include patients with complex medical problems at the extremes of age, complication rates have remained relatively stable. To avoid complacency, it is important to emphasize that the spectrum of complications encountered in the outpatient setting is all encompassing. Despite relatively low complication rates, ambulatory surgery facilities need to be prepared to manage life-threatening emergencies. In an effort to minimize complications, educate personnel, and continuously improve care, ongoing quality assessment programs must remain an integral part of the ambulatory surgery center.

References

1. Gold BS: Unanticipated admissions. In McGoldrick KE, editor: Ambulatory anesthesiology: a problem oriented approach, Baltimore, in press, William & Wilkins.

2. Patel RI, Hannallah RS: Anesthetic complications following pediatric ambulatory surgery: a 3-year study. Anesthesiology 1988; 69:1009-12.

3. Postuma R, Ferguson CC, Stanwick RS, Horne JM: Pediatric day-care surgery: a 30-year hospital experience. J Pediatr Surg 1987; 22:304-7.

4. Moir CR, Blair GK, Fraser GC, Marshall RH: The emerging pattern of pediatric day-care surgery. J Pediatr Surg 1987; 22:743-5.

5. Patel RI, Hannallah RS: Complications following pediatric ambulatory surgery—less of the same? Anesthesiology 1993; 79:3A.

6. Fancourt-Smith PF, Hornstein J, Jenkins LC: Hospital admissions from the Surgical Day Care Centre of Vancouver General Hospital 1977-1987. Can J Anaesth 1990; 37:699-704.

7. Gold BS, Kitz DS, Lecky JH, Neuhaus JM: Unanticipated admission to the hospital following ambulatory surgery. JAMA 1989; 262:3008-10.

8. Levin P, Stanziola A, Hand R: Postoperative hospital retention following ambulatory surgery in a hospital-based program. Am Coll Utilz Rev Physicians 1990; 5:90-4.

9. Freeman LN, Schachat AP, Manolio TA, Enger C: Multivariate analysis of factors associated with unplanned admission in "outpatient" ophthalmic surgery. Ophthalmic Surg 1988; 19:719-23.

10. Strong NP, Wigmore W, Smithson S et al: Daycase cataract surgery. Br J Ophthalmol 1991; 75:731-3.

11. Meeks GR, Waller GA, Meydrech EF, Flautt FH: Unscheduled hospital admission following ambulatory gynecologic surgery. Obstet Gynecol 1992; 80:446-50.

12. Thompson EM, Mathews HML, McAuley DM: Problems in day care surgery. Ulster Med J 1991; 60:176-82.

13. Biswas TK, Leary C: Postoperative hospital admission from a day surgery unit: a seven-year retrospective survey. Anaesth Intens Care 1992; 20:147-50.

14. Johnson CD, Jarrett PEM: Admission to hospital after day case surgery. Ann R Coll Surg Engl 1990; 72:225-8.

15. Colclasure JB, Graham SS: Complications of outpatient tonsillectomy and adenoidectomy: a review of 3340 cases. Ear Nose Throat J 1990; 69:155-60.

16. Hanson, CW: Asymptomatic cardiomyopathy presenting as cardiac arrest in the day surgical unit. Anesthesiology 1989; 71:982-4.

17. Duncan PG, Cohen MM, Tweed WA et al: The Canadian four-centre study of anaesthetic outcomes: III. Are anaesthetic complications predictable in day surgical practice? Can J Anaesth 1992; 39:440-8.

18. Warner MA, Shields, SE, Chute CG: Major morbidity and mortality within 1 month of ambulatory surgery and anesthesia. JAMA 1993; 270:1437-41.

19. Philip BK: Patients' assessment of ambulatory anesthesia and surgery. J Clin Anesth 1992; 4:355-8.

20. Thompson GE, Remington JM, Millman BS, Bridenbaugh LD: Experiences with outpatient anesthesia. Anesth Analg 1973; 52:881-7.

21. Heneghan C, McAuliffe R, Thomas D, Radford P: Morbidity after outpatient anaesthesia. Anaesthesia 1981; 36:4-9.

22. Fahy A, Marshall M: Postanesthetic morbidity in out-patients. Br J Anaesth 1969; 41:433-8.

23. Ogg TW: An assessment of postoperative outpatient cases. Br Med J 1972; 4:573-6.

24. Brindle GF, Soliman MG: Anesthetic complications in surgical outpatients. Can Anaesth Soc J 1975; 22:613-9.

25. Watcha MF, White PF: Postoperative nausea and vomiting. Anesthesiology 1992; 77:162-84.

26. Kapur PA: The big "little problem." Anesth Analg 1991; 73:243-5.

27. Abramowitz MD, Oh TH, Epstein BS et al: The antiemetic effect of droperidol following outpatient strabismus surgery in children. Anesthesiology 1983; 59:579-83.

28. White PF, Shafer A: Nausea and vomiting: causes and prophylaxis. Semin Anesthesia 1987; 6:300-8.

29. Beattie WS, Lindblad T, Buckley DN, Forrest JB: The incidence of postoperative nausea and vomiting in women undergoing laparoscopy is influenced by the day of menstrual cycle. Can J Anaesth 1991; 38:298-302.

30. Beattie WS, Lindblad T, Buckley DN, Forrest JB: Menstruation increases the risk of nausea and vomiting after laparoscopy. Anesthesiology 1993; 78:272-6.

31. Eger EI: MAC. In Eger EI, editor: Nitrous oxide, New York, 1985, Elsevier, pp. 58-9.

32. Lonie DS, Harper JN: Nitrous oxide anaesthesia and vomiting. Anaesthesia 1986; 41:703-7.

33. Muir JJ, Warner MA, Offord KP et al: Role of nitrous oxide and other factors in postoperative nausea and vomiting: a randomized and blinded prospective study. Anesthesiology 1987; 66:513-8.

34. Korttila K, Hovorka J, Erkola O: Nitrous oxide does not increase the incidence of nausea and vomiting after isoflurane anesthesia. Anesth Analg 1987; 66:761-5.

35. Doze VA, Shafer A, White PF: Propofol-nitrous oxide versus thiopental-isoflurane-nitrous oxide for general anesthesia. Anesthesiology 1988; 69:63-71.

36. Korttila K, Ostman P, Faure E et al: Randomized comparison of recovery after propofol-nitrous oxide versus thiopentone-isoflurane-nitrous oxide anaesthesia in patients undergoing ambulatory surgery. Acta Anaesthesiol Scand 1990; 34:400-3.

37. Raftery S, Sherry E: Total intravenous anaesthesia with propofol and alfentanil protects against postoperative nausea and vomiting. Can J Anaesth 1992; 39:37-40.

38. Watcha MF, Simeon RM, White PF, Stevens JL: Effect of propofol on the incidence of postoperative vomiting after strabismus surgery in pediatric outpatients. Anesthesiology 1991; 75:204-9.

39. Martin TM, Nicolson SC, Bargas MS: Propofol anesthesia reduces emesis and airway obstruction in pediatric outpatients. Anesth Analg 1993; 76:144-8.

40. McCollum JSC, Milligan KR, Dundee JW: The antiemetic action of propofol. Anaesthesia 1988; 43:239-40.

41. Olsson GL, Hallen B, Hambraeus-Jonzon K: Aspiration during anaesthesia: a computer-aided study of 185,358 anaesthetics. Acta Anaesthesiol Scand 1986; 30:84-92.

42. Tiret L, Desmonts JM, Hatton F, Vourc'h G: Complications associated with anaesthesia—a prospective survey in France. Can Anaesth Soc J 1986; 33:336-44.

43. Kallar SK: Aspiration penumonitis: fact or fiction? Probl Anesthesia 1988; 2:29.

44. Caplan RA, Posner KL, Ward RJ, Cheney FW: Adverse respiratory events in anesthesia: a closed claims analysis. Anesthesiology 1990; 72:828-33.

45. Tiret L, Nivoche Y, Hatton F et al: Complications related to anaesthesia in infants and children. Br J Anaesth 1988; 61:263-9.

46. Manchikanti L, Colliver JA, Marrero TC, Roush JR: Assessment of age-related acid aspiration risk factors in pediatric, adult, and geriatric patients. Anesth Analg 1985; 64:11-7.

47. Coté CJ, Goudsouzian NG, Liu LM et al: Assessment of risk factors related to the acid aspiration syndrome in pediatric patients—gastric pH and residual volume. Anesthesiology 1982; 56:70-2.

48. Kallar SK, Everett LL: Potential risks and preventive measures for pulmonary aspiration: new concepts in preoperative fasting guidelines. Anesth Analg 1993; 77:171-82.

49. Ong BY, Palahniuk RJ, Cumming M: Gastric volume and pH in outpatients. Can Anaesth Soc J 1978; 25:36-9.

50. Haavik PE, Soreide E, Hofstad B, Steen PA: Does preoperative anxiety influence fluid volume and acidity? Anesth Analg 1992; 75:91-4.

51. Maltby JR, Sutherland AD, Sale JP, Shaffer EA: Preoperative oral fluids: is a five-hour fast justified prior to elective surgery? Anesth Analg 1986; 65:1112-6.

52. Sutherland AD, Stock JG, Davies JM: Effects of preoperative fasting on morbidity and gastric contents in patients undergoing day-stay surgery. Br J Anaesth 1986; 58:876-8.

53. Maltby JR, Lewis P, Martin A, Sutherland LR: Gastric fluid volume and pH in elective patients following unrestricted oral fluid until three hours before surgery. Can J Anaesth 1991; 38:425-9.

54. Talke PO, Solanki DR: Dose-response study of oral famotidine for reduction of gastric acidity and volume in outpatients and inpatients. Anesth Analg 1993; 77:1143-8.

55. Strunin L; How long should patients fast before surgery? Time for new guidelines (editorial). Br J Anaesth 1993; 70:1-3.

56. Sandhar BK, Goresky GV, Maltby JR, Shaffer EA: Effect of oral liquids and ranitidine on gastric fluid volume and pH in children undergoing outpatient surgery. Anesthesiology 1989; 71:327-30.

57. Schreiner MS, Triebwasser A, Keon TP: Ingestion of liquids compared with preoperative fasting in pediatric outpatients. Anesthesiology 1990; 72:593-7.

58. Splinter WM, Schaefer JD, Zunder IH: Clear fluids three hours before surgery do not affect the gastric fluid contents of children. Can J Anaesth 1990; 37:498-501.

59. Crawford M, Lerman J, Christensen S, Farrow-Gillespie A: Effects of duration of fasting on gastric fluid pH and volume in healthy children. Anesth Analg 1990; 71:400-3.

60. Coté CJ: NPO after midnight for children: a reappraisal. Anesthesiology 1990; 72:589-92.

61. Ryan J: Malignant hyperthermia. In Coté CJ, Ryan JF, Todres ID, Goudsouzan NG, editors: A practice of anesthesia for infants and children, ed 2, Philadelphia, 1993, WB Saunders, pp. 417-28.

62. Gronert GA: Malignant hyperthermia. In Barash PG, editor: Refresher courses in anesthesiology, Philadelphia, 1989, JB Lippincott, pp. 107-15.

63. Beebe JJ, Sessler DI: Preparation of anesthesia machines for patients susceptible to malignant hyperthermia. Anesthesiology 1988; 69:395-400.

64. Yentis SM, Levine MF, Hartley EJ: Should all children with suspected or confirmed malignant hyperthermia susceptibility be admitted after surgery? A 10-year review. Pediatr Anesthesia 1992; 75:345-50.

65. McGoldrick K: Is malignant hyperthermia a contraindication for outpatient surgery? Soc Ambul Anesth News 1992; 11.

66. Kallar SK, Jones GW: Postoperative complications. In White PF, editor: Outpatient anesthesia, New York, 1990, Churchill Livingstone, pp. 397-415.

67. Fraser I: American Hospital Association (personal communication), 1993.

68. Tait AR, Knight PR: The effects of general anesthesia on upper respiratory tract infections in children. Anesthesiology 1987; 67:930-5.

69. DeSoto H, Patel RI, Soliman IE, Hannallah RS: Changes in oxygen saturation following general anesthesia in children with upper respiratory infection signs and symptoms undergoing otolaryngological procedures. Anesthesiology 1988; 68:276-9.

70. Cohen MM, Cameron CB: Should you cancel the operation when a child has an upper respiratory tract infection? Anesth Analg 1991; 72:282-8.

71. Colclasure JB, Graham SS: Complications of outpatient tonsillectomy and adenoidectomy. A review of 3340 cases. Ear Nose Throat J 1990; 69:155-60.

72. Tom LW, DeDio RM, Cohen DE et al: Is outpatient tonsillectomy appropriate for young children? Laryngoscope 1992; 102:277-80.

73. Reiner SA, Sawyer WP, Clark KF, Wood MW: Safety of outpatient tonsillectomy and adenoidectomy. Otolaryngol Head Neck Surg 1990; 102:161-8.

74. Haberman RS, Shattuck TG, Dion NM: Is outpatient suction cautery tonsillectomy safe in a community hospital setting? Laryngoscope 1990; 100:511-5.

75. Richmond KH, Wetmore RF, Baranak CC: Postoperative complications following tonsillectomy and adenoidectomy—who is at risk? Int J Pediatr Otorhinolaryngol 1987; 13:117-24.

76. Twersky RS: How to assess quality in ambulatory surgery. J Clin Anesth 1992; 4:25S-32S.

77. Joint Commission on Accreditation of Healthcare Organizations: Accreditation manual for hospitals, Oakbrook Terrace, Ill, 1993, JCAHO.

78. Donabedian A: The quality of care: how can it be assessed? JAMA 1988; 260:1743-8.

79. Joint Commission on Accreditation of Healthcare Organizations: Joint Commission indicators for the indicator monitoring system, betaphase testing, and hospital internal use only. In 1994 Accreditation manual for hospitals, Oakbrook Terrace, Ill, 1993, JCAHO, pp. 1-13.

80. Tinker JH, Jensen NF: CQI—Continuous quality improvement. In International Anesthesia Research Society: Review course lectures, Baltimore, 1993, Williams & Wilkins, pp. 40-5.

Cost Containment in Ambulatory Surgery

14

Yung-Fong Sung

Cost saving for management
    Personnel
    Supplies
    Equipment
    Other savings
Cost saving for medical professionals
    Laboratory tests
    Anesthetic techniques and agents of choice
    Patient care
    Prevention of complications
Summary

Cost Saving for Management

Each dollar spent on ambulatory surgery health care can be divided into several categories: medical personnel costs, ancillary personnel salary, administrative spending, laboratory tests, supplies, advanced technology, insurance, etc.

Each category of health care spending should be looked into with the aim to make it more cost-effective. It was recently reported by Woodhandler et al.[1] that in 1990 the U.S. hospitals employed about 4.5 times more managers and clerks than in 1968. U.S. hospital expenditures on administration vary widely from

20% to 30%, with an average of 24.8%. In 1993, U.S. hospitals billed consumers for an estimated $81.7 billion in administrative costs.[2] By comparison, Canada spends only 9% to 11% of hospital expenditures on administration. In other words, hospitals in the United States spend about 2.5 times more for administration than do the Canadians. If U.S. hospitals could cut administrative expenses to the levels reached in Canada, they could trim their bills by 60%, or $49.1 billion, which could be used to improve patient care. Increasing management cost and increasing the number of administrators in the hospital will not improve patient care; it only increases the bureaucracy. However, new developments in health care technology are important and provide safer patient care, especially when surgery is performed in an ambulatory setting, where the charges are about 30% to 50% lower than those for surgery performed in a hospital setting.[3] Appreciation of the various factors that play a role in the operating costs of an ambulatory surgery facility is vital to adopting any cost-containment measures. Additionally, regional variation in costs, participation in pharmaceutical and equipment consortiums, and other contractual arrangements may explain differences in ambulatory surgery costs described in this Chapter.

Personnel (Box 14-1)

Personnel expense occupies a large portion of the health budget, and hiring multitalented individuals who can work in different areas will save money.

Management personnel in an ambulatory surgery center should consist of a medical director, an operating room (OR) manager, and an administrator.

The medical director should be actively practicing medicine and, preferably, an anesthesiologist[4] who is in the unit on a daily basis caring for patients preoperatively, during surgery, and postoperatively. Anesthesiologists play an important leadership role with economic issues and quality of improvement in outpatient surgical care. This is due to the fact that anesthesiologists are among the prime motivators in the development of ambulatory surgical care.

The OR manager should, preferably, be a registered nurse (RN) with business knowledge and who still practices nursing. The administrator should take care of legal issues, space, budget, planning, quality assurance, policy and procedures, and so forth.

Box 14-1 *Personnel Required for Ambulatory Surgery Center*

Administrator (part-time)
Medical director (anesthesiologist)
Anesthesiologists
Anesthetists
Anesthesia technical assistants
Nurse manager or nurse coordinator
Nurses for holding area, operating room, and post-anesthesia care unit
Clerks for holding area, operating room, and post-anesthesia care unit
Instrumentation specialists for operating room
Anesthesia laboratory technologist for both laboratory and anesthesia equipment
Housekeeping
Transporter
Operating room supply storage caretaker

Part-time anesthesiologists, anesthetists, and nurses should be hired to provide needed coverage for the inevitable peaks and valleys of patient population.

All of the RNs should be capable of working in all of the different areas of the ambulatory surgery center, such as the preoperative area, operating room, and postanesthesia care unit (PACU). These individuals need to be multitalented and should learn from each other and be prepared to take care of all different services as needed. Preoperative area nurses should have the ability to assist the anesthesiologist in patient screening. This would save physician time and would reduce cost by allowing the anesthesiologist to devote more time to patient care in the preoperative, operative, and postoperative area. PACU nurses should make the follow-up postoperative calls to the patients. Any patient comments and/or complications should be recorded by these nurses and reported to the pertinent party, i.e., the surgeon, the anesthesiologist, or the manager.

All personnel should be educated in the team approach, with the philosophy that the patient comes first. This is the most important philosophy for the practice of medicine anywhere. The ambulatory surgery center is no exception. It takes a team effort to get the job done and to maintain cost-effectiveness.

Supplies

Supplies can easily get out of hand, resulting in waste and spiraling costs. Continuous awareness and control of inventory by all personnel is the obvious course to follow.

Each person should learn how to take care of supplies and inventory in his or her own section. This would include being responsible for ordering supplies with minimal clerk assistance. Inventories should be assessed often, at least every 2 to 4 weeks to prevent excessive ordering and to eliminate waste resulting from expired drugs or stock, i.e., a box of 12 bags of expired Hespan would cost the unit $696.00, a box of four bottles of ondansetron (20 cc per bottle) would cost $691.68, throwing out a laryngeal mask airway (LMA) would cost $200.00.

Often, decreased inventory will also decrease the space required for supplies, thereby decreasing administrative costs. Keeping a smaller inventory offers more flexibility in keeping up with new technology and in trying new items. It also decreases waste from overstocking and from having older supplies on hand that are not being used.

Equipment

Anesthesiology and OR equipment is also a major expenditure for the ambulatory surgical center. A piece of well cared for equipment will last a long time.

When purchasing equipment, one must take into consideration the advanced technology of the equipment, as well as the need to analyze the frequency of its usage and its importance to patient care. Examples of costs of commonly used anesthesia equipment are given in Table 14-1. Well maintained equipment will remain useful for a longer time than will equipment that is not cared for properly. Maintaining equipment should not be the responsibility of only the trained technologist; rather, the principal responsibility for proper maintenance of equipment resides with the daily user of the equipment. Therefore, the physicians, anesthetists, and trainees should be educated continuously about the proper care and maintenance of all of the equipment, thus decreasing the cost involved in repairing or replacing equipment.

***Table* 14-1**   Anesthesia Equipment Costs*

Equipment	Costs
Anesthesia cart (Blue Bell)	$ 229.99
Datex AS/3 monitor (with 14-inch display modules: ECG, temp, pulse oximeter, gas analyzer, etc.)	$28,700.00
Ohmeda Modulus II Plus (anesthesia system including freight cost)	$40,532.00
Vaporizers	
Isoflurane	$ 3,275.00
Halothane	$ 3,275.00
Enflurane	$ 3,275.00
Desflurane	$ 9,240.00

*Costs to author's ASU.

For example, replacing a broken Bard InfusOR pump would cost $2,000. A $100,000 piece of equipment ordinarily can last for 10 years. If it lasts for 2 extra years because of good care, $20,000 can be saved. When multiplied by the number of major pieces of equipment in the facility, the potential savings can be substantial.

When necessary, monitoring equipment in the OR should be upgraded first. The used OR equipment can then be moved to the PACU, and the used PACU equipment can then be transferred to the preoperative area. This provides efficient and continuous use of the equipment.

Other Savings

Operating room time is expensive. Saving operating room time will save money. Great efficiencies in this area can be achieved by improving communication among OR personnel and between OR personnel and patients. The surgeon, anesthesiologists, patients and their family all need to be educated to improve communications, which result in improvement in the usage of both OR and PACU time.

Communication

Surgeon, anethesiologist, and OR coordinator should always communicate well with each other. This decreases delays and improves turnover time.

Communication with patients

Be sure the patient arrives on time before the scheduled surgical procedure. Patients scheduled for a procedure late in the day should be able to be contacted if the schedule unexpectedly changes so that the patient can be seen earlier, thereby preventing unproductive gaps in the OR schedule.

Avoid cancellation

Last minute cancellations waste OR time; therefore, the pre-anesthetic screening is very important to ensure that the patient is ready for the operative procedure. Cancellation also wastes the time of the patient's family, who may have taken time from their work to care for the patient, so-called "indirect costs."[5]

Prime time in the OR is from 7:00 A.M. until 3:30 P.M. Within this 8½-hour period, assume that a minimum of six 1-hour cases can be done easily with a turnaround time of 15 minutes for each case. This allows enough time for clean up. However, if each case is delayed by only 10 minutes, 1 hour will be wasted per day. If this occurred in six rooms, the waste would be 6 hours. This daily rate multiplied by 251 working days results in 1506 hours wasted per year.

It is customary that after an 8-hour work day, OR nurses, PACU nurses, and anesthetists (CRNA) are paid overtime. The overtime for 1506 hours at time and a half will be 2259 hours per year for each one of those groups. Additionally, there will be technical assistants and cleaning people working overtime. There-fore, if 1 hour is wasted in each OR every day for a six operating room facility, the result is a tremendous waste in overtime pay for personnel. There are additional costs and expenses related to these delays as well.

Using the above data and an average hourly wage (OR nurse: $2259 \times \$20 = \$45,180$; PACU nurses: $2259 \times \$20 = \$45,180$; CRNA: $2259 \times \$35 = \$79,065$), a total of $169,425 per year is wasted. It is even more expensive if including time for surgeons, anesthesiologists, business office staff, and other nontechnical personnel.

Cost Saving for Medical Professionals

Within the last 20 years, anesthesia and surgery have become more symbiotic. Due to the development of new surgical proce-dures, anesthesiology has had to make comparable advances in technology. Subsequently, the advances made in anesthesia

Table 14-2   Cost of Laboratory Tests*

Test	Cost
Pregnancy Tests	
Serum	$25.00
Urine	$25.00
CBC + DIF	$26.00
SMA 18	$46.00
ECG	$64.00
Chest x-ray	
1 view	$75.00
2 views	$92.00

*Costs to author's ASU.

technology caused more advances in surgery, e.g., laser surgery, microsurgery, transplantation. These advances also increased the quality of patient care. Ambulatory surgery is no exception. Advances in technology allow ambulatory surgery centers to do more complicated procedures than were previously possible in an outpatient setting. Now this type of patient can be discharged to home, shifting part of the nursing care to the relatives (e.g., pediatric patients; patients undergoing bone marrow harvest, face lifts, reduction mammoplasty).[6,7] Advances in technology and highly trained personnel are costly; however, under the current health care environment, the health care spending is out of hand. We must decrease the cost, yet maintain the high quality of care.

Laboratory Tests (Table 14-2)

Blue Cross/Blue Shield estimated 10 years ago that 30 billion dollars were spent for preanesthetic laboratory tests. It was believed that 12 to 18 billion dollars could be saved if laboratory tests are ordered after the history and physical or, at the least, after taking an oral history from the patient.[8]

The laboratory package became a must before anesthesia administration. This situation stems from several factors. One of these is the fear of halothane hepatitis, first reported in the 1950s. Another factor is that a third party pays the money. Not to be overlooked is the general attitude that Americans demand the best medical care. Gradually, the majority of authors found that most laboratory tests before anesthesia were normal and that the majority of the anesthesiologists did not pay much attention to the preoperative laboratory tests, especially in healthy patients. Therefore, the question was raised, are laboratory tests necessary before anesthesia? Laboratory studies should only be considered after acquiring the patient's history or after completing a physical examination. An algorithm for recommended laboratory tests is provided in Chapter 1.

Anesthetic Techniques and Agents of Choice

Early patient discharge from ambulatory surgery center PACU is closely related to anesthetic management. By carefully choosing anesthetic agents and/or techniques tailored to the patient's operative procedure, prompt discharge is assured. Decreasing the PACU time will permit commensurate reduction in the size of the PACU team and will reduce medical costs.

In the past, anesthesia research has looked at the effects of an anesthetic agent from the viewpoint of outcome and the high quality of patient care. In recent years, the anesthetic agents of choice not only have to possess those features that lend themselves to high quality of care for the patient's well being and to a good case outcome, but they must also possess the characteristics that make them cost-effective.

Anesthetic techniques of choice

Regional

Regional anesthesia (Table 14-3) is often used in ambulatory surgery because it is associated with a rapid recovery and discharge of the patient, thereby decreasing costs. The patient usually can return to normal functions earlier than one who undergoes other anesthetic techniques. Regional anesthesia for eye procedures, such as retrobulbar and peribulbar block, is often used in the elderly or debilitated patient. It is sometimes combined with monitored anesthesia care (MAC) to decrease hospitalization time and prompt earlier discharge to home. Regional anesthesia, such as intravenous regional and ankle blocks for surgery of the upper or lower digits, is often used and is relatively safe and effective, as well as less costly compared with general anesthesia. Often, spinal and epidural injections can be done in ambulatory surgery, which also results in early recovery of the patient. However, for spinal and epidural anesthesia, attention must be paid to several points. For example, for spinal anesthesia, a small-bore needle (25-gauge or less) or a dull-tip needle should be used to reduce the incidence of postdural

***Table* 14-3**   Cost of Regional Anesthesia Trays*

Trays	Cost
Spinal (with agents)	$23.00
Nerve block (without agents)	$23.42
Epidural (without agents)	$29.14

*Cost to author's ASU.

puncture headache. To further prevent this, the fibers of the dura mater must be split (parallel insertion)[9] rather than cut (vertical insertion). In epidural cases, good techniques should be applied to avoid penetration of the dura, which will cause postepidural headache. Such a headache can debilitate a patient for up to a week, delaying the patient's return to normal daily activities and increasing both direct (medical care) and indirect costs (patient lost wages). The agent of choice is also a very important consideration in spinal anesthesia. Short-acting agents (e.g., lidocaine) should be used instead of long-acting agents (e.g., tetracaine) so that the patient's PACU stay will not be prolonged. Of the postspinal patients who have a problem with recovery of motor functions of the extremities, the majority also have a problem with urination, especially after a long-acting local anesthetic.

Postepidural back pain caused by muscle spasm following chloroprocaine anesthesia may limit its use in ambulatory surgery.[10] For lengthy procedures, a regional block is often combined with MAC to make the patient relaxed and comfortable on the OR table. Most patients have a good experience with MAC anesthesia. A more detailed discussion of regional anesthesia and recovery are found in Chapters 8 and 11.

MAC combined with local

In our facility, for MAC for eye procedures in elderly patients, we often use a Bard pump loaded with a low dose of alfentanil, which is diluted from 500 μg per cc to 50 μg per cc (one decimal point to the left of the calibration on the pump) combined with propofol. Just before the eye block, we use a few bolus doses of alfentanil (2.5 μg/kg) plus a bolus dose of propofol, 20 to 40 mg. During the actual operation, we use an alfentanil drip only (0.1 to 0.2 μg per kilogram per minute). Immediately after the procedure, the patient can sit up, eat, drink, and is ready to be discharged.

Low dosage opioids combined with propofol infusion are also used as MAC, with local infiltration for superficial operative procedures. The patient is very comfortable during the operation and has very few problems with respiratory depression. Following the operation, the patient quickly becomes alert, and the PACU stay is shortened.

We also use MAC for genitourinary procedures, especially for cystoscopies in elderly patients, i.e., MAC combined with lidocaine jelly urethral injections. This is often used in our institution for elderly patients who return every 3 to 6 months to have bladder cancer follow-up examinations. Because it is a pleasant experience for them, MAC anesthesia is often requested by these patients when they return. MAC anesthesia also shortens the recovery time and promotes early discharge.

General

In the ambulatory surgery setting, a mask is often used to administer general anesthesia in *elective cases* that are less than 1 hour in length. If the procedure is longer than 1 hour, a LMA is used in place of the endotracheal tube. This decreases postoperative complications (i.e., sore throat, laryngospasm).[11] In certain operative procedures, owing to necessity, endotracheal intubation is still used often as a general anesthesia technique.

Anesthetic agents of choice

Preoperative medication

Preoperative sedation is rarely used in the ambulatory surgery center in contrast to H_2 histamine receptor blockers (Table 14-4), which are used often. The indications for either use are discussed in Chapter 6. Certain sedation may be given in the OR before induction of anesthesia, such as short-acting opioids, benzodiazepines, 10 to 20 mg of propofol or 1.0 to 2.0 cc of thiopental, to make the patient slightly sedated and comfortable (Table 14-5). In our experience, some patients even find 3.0 mg IV d-tubocurare, the pretreatment dosage for succinylcholine, very relaxing mentally.

Intravenous induction agents (Table 14-6)

Since propofol was introduced to the market in 1989, it has become very popular because of its smooth, pleasant induction and because of the speed of recovery from propofol-induced

Table 14-4   Cost Comparison of Frequently Used Antacids and H$_2$ Antagonists*

	Dosage	Price
Metoclopramide (PO)	10 mg	$0.08
Bicitra (PO)	30 cc	$0.40
Metoclopramide (IV)	10 mg	$0.88
Ranitidine (PO)	150 mg	$1.30
Ranitidine (IV)	50 mg	$3.33
Cimetidine (PO)	400 mg	$1.38

*Costs to author's ASU.

Table 14-5   Cost Comparison of Preinduction Sedation*

	Concentration/volume	Price/cc
Thiopental (to reconstitute)	25 mg/cc	$0.17
Thiopental (syringe premixed)	25 mg/cc	$0.46
Propofol	10 mg/cc	$0.49
Fentanyl	50 mcg/cc	$1.29
Midazolam	1 mg/cc	$1.45
Alfentanil	500 mcg/cc	$3.42

*Costs to author's ASU.

anesthesia. Propofol also decreases postoperative nausea and vomiting. However, the older agents, thiopental and methohexital, are still good agents of choice for smooth induction, despite the fact that methohexital often causes hiccuping. Some induction agents, such as ketamine, which causes postoperative confusion, are not often used in ambulatory surgery anesthesia. Etomidate is rarely used in the ambulatory surgery center setting because it causes postoperative nausea and vomiting and prolongs PACU time and delays discharge to home. All of these side effects contribute to increased costs.

Maintenance agents

Propofol is commonly used as an intravenous maintenance agent. Propofol can be conveniently administered with an automated infusion pump providing early awakening and decreased nausea and vomiting. There is also less hangover effect, resulting in a decrease in the length of the PACU stay and earlier

Table 14-6   Cost Comparison of Frequently Used
Intravenous Agents*

	Concentration/volume	Price
Fentanyl	100 mcg/amp	$2.58
Thiopental	500 mg/20 cc	$3.44
Thiopental	500 mg/premixed syringe	$9.29
Alfentanil	1000 mcg/amp	$6.84
Midazolam	5 mg/amp	$7.25
Methohexital	500 mg/vial	$9.40
Propofol	200 mg/amp	$9.90

*Costs to author's ASU.

resumption of normal daily activities.[12] Thiopental and methohexital are not as good maintenance agents as propofol because of
their long elimination times and consequent hangover effects.
Ketamine and etomidate are not used as maintenance agents at all.

When using inhalation agents for the maintenance of anesthesia, especially in the case of desflurane, low inflow is highly
recommended, not only for decreasing pollution but also for
saving costs.[13] The inhalation maintenance agents (Table 14-7)[14]
most often used are isoflurane, in adults, and halothane, in
children. Recently developed inhalation agents, such as desflurane, are gaining in popularity for use in outpatients, especially
when combined with propofol induction. Desflurane has a low
blood/gas solubility coefficient, so the patient returns to consciousness early.[15] However, a high incidence of nausea and
vomiting,[16] especially in outpatients, is still a problem.

Muscle relaxants

Current cost data (Table 14-8) suggest that when nondepolarizing muscle relaxants are used for intubation, atracurium is the
most expensive, vecuronium and rocuronium are intermediate,
and mivacurium is the least expensive. Succinylcholine still
remains the least expensive, even when maintenance with nondepolarizing agents is used. Succinylcholine provides a rapid onset
of action that is reliable and is still often used in ambulatory
surgery, especially in private practice. However, succinylcholine
is not a perfect muscle relaxant; it also has its faults. Succinylcholine cannot be used for lengthy procedures, and, if used improp-
erly, prolonged apnea will occur. Also, in certain patients,

Table 14-7   Cost Comparison of Inhalational Agents (In 3 L Flow)

	MAC	$/ml	$/hr
Halothane	0.78	0.069	0.46
Isoflurane	1.15	0.86	8.90
Enflurane	1.68	0.59	8.92
Desflurane	6.00	0.29	15.66

*Costs provided directly by company.

ml liquid/hr = 3 × L/min × 1 MAC

Modified from Wetchler BV: Economic impact of anesthesia decision making: they pay the money, we make the choice. J Clin Anesth 1992; 4(Suppl 1):20S-24S.

Table 14-8   Cost Comparison of Frequently Used Muscle Relaxants*

	Concentration/volume	Price/cc
Succinylcholine	20 mg/cc	$0.044
Rocuronium	10 mg/cc	$3.32
Vecuronim	1 mg/cc	$1.90
Mivacurium	2 mg/cc	$1.50
Atracurium	10 mg/cc	$4.60

*Costs to author's ASU.

succinylcholine will cause postanesthesia myalgia, which delays return to daily activities. It is also suspected that succinylcholine contributes to malignant hyperthermia.

The other muscle relaxants that are good alternatives for use in outpatients are mivacurium, atracurium, vecuronium, and now, rocuronium. Mivacurium is considered to be an intermediate duration nondepolarizing muscle relaxant. The advantage of mivacurium is that it often does not require a reversal agent (Table 14-9), which decreases postoperative nausea and vomiting[17] and also saves the costs of muscle relaxant reversal agents. However, mivacurium increases histamine release and, like succinylcholine, can develop a more prolonged block in the presence of cholinesterase deficiency and when followed by other nondepolarizing muscle relaxants.[18,19] When using the intermediate acting muscle relaxants atracurium or vecuronium in ambulatory surgery, one should communicate with the surgeon regarding the length of the procedure. Occasionally, an error in the estimation of the case

Table 14-9   Cost Comparison of Reversal Agents*

	Dose	Price
Glycopyrrolate	0.6 mg	$1.38
Neostigmine	3 mg	$1.89
Edrophonium	10 mg	$3.40

*Costs to author's ASU.

length will cause a problem in reversal of the patient. Therefore, turnover time is prolonged. The role of rocuronium for ambulatory surgery will be determined as wider clinical experience is gained.

Patient Care

Patient care starts with the preanesthetic interview and continues to the postanesthetic discharge and follow-up. Each step should bear cost savings in mind.

Preoperative evaluation

Determination of laboratory studies

Preoperative history and/or physical examinations are very important factors in determining needed laboratory tests. As noted in Table 14-2, costs of preoperative laboratory tests can be significant. Females less than 50 years old and males less then 40 years old who are active, undergo a physical examination each year, and eat a normal diet rarely need an ECG or laboratory tests, unless symptoms indicate otherwise.[20,21] Specific recommendations for laboratory testing are addressed in Chapter 1. The use of written or automated health questionnaires may result in cost savings to an ASC by cutting personal time and enhancing the professional visit. The use of Health Quiz Prescreen, an automated preanesthetic medical history system, has been shown to be as accurate as a personal interview and, through standardized questions, provides a patient summary with patient-specific preoperative laboratory tests. Apfelbaum and colleagues reported an average savings of $68.70 per patient when unnecessary tests would not be ordered.[22]

Patient preparation for surgery

Because of advances in anesthesiology, patients with multisystemic diseases can also be managed in the outpatient setting and can be discharged as long as the patient has someone to provide home care. A careful preoperative evaluation is very important to bring the patient to a stable condition. When indicated, specialty consultations will assist in optimizing the patient's condition for surgery.

Preoperative instructions
For the patient with multisystemic disease or multimedications, preoperative instruction should be given very carefully. Proper preoperative instructions are important in ensuring patient safety and reducing unnecessary cancellations, the latter of which can result in increased costs of operation and reduce efficiency.

Postoperative planning for home readiness
Escort and home supervision
The patient's home readiness after anesthesia and surgery does not rely only on the patient's recovery, but also on the patient escort. Escort availability must be determined during the preoperative evaluation before the patient is taken to the OR and is anesthetized. If the patient has no escort or if the escort is incapacitated, then the patient should be preadmitted to the 23-hour postanesthesia care unit. If the patient lives alone, provisions should be explored preoperatively for home care.

Prevention of Complications
Any complications will cost money, whether major or minor (i.e., prolonged PACU stay, unexpected admission to the hospital). It is a good principle for both the anesthesiologist and the surgeon to practice preventive medicine in the ambulatory surgery center. Major complications occur infrequently.[23] A more detailed discussion is covered in Chapter 13. The majority of complications that prolong PACU stays and sometimes result in hospital admissions are intractable pain, nausea and vomiting, inability to void, and postsurgical bleeding. For pain and nausea and vomiting, a detailed history should be obtained preoperatively. Patients should be questioned regarding their sensitivity to pain and what type of analgesia worked for them in past surgical procedures. The patient should be asked if there is a history of nausea and vomiting or motion sickness and what type of antiemetic works the best for the patient. Preoperative sedation and intraoperative analgesia may relieve patient anxiety and pain, and it will probably also help

postoperative pain management. The combination of long- and short-acting opioids with nonsteroidal antiinflammatory analgesia, such as ketorolac, will provide good pain relief. Nausea and vomiting should be pretreated with antiemetics, especially patients susceptible to nausea and vomiting or motion sickness. Occasionally, stomach suction will be required to relieve postoperative nausea and vomiting.

The inability to void postoperatively may be related to surgical or anesthetic characteristics; however, adequate hydration is a very important factor and can decrease such complications. To help decrease postoperative bleeding, the anesthesiologist can contribute by getting the patient's blood pressure up to normal range or slightly above the normal range before the surgeon closes the wound. This will enable the surgeon to find the bleeding before closing and decrease postoperative bleeding considerably.

For the prevention of complications, there needs to be good communication among the surgeon, the anesthesiologist, and the patient. The impetus to save medical expenses will result in more complicated operative procedures being performed in ASCs. It is our obligation to maintain the high standards and continue minimizing complications.

23-hour recovery facility

The 23-hour facility is an extension of ambulatory surgery care, especially for more complicated procedures. This allows the patient to be observed overnight or up to 23 hours following surgery. This type of recovery unit provides observation for complications, e.g., laparoscopic gall bladder procedures, total mastectomy, reconstructive knee surgery, prolonged plastic surgical procedure. It can be used for the individual who is not able to take care of him- or herself and has no one to care for them (i.e., family lives out of town, or too many children at home and the patient cannot get any rest). It is also useful to those who come from out of town to undergo operative procedures. Others who need 23-hour care are the patients who have had plastic surgery and some other types of procedures that they would prefer to keep confidential from some of their family members or friends. The 23-hour care unit also brings convenience and safety for patients who are discharged late in the day from ambulatory surgery. The indirect cost of having family or friends travel a long distance to provide the needed care is also saved. After the stay in the

23-hour care unit, the majority of the patients are ready for self care when they are discharged, as well as ready to resume productive activities.

There are three ways to operate the 23-hour care unit:

1. To operate the unit by the ambulatory surgery center. It would be more cost-effective if the 23-hour care facility is combined with a home care team, which allows for arrangement of the most efficient personnel coverage.

2. To contract with an adjacent hospital, e.g., in our facility we contract with Emory Hospital for 23-hour care and the charge is reasonable for the patient. The price is $71.00 for the first hour or fraction, each additional hour or fraction is $41.00. The total observation bed charges, exclusive of ancillaries, shall not exceed the daily inpatient routine service charge for the accommodations used ($399).

3. To utilize adjacent progressive care or personal care homes. This type of home is for the elderly, where they own their own apartment and there is space designated for personal care. Patients in these homes are not quite ready to be placed in a nursing home but still need some assistance, i.e., preparing food, taking medication, and so forth. The individuals are semiambulatory. Nurses and nursing assistants are provided to care for these semiambulatory individuals. For a fee, the empty beds in this type of facility could be used for ambulatory surgery patients. This is more cost-effective than having the patient stay in a hotel setting, and it allows the family to stay with the patient. This should be the most cost-effective and convenient of all the 23-hour care facilities.

Home care team

The home care team would be able to take care of relatively complicated surgical procedures done in the ambulatory surgery center in the future. The team can provide administration of medication, as well as watch for complications for a few days until the patient recuperates. This would be an indirect cost savings for the family also. An analysis of the costs of home care following ambulatory surgery must factor the different levels of care ranging from complete technical nursing by registered nurses to nonprofessional care rendered by a relative. Home care is less costly only when the value of services provided by the relatives is not included. Ancona-Berk et al.[6] reported a mean difference between the cost of hospital care and various home care models to range from $69 to $335 per patient.

Transportation

Americans are growing older. In recent years, most elderly couples are able to care for themselves, but they do depend on others for transportation. The lost income by those who must take time off from their own employment to provide such transportation is another example of the indirect cost of medical care. If transportation is provided by the ambulatory surgery facility, this cost can be lowered. Additionally, some insurance carriers reimburse for ambulette transportation service. The costs vary according to distance travelled, but are not excessive. Accompanied by an escort, a livery or taxi service is a less expensive alternative.

Summary

The major concerns facing health care professionals today are the spiraling costs of health care and the need to contain costs while maintaining quality of services. Although anesthesia costs only represent a fraction of expenditures, cost containment impacts on the successful organization of an ambulatory surgery unit. Reduction in diagnostic tests can yield substantial savings in the area of ambulatory surgery. Clinicians are becoming extremely aware of the financial impact of drug selection in the perioperative period. It is no longer sufficient to introduce a new drug that has a high benefit low-risk ratio; the cost-benefit must be considered. Outpatient surgery managers and medical directors must enforce the need to be more efficient in the use of operating room time, control of inventory and supplies, and effective use of medical personnel. The development of 23-hour recovery units provides postoperative care for relatively more complicated procedures or patients requiring additional postoperative observation. These type of facilities have been expanded to include the demands of growing ambulatory services to contain costs and avoid the use of hospital beds. The savings in ambulatory surgery has not factored in the costs to the family or caretaker postoperatively. Various alternatives for home care need to be considered especially in the elderly population. While ambulatory surgery may be an overall cost saving to hospitals, facilities must adopt cost containment measures to preserve this economic benefit.

References

1. Woodhandler S, Himmelstein DU, Lewontin JP: Administrative costs in U.S. Hospitals. N Engl J Med 1993; 329(6):400-3.
2. Sternbert S: Paperwork pushing up health costs. Atlanta Constitution August 5,1993; A1, D1.
3. Stephen SV: Ambulatory surgical centers. JAMA 1985; 253(3):342-3.
4. Apfelbaum JL, Schreider BD: Outpatient facility and personnel. In White PF, editor: Outpatient anesthesia, New York, 1990, Churchill Livingstone, pp. 57-81.
5. Gold B, Orkin FK: Cost-effectiveness of outpatient surgery. Anesthesiology 1988; 1:76-80.
6. Ancona-Berk VA, Chalmers TC: An analysis of the costs of ambulatory and inpatient care. AJPH 1986; 76(9):1102-4.
7. Stanwick RS, Horne JM, Peabody DM, Postuma R: Day-care versus inpatient pediatric surgery: a comparison of costs incurred by parents. Can Med Assoc J 1987; 137:21-6.
8. Apfelbaum JL: Preparation evaluation, laboratory screening, and selection of adult surgical outpatients in the 1990s. Anesth Rev 1990; 17(2):4-12.
9. Mihic DN: Postspinal headache and relationship of needle bevel to longitudinal dural fibers. Regional Anaesth 1985; 10:76-81.
10. Stevens RA, Urmey WF, Urquhart BL, Kao TC: Back pain after epidural anesthesia with chloroprocaine. Anesthesiology 1993; 78:492-7.
11. Smith I, White PF: Use of the laryngeal mask airway as an alternative to a face mask during outpatient arthroscopy. Anesthesiology 1992; 77:850-5.
12. Sung YF, Reiss N, Tillette T: The differential cost of anesthesia and recovery with propofol-nitrous oxide anesthesia versus thiopental sodium-isoflurane-nitrous oxide anesthesia. J Clin Anesth 1991; 3:391-4.
13. Weiskopf RB, Eger EI: Comparing the costs of inhaled anesthetics. Anesthesiology 1993; 79:1413-8.
14. Wetchler BV: Economic impact of anesthesia decision making: they pay the money, we make the choice. J Clin Anesth 1992; 4(Suppl 1):20S-24S.

15. Lebenbom-Mansour MH, Pandit SK, Kothary SP et al: Desflurane versus propofol anesthesia: a comparative analysis in outpatients. Anesth Analg 1993; 76:936-41.

16. White PF: Studies of desflurane in outpatient anesthesia. Anesth Analg 1992; 75:S47-54.

17. King MJ, Milazkiewicz R, Carli F, Deacock AR: Influence of neostigmine on postoperative vomiting. Br J Anaesth 1988; 61:403-6.

18. Goudsouzian NG, d'Hollander AA, Viby-Mogensen J: Prolonged neuromuscular block from mivacurium in two patients with cholinesterase deficiency. Anesth Analg 1993; 77:183-5.

19. Bevan DR: Prolonged mivacurium-induced neuromuscular block. Anesth Analg 1993; 77:4-6.

20. Gold BS, Young ML, Kinman JL et al: The utility of preoperative electrocardiograms in the ambulatory surgical patient. Arch Intern Med 1992; 152:301-5.

21. Paraskos JA: Who needs a preoperative electrocardiogram? Arch Intern Med 1992; 152:261-3.

22. Apfelbaum J, Robinson D, Murray J et al: An automated method to validate preoperative test selection: first results of a multicenter study. Anesthesiology 1989; 71:A928.

23. Warner MA, Shields SE, Chute CG: Major morbidity and mortality within 1 month of ambulatory surgery and anesthesia. JAMA 1993; 270:1437-41.

Appendix 1   Preoperative Cardiac Evaluation Algorithm

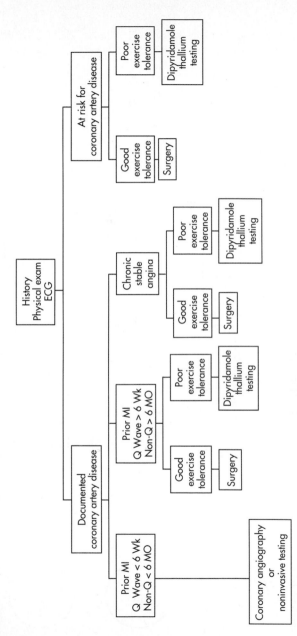

(From Fleischer LA, Barash PG. Anesth Analg 1992; 74:586-98.)

Appendix 2 Subcutaneous Insulin Regimen for Outpatients Algorithm

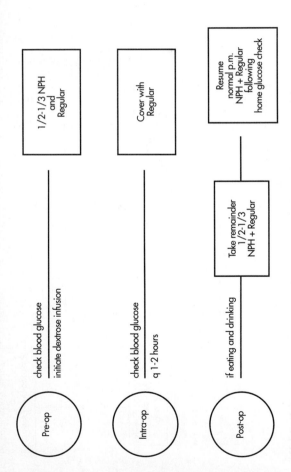

Pre-op
- check blood glucose
- initiate dextrose infusion

→ 1/2–1/3 NPH and Regular

Intra-op
- check blood glucose
- q 1-2 hours

→ Cover with Regular

Post-op
- if eating and drinking

→ Take remainder 1/2–1/3 NPH + Regular

→ Resume normal p.m. NPH + Regular following home glucose check

Appendix 3 Preoperative Testing Algorithm

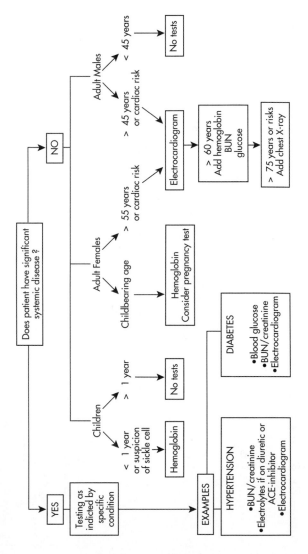

Appendix 4 *American Society of Anesthesiologists Difficult Airway Algorithm*

1. Assess the likelihood and clinical impact of basic management problems:
   A. Difficult Intubation
   B. Difficult Ventilation
   C. Difficulty with Patient Cooperation or Consent

2. Consider the relative merits and feasibility of basic management choices:

   A. Nonsurgical Technique for Initial Approach to Intubation   vs.   Surgical Technique for Initial Approach to Intubation

   B. Awake Intubation   vs.   Intubation Attempts After Induction of General Anesthesia

   C. Preservation of Spontaneous Ventilation   vs.   Ablation of Spontaneous Ventilation

3. Develop primary and alternative strategies:

   A. AWAKE INTUBATION

   Airway Approached by Nonsurgical Intubation → Succeed* / FAIL
   Airway Secured by Surgical Access*

   FAIL → Cancel Case / Consider Feasability of Other Options[a] / Surgical Airway*

   B. INTUBATION ATTEMPTS AFTER INDUCTION OF GENERAL ANESTHESIA

   Initial Intubation Attempts Successful* / Initial Intubation Attempts UNSUCCESSFUL

   FROM THIS POINT ONWARD REPEATEDLY CONSIDER THE ADVISABILITY OF:
   1. Returning to spontaneous ventilation.
   2. Awakening the patient.
   3. Calling for help.

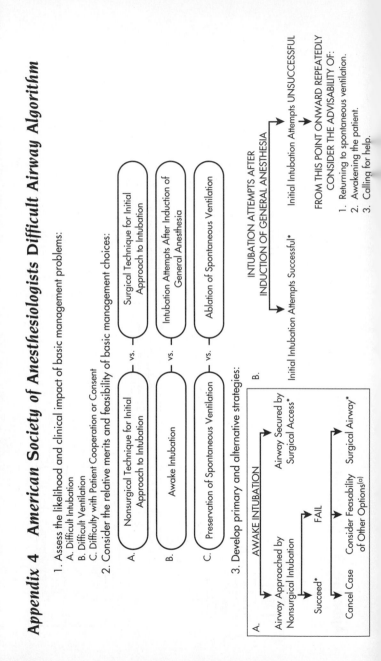

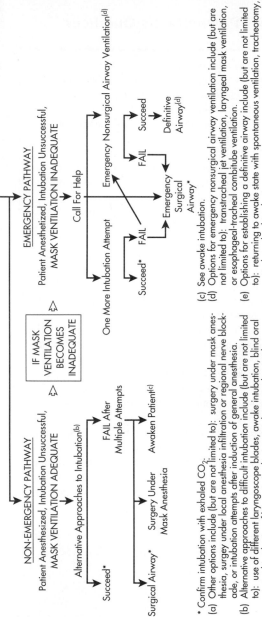

NON-EMERGENCY PATHWAY
Patient Anesthetized, Intubation Unsuccessful,
MASK VENTILATION ADEQUATE

Alternative Approaches to Intubation[b]

Succeed*

Surgical Airway*

FAIL After Multiple Attempts

Surgery Under Mask Anesthesia

Awaken Patient[c]

⇔ IF MASK VENTILATION BECOMES INADEQUATE ⇔

EMERGENCY PATHWAY
Patient Anesthetized, Intubation Unsuccessful,
MASK VENTILATION INADEQUATE

One More Intubation Attempt

Call For Help

Emergency Nonsurgical Airway Ventilation[d]

Succeed*

FAIL

Emergency Surgical Airway*

FAIL

Succeed

Definitive Airway[d]

* Confirm intubation with exhaled CO_2.

(a) Other options include (but are not limited to): surgery under mask anesthesia, surgery under local anesthesia infiltration or regional nerve blockade, or intubation attempts after induction of general anesthesia.

(b) Alternative approaches to difficult intubation include (but are not limited to): use of different laryngoscope blades, awake intubation, blind oral or nasal intubation, fiberoptic intubation, intubating stylet or tube changer, light wand, retrograde intubation, and surgical airway access.

(c) See awake intubation.

(d) Options for emergency nonsurgical airway ventilation include (but are not limited to): transtracheal jet ventilation, laryngeal mask ventilation, or esophageal-tracheal combitube ventilation.

(e) Options for establishing a definitive airway include (but are not limited to): returning to awake state with spontaneous ventilation, tracheotomy, or endotracheal intubation.

Appendix 5   Preanesthetic Questions

- What operation are you having?
- Do you have any medical problems other than the condition for which you are having surgery?
- Do you feel sick at this time?
- Have you ever had a problem with your heart, such as chest pain, palpitation, or heart attack?
- How much physical activity can you endure?
- Do you get short of breath during normal activities?
- Do you have any problems with your blood pressure?
- Do you smoke or drink alcohol?
- Do you use any nonprescription drugs or other chemicals?
- Have you ever had bronchitis, pneumonia, or asthma?
- Do you wear dentures, eyeglasses, or contact lenses?
- Do you have any symptoms suggestive of obstructive sleep apnea, like snoring?
- Do you have any neurological problems, such as convulsions, severe headaches, or memory loss?
- Have you had a cough or cold recently?
- Have you ever had any jaundice or problem with your liver?
- Do you have reflux, hiatal hernia, or gastritis?
- Have you ever had a problem with your kidneys?
- Do you have any problems with your thyroid or adrenal glands?
- Do you bleed easily or have any problems with blood clotting?
- Do you have sickle cell disease or any other hemoglobin problems?
- Have you ever received a blood transfusion? Would you accept a blood transfusion if it were medically necessary?
- Do you take any medications on a regular basis? Have you taken any other medications in the last year?
- Have you ever had an operation?

Appendix 5   Preanesthetic Questions—cont'd

- Was there any problem with the anesthetic that you know of?
- Have you or anyone in your family ever had a problem with an anesthetic?
- Are you allergic to any medications?
- Is there anything else about your health that you think I should know?
- And to menstruating females ask:
  - When was your last menstrual period?
  - Could you possibly be pregnant?
  - Do you use any birth control?
    - For the parents of pediatric patients:
  - Was your child's delivery premature or at term?
  - Did your child experience any neonatal complications?
  - Does your child have a history of bradycardia or apnea?
  - Is there any history of sudden infant death syndrome (SIDS) in your family?

Appendix 6 Indications for Laboratory Testing

No laboratory test is indicated merely because the patient is undergoing anesthesia or surgery. Laboratory tests should be chosen according to specific indications, based on a comprehensive history and physical examination. Some guidelines are listed below.

Test	Indications
Hemoglobin	Menstruating females, children less than 1 year old or with suspected sickle cell disease, history of anemia, blood dyscrasia or malignancy, congenital heart disease, chronic disease states, age greater than 60 years
WBC count	Suspected infection or immunosuppression
Platelet count	History of abnormal bleeding or bruising, liver disease, blood dyscrasias, chemotherapy, hypersplenism
Coagulation studies	History of abnormal bleeding, anticoagulant drug therapy, liver disease, malabsorption, poor nutritional status
Electrolytes, blood glucose, BUN/creatinine	Patients with hypertension, diabetes, heart disease, or disease states with the potential for fluid-electrolyte abnormalities. Patients taking digoxin, diuretics, steroids, or ACE-inhibitors
Liver function tests	Patients with liver disease, history of or exposure to hepatitis, history of alcohol or drug abuse, drug therapy with agents that may affect liver function
Pregnancy test	Patients in whom pregnancy cannot be reliably ruled out by history (some suggest all females of childbearing years)

Test	Indications
Urinalysis	No indication in preanesthetic evaluation; surgeon may request to rule out infection before certain surgical procedures, particularly those involving prosthetic implants
Electrocardiogram	Males more than 45 years old, females more than 55 years old, history or symptoms of cardiac disease, history of hypertension, diabetes, morbid obesity, significant pulmonary disease, cocaine abuse
Chest x-ray	Patients with symptoms of pulmonary disease, airway obstruction, cardiac disease, malignancy, history of heavy smoking, age greater than 75 years
Cervical spine flexion/extension	Patients with rheumatoid arthritis or Down's syndrome

Appendix 7   Standard Prophylactic Regimen Recommendations for Dental, Oral, or Upper Airway Procedures in Adult Patients at Risk

Standard Regimen

Amoxicillin	3.0 g orally, 1 hour before procedure; 1.5 g 6 hours after initial dose

In Amoxicillin/Penicillin-Allergic Patients

Erythromycin	Erythromycin ethyl succinate 800 mg, or erythromycin stearate 1.0 g orally 2 hours before procedure; then half the dose 6 hours after the initial dose
or	
Clindamycin	300 mg orally 1 hour before procedure; then 150 mg 6 hours after the initial dose

Appendix 8   Alternate Prophylaxis Regimen for Adult Patients Unable to Take Oral Medications

Standard Regimen

Ampicillin: 2.0 g intravenously or intramuscularly 30 minutes before procedure, then amoxicillin 1.0 g orally, 6 hours after initial dose

Ampicillin/Amoxicillin/Penicillin-Allergic Patients

Clindamycin: 300 mg intravenously 30 minutes before the procedure; then 150 mg orally, 6 hours after the initial dose

Patients Who Are Considered High Risk

Ampicillin, gentamicin, and amoxicillin: Ampicillin 2.0 g intravenously and gentamicin 1.5 mg/kg (not to exceed 80 mg) 30 minutes prior to procedure; then amoxicillin 1.5 g orally 6 hours after the initial dose (Alternatively, the parenteral dose may be repeated 8 hours later.)

Ampicillin/Amoxicillin/Penicillin-Allergic Patients

Vancomycin 1 g infused intravenously over 1 hour starting 1 hour before procedure; no repeated dose necessary

Appendix 9   Prophylaxis Regimen for Genitourinary and Gastrointestinal Procedures in Adults

Standard Regimen

Ampicillin, gentamicin, and amoxicillin
  Ampicillin 3 g intravenously plus gentamicin 1.5 mg/kg
  (not to exceed 80 mg), then amoxicillin 1.5 g orally 6
  hours after initial dose (Alternatively, the parenteral regimen can be repeated 8 hours after the initial dose.)

Ampicillin/Amoxicillin/Penicillin-Allergic Patients

Vancomycin and gentamicin
  Vancomycin 1.0 g infused intravenously over 1 hour, plus
  gentamicin 1.5 mg/kg (not to exceed 80 mg), 1 hour before
  procedure; may be repeated 8 hours after initial dose

Alternate Low-Risk Patient Regimen

Amoxicillin
  3 g orally 1 hour before procedure; then 1.5 g 6 hours
  after initial dose

Appendix 10   Treatment Modalities for Postoperative Hypertension

Drug	Dose range	$t_{1/2}\beta^*$
β Blockers		
Propranolol (Inderal)	0.5-1.0 mg IV	2-4 hours
Labetalol (mixed α&β) (Trandate, Normodyne)	5-10 mg bolus IV	4-6 hours
Esmolol (β_1 selective) (Brevibloc)	0.25-0.5 mg/kg bolus IV; may be followed by an infusion of 50-200 ug/kg/ min	9 minutes
Metoprolol (β_1 selective) (Lopressor)	5-25 mg IV increments	2.5-4.5 hours
Smooth-muscle Vasodilators		
Hydralazine (Apresoline)	2.5-5.0 mg IV increments	4-6 hours
Nitroglycerin	50-100 µg IV bolus; 0.1 ug/kg/min	
Calcium Channel Blockers		
Nifedipine (Procardia)	10-20 mg PO, SL	4-6 hours
Nicardipine (Cardene)	2.5 mg IV	6 hours
ACE Inhibitors		
Enalapril/ Enalaprilat (Vasotec)	2.5 mg IV	4-6 hours

* β half-life may not predict clinical duration of action.

Adjust dosing recommendations in presence of impaired renal/liver function.

Appendix 11   Postoperative Antiemetic Therapy

Drug	Dose	Side effects
Butyrophenones		
Droperidol (Inapsine)	0.625-1.25 mg IV, IM	Extrapyramidal effects, dysphoria, drowsiness, dizziness
Phenothiazines		
Prochlorperazine (Compazine)	5-10 mg IV, IM, PO; 25 mg rectal suppos.	Sedation, drowsiness, hypotension
Antihistamines (H_1 Antagonists)		
Promethazine (a phenothiazine) (Phenergan)	25-50 mg PO, IV 12.5-50 mg rectal suppos.	Sedation
Hydroxyzine (Vistaril)	25-50 mg IV, IM	
Diphenhydramine (Benadryl)	10-50 mg IV, IM, PO	
Benzamides		
Metoclopramide (Reglan)	0.15 mg/kg or 10 mg IV, IM	Extrapyramidal effects, dysphoria, drowsiness, anxiety, dizziness
Trimethobenzamide (Tigan)	100-200 mg IV, IM; 200 mg rectal suppos.	
Anticholinergics		
Scopolamine patch (Transderm Scop)	1.5 mg transdermal	Delayed onset, diplopia, hallucinations, dry mouth
5-HT$_3$ Serotonin Antagonist		
Ondansetron (Zofran)	4-8 mg IV	Headache, dizziness

Appendix 12 Commonly Used Analgesic Drugs and Dosages

Drug	Route	Dose	Duration of action (hrs)
Acetaminophen	PR/PO	10-15 mg/kg*	4-6
Ketorolac	IM/?IV	1 mg/kg (max 30 mg)	6-8
	PO	1 mg/kg (max 10 mg)	4-6
Ibuprofen	PO	5 mg/kg	6-8
Codeine	PO	0.5-1 mg/kg	4-6
Naproxen	PO	10 mg/kg	6-8
Fentanyl	IV	1-2 mcg/kg	0.5-1
Meperidine	IV/IM	0.5-1 mg/kg	2-4
Morphine	IV/IM	0.05-0.1 mg/kg	2-4

*Acetaminophen suppositories are available in 120 mg, 325 mg, and 650 mg sizes. Usually the calculated dose is rounded up or down to the nearest whole or half size suppository.

Appendix 13 Regional Techniques for Pediatric Ambulatory Surgery

Surgical procedure	Block	Drug	Dose
Inguinal hernia, hydrocelectomy, orchiopexy	Caudal	Bupivacaine 0.25%-0.125%	0.75-1.0 ml/kg
	Ilioinguinal/iliohypogastric	Bupivacaine 0.25%	0.3-0.5 ml/kg
	Instillation	Bupivacaine 0.25%	0.5 ml/kg
		Bupivacaine 0.25%	0.5 ml/kg
Umbilical hernia	Infiltration	Bupivacaine 0.25%	0.3-0.5 ml/kg
	Caudal	Bupivacaine 0.125%	1.25 ml/kg
Circumcision, hypospadias	Caudal	Bupivacaine 0.25%	0.5 ml/kg
	Dorsal nerve	Bupivacaine 0.25%	4-6 ml
	Ring block	Bupivacaine 0.25%	4-6 ml
	Topical (end of surgery)	Lidocaine jelly or ointment (2%)	
T & A	Infiltration	Bupivacaine 0.25% with epinephrine 1:200,000	0.5 ml/kg
	Topical	Lidocaine 10% spray	
Extremities	Peripheral nerve blocks, e.g., axillary	Bupivacaine	4 mg/kg
		Lidocaine	2.5 mg/kg
Airway endoscopy	Topical	Lidocaine	5 mg/kg
			2 mg/kg

Appendix 14   A Modified Postanesthetic Discharge Scoring System (MPADSS)

1. Vital signs
   2 = Within 20% of preoperative value
   1 = 20% to 40% of preoperative value
   0 = 40% of preoperative value
2. Ambulation
   2 = Steady gait/no dizziness
   1 = With assistance
   0 = None/dizziness
3. Nausea/vomiting
   2 = Minimal
   1 = Moderate
   0 = Severe
4. Pain
   2 = Minimal
   1 = Moderate
   0 = Severe
5. Surgical bleeding
   2 = Minimal
   1 = Moderate
   0 = Severe

*The total score is 10. Patients scoring ≥ 9 are considered fit for discharge.

Appendix 15   Malignant Hyperthermia Treatment Regimen

1. Stop anesthesia and surgery immediately.
2. Hyperventilate patient with 100% oxygen.
3. Administer dantrolene (Dantrium), 2.5 mg/kg IV, and procainamide (up to 15 mg/kg IV slowly if required for dysrhythmias) as soon as possible.
4. Initiate cooling.
5. Correct acidosis.
6. Secure monitoring lines: electrocardiogram, temperature, urinary catheter, arterial pressure, central venous pressure.
7. Maintain urine output.
8. Monitor patient until danger of subsequent episodes is past (48 to 72 hours).
9. Administer dantrolene PO or IV for 48 to 72 hours.

From Ryan JF: Malignant hyperthermia. In Coté CJ, Ryan JF, Todres ID, Goudsouzian NG, editors: A practice of anesthesia for infants and children, ed 2, Philadelphia, 1993, WB Saunders, pp. 417-28.

Appendix 16   Premedication and Preinduction Agents

Drug	Route	Usual dose (mg/kg)
Midazolam	Oral	0.5
	Nasal	0.2
	Rectal	1
Methohexital (10%)	Rectal	25
Ketamine	Oral	6
	Rectal	3
	Intramuscular	2
OTFC (Oralet)	Transmucosal	0.005-0.015

Appendix 17 Intravenous Anesthesia Infusions

Intravenous anesthesia component	Loading dose (µg/kg)	Maintenance infusion (µg/kg/min)	Stop infusion prior end of case (min)	Plasma drug concentration (minor surgery)
Analgesic				
Alfentanil	10-30	0.5-2.0	15-30	100-300 ng/ml
Fentanyl	2-4	0.02-0.08*	45-60	2-5 ng/ml
Sufentanil	0.25-0.75	0.005-0.01	15-30	0.3-1.5 ng/ml
Sedative/hypnotic[†]				
Propofol	1000-2000	120-200	5-10	3-5 µg/ml
Midazolam	100-250	0.25-1.0	15-30	50-250 ng/ml
Methohexital	1000-2000	50-150	10-15	5-10 mg/ml

Recommended infusion schemes are when combined with 65% to 70% N_2O.

*Recommended for long cases *only*.

[†]Titrated to loss of consciousness.

Adapted from Glass PSA, Shafer SL, Jacobs JR, Reves JF: Intravenous drug delivery systems. In Miller RD, editor: Anesthesia, ed 4, New York, 1994, Churchill Livingstone, pp. 389-416.

Index